T0382690

Atlas of Pediatric Hematopathology

Atlas of Pediatric Hematopathology

Edited by

Silvia T Bunting
Cleveland Clinic Florida

Xiayuan Liang
University of Colorado

Michele E. Paessler
University of Pennsylvania School of Medicine

Satheesh Chonat
Emory University

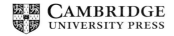

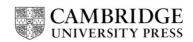

Shaftesbury Road, Cambridge CB2 8EA, United Kingdom

One Liberty Plaza, 20th Floor, New York, NY 10006, USA

477 Williamstown Road, Port Melbourne, VIC 3207, Australia

314–321, 3rd Floor, Plot 3, Splendor Forum, Jasola District Centre,
New Delhi – 110025, India

103 Penang Road, #05–06/07, Visioncrest Commercial, Singapore 238467

Cambridge University Press is part of Cambridge University Press & Assessment,
a department of the University of Cambridge.

We share the University's mission to contribute to society through the pursuit of
education, learning and research at the highest international levels of excellence.

www.cambridge.org
Information on this title: www.cambridge.org/9781108696951
DOI: 10.1017/9781108696944

© Cambridge University Press & Assessment 2023

First published 2023

Printed in the United Kingdom by TJ Books Limited, Padstow Cornwall

A catalogue record for this publication is available from the British Library.

Library of Congress Cataloging-in-Publication Data

ISBN 978-1-108-48258-5 Hardback
ISBN 978-1-108-69694-4 Cambridge Core
ISBN 978-1-108-69695-1 Print online bundle

Cambridge University Press & Assessment has no responsibility for the persistence
or accuracy of URLs for external or third-party internet websites referred to in this
publication and does not guarantee that any content on such websites is, or will
remain, accurate or appropriate.

....

Every effort has been made in preparing this book to provide accurate and up-to-
date information that is in accord with accepted standards and practice at the time
of publication. Although case histories are drawn from actual cases, every effort
has been made to disguise the identities of the individuals involved. Nevertheless,
the authors, editors, and publishers can make no warranties that the information
contained herein is totally free from error, not least because clinical standards are
constantly changing through research and regulation. The authors, editors, and
publishers therefore disclaim all liability for direct or consequential damages
resulting from the use of material contained in this book. Readers are strongly
advised to pay careful attention to information provided by the manufacturer of
any drugs or equipment that they plan to use.

Contents

Section V Histiocytic Neoplasm and Miscellaneous Bone Marrow Diseases

Contributors

Caroline An, MD
Associate Director, Hematopathology
CSI Laboratories

Nicole Arva, MD, PhD
Pediatric Pathologist, Ann and Robert H. Lurie
Children's Hospital of Chicago
Associate Professor, Department of Pathology,
Feinberg School of Medicine, Northwestern
University

Silvia T Bunting, MD, MSc
Staff Pathologist
Director, Hematopathology, Hematology, Flow
Cytometry
Department of Pathology and Laboratory Medicine
Cleveland Clinic Florida

Katherine R. Calvo, MD, PhD
Senior Research Physician
Hematology Section
Department of Laboratory Medicine
National Institutes of Health Clinical
Center

Billie Carstens, BSc
Instructor of Pathology
Department of Pathology
Colorado Genetics Laboratory
University of Colorado School of Medicine

Kudakwashe Chikwava, MBChB, MScEd
Associate Professor of Pathology
Sidney Kimmel Medical College of Thomas Jefferson
University
Nemours Children's Hospital, Delaware
Department of Pathology

Karen M. Chisholm, MD, PhD
Medical Director of Hematopathology
Seattle Children's Hospital
Clinical Associate Professor, University of Washington

Satheesh Chonat, MD
Assistant Professor, Pediatric Hematology
Emory University School of Medicine
Aflac Cancer and Blood Disorders Center, Children's
Healthcare of Atlanta

Alina Dulau-Florea, MD
Assistant Research Physician
Director of Coagulation
Department of Laboratory Medicine
National Institutes of Health Clinical Center

Tracy I. George, MD
President and Chief Scientific Officer
ARUP Laboratories
Professor of Pathology
University of Utah

Shunyou Gong, MD, PhD
Director of Hematology and Hematopathology, Ann and
Robert H. Lurie Children's Hospital of Chicago
Associate Professor of Pathology, Northwestern
University Feinberg School of Medicine

Sara Graciaa, MSN, CPNP
Pediatric Nurse Practitioner, Pediatric Hematology
Aflac Cancer and Blood Disorders Center, Children's
Healthcare of Atlanta

Jeffrey Jacobsen, MD
Phoenix Children's Hospital
Department of Pathology and Laboratory Medicine
Section Medical Director, Hematology and Flow
Cytometry
Clinical Assistant Professor of Child Health and
Pathology, University of Arizona College of Medicine–
Phoenix

Soma Jyonouchi, MD
Attending Physician
Division of Allergy and Immunology, Children's Hospital
of Philadelphia

Associate Professor of Pediatrics, Perelman School of Medicine, University of Pennsylvania

Virginia Knez, MD
Assistant Professor of Pathology
Department of Pathology
University of Colorado School of Medicine

Xiayuan Liang, MD
Professor of Pathology
University of Colorado School of Medicine
Director, Hematopathology,
Flow Cytometry
Department of Pathology
Children's Hospital Colorado

Brian Lockhart, BS
Coordinator
Division of Hematopathology
Children's Hospital of Philadelphia

Rachel A. Mariani, MD
Assistant Professor, University of Arizona College of Medicine – Phoenix
Department of Pathology and Laboratory Medicine
Staff Pathology, Child Health and Pathology, Phoenix Children's Hospital

Aurelia Meloni-Ehrig, PhD, DSc
Genetic Director
CSI Laboratories

Michele E. Paessler, DO
Associate Professor of Clinical Pathology and Laboratory Medicine
Perelman School of Medicine at the University of Pennsylvania
Division Chief, Hematopathology
The Children's Hospital of Philadelphia

Kristian T. Schafernak, MD, MPH
Staff Pathologist, Phoenix Children's Hospital
Associate Professor of Child Health and Pathology, University of Arizona College of Medicine – Phoenix
Associate Clinical Professor of Pathology, Creighton University School of Medicine
Assistant Professor of Laboratory Medicine and Pathology, Mayo Clinic College of Medicine

Stephanie D. Schniederjan, MD
Associate Director, Hematopathology
CSI Laboratories

Dehua Wang, MD, MSc
Clinical Associate Professor
Department of Pathology and Laboratory Medicine
Rady Children's Hospital
University of California San Diego

Gerald Wertheim, MD, PhD
Associate Professor of Clinical Pathology and Laboratory Medicine
Perelman School of Medicine at the University of Pennsylvania
The Children's Hospital of Philadelphia

Chapter

1

Peripheral Blood Smear Review

Satheesh Chonat, Brian Lockhart, Sara Graciaa, Michele E. Paessler

Despite all the advances in laboratory medicine, microscopic review of the peripheral blood smear is still highly informative and clinically relevant and remains an indispensable diagnostic tool. In a pediatric hospital, a common and challenging request is the evaluation of a newborn blood smear. This chapter provides an overview of some of the characteristics of a newborn smear and common reactive conditions.

Blood smear evaluation is often performed for three essential reasons: first, to clarify a flagged result such as immature cells or a low platelet count to rule out pseudo-thrombocytopenia from platelet clumping; second, to evaluate the morphology of red blood cells, white blood cells, and platelets; and, third, to confirm morphologic findings identified by lab staff or an instrument [1]. The latter may be requested by a physician due to a clinical suspicion or by members of the laboratory staff for review of an abnormal finding. Common reasons for peripheral smear review include cytopenias or cytoses, abnormal cells, malignancy, and infections [2]. The criteria for when evaluation is performed also depend on national and institutional guidelines.

Examination of a well-prepared blood smear is essential in many clinical situations. Peripheral blood smear preparation should be performed by a laboratory professional and controlled for preanalytical variables in order to ensure optimal quality. Blood should be sampled correctly and is commonly drawn from a peripheral vein and placed in an anticoagulant tube. It is essential to have the blood-to-anticoagulant ratio in the correct proportion or this can affect the cytology. In the pediatric population, particularly in neonates, the lab routinely receives microcapillary containers from heel sticks. Ethylene diamine tetra-acetic acid (EDTA) is the most common anticoagulant used. Specimens should be sent to the laboratory as soon as possible and are best analyzed within 2 hours. This is not always possible, but delay in preparation can result in degeneration of the cells and pseudo-thrombocytopenia. Morphology of the cells is best viewed

in the monolayer part of the smear. It is best to avoid the thickest part of the smear when reviewing cell morphology, but it may be useful when searching for parasites. The feathered edge of the slide is an ideal place to look for platelet clumps and large cells such as blasts.

Slide preparation should be performed by a trained laboratory medical technologist. The quality of the slide depends on proper smearing technique and the quality of the staining process so there is no over- or under-staining of the cells. These processes require good quality control and are essential for a quality blood smear review and differential count. Many labs now use automated analyzers that prepare stained slides.

Interpreting a peripheral blood smear requires a skilled approach and should be done by a trained medical technologist. Review of the peripheral blood smear should follow a systemic approach. It is essential to review all lineages and assess the size, shape, maturation, and morphology. Findings on the peripheral blood smear should be interpreted in the context of the patient's clinical history and other laboratory information. Anemia is a frequently encountered problem in the newborn nursery or intensive care unit, and the presence of other cellular abnormalities related to neutrophils and platelets is not uncommon, especially if the neonate is sick or has medical issues.

Once the decision is made to evaluate the smear, a well-mixed drop of blood of about 2–3 mm in diameter is placed about one quarter of an inch from one end of the slide. Then a "spreader" slide is placed with its edge in front of this drop of blood at an angle of approximately 35–45°. This slide is gently moved back to touch the blood and then, with one smooth motion, this "spreader" slide is pushed to the other end of the slide, maintaining the angle until a wedge is created (Figure 1.1). Hence, this method is often referred to as the wedge method. The slide is air dried and fixed with methanol or ethyl alcohol and stained. The thin portion of the blood smear 1–2 mm from the feathered edge is used to examine the morphology of the cells as they are likely

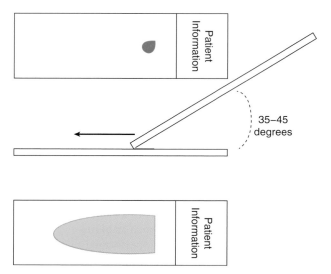

Figure 1.1 Diagram of the wedge method of peripheral blood smear preparation. The edge of the "spreader" slide is placed at an angle of approximately 35–45°. This slide is gently moved back to touch the blood and then, with one smooth motion, the "spreader" slide is pushed to the other end of the slide maintaining the angle.

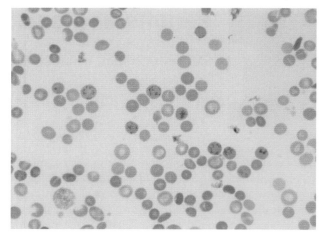

Figure 1.2 (Supravital stain, 50x) Immature RBCs show reticulofilamentous precipitates of ribosomes. The stain causes clumping and staining of residual nucleic acid present in immature cells. The stained cells represent reticulocytes and are counted as a percentage of total red blood cells.

separated from one another and not overlapping. A thick smear is used to evaluate for malarial parasites with low levels of viremia.

The frequently used stains are Wright or Wright-Giemsa stains; the latter ensures adequate staining of nuclear features and granular components. A Wright stain is a polychromatic stain consisting of a mixture of eosin and methylene blue. The Wright stain is methanol based; therefore, the slides do not need to be fixed. However, fixation helps reduce water artifact that can occur on humid days or with aged stain. Eosin Y is an acidic anionic dye and methylene blue is a basic cationic dye. Eosin stains the basic components such as hemoglobin and eosinophilic granules an orange to pink color. Methylene blue stains acidic cellular components such as nucleic acid and basophilic granules in varying shades of blue. The neutral components of the cells are stained by both components of the dye, producing variable colors. Another special stain used is a supravital stain. The supravital stain is performed to detect the reticulofilamentous pattern of ribosomal RNA in immature red blood cells (RBCs) using new methylene blue (Figure 1.2). The result provides information into bone marrow erythropoiesis. Another utility of a supravital stain is to detect Heinz bodies, which is not visible on a Wright-Giemsa stain. Heinz bodies are denatured hemoglobin seen in persons with glucose-6-phosphate dehydrogenase deficiency or unstable hemoglobin when their RBCs undergo oxidative damage. Reticulocyte counts are often automated but manual counts are still performed. The Reticulocyte Index (RI) is a calculated value in the diagnosis of anemia (see the following formula).

Reticulocyte Index (RI) = Retic percentage (%) × (Patient's hematocrit/Normal hematocrit)/2

Reticulocyte index interpretation:

RI should be between 0.5% and 2.5% for a healthy individual.

RI < 2% with anemia indicates maturation disorder – an inappropriate response to correct the anemia, such as iron deficiency anemia or myelodysplastic syndrome.

RI > 3% with anemia indicates an increased compensatory production of reticulocytes such as hemolytic anemia.

A common and challenging request is the evaluation of a newborn blood smear. Anemia is a frequently encountered problem in the newborn nursery or intensive care unit, and the presence of other cellular abnormalities related to neutrophils and platelets is not uncommon, especially if a neonate is sick or has medical issues. The next portion of this chapter provides an overview of the characteristics of a newborn smear.

Erythrocyte

As erythropoiesis switches from the fetal to the newborn period, the rate of hemoglobin synthesis and RBC production decreases drastically, secondary to the sudden increase in tissue oxygenation and marked decrease of erythropoietin. There is a period of physiologic anemia in the second week of life as RBC production reaches a nadir. Due to these changes, RBCs in the neonatal period have different indices compared to adult RBCs (Table 1.1). Neonatal RBCs demonstrate unique metabolic features due to enzymatic activities. Examination and familiarization of newborn smears are encouraged as they often exhibit variation in shapes including acanthocytes, echinocytes, schistocytes, stomatocytes, or target cells, which leads to decreased deformability in the first few weeks of life. Normal newborn RBC hemoglobin content is comprised of more than 70% fetal hemoglobin, and the remainder is adult hemoglobin. Additionally, RBC enzyme levels are lower in mature newborns. These characteristics of newborn RBCs make a diagnosis of an RBC membrane disorder very challenging. They also reduce the life span to 60 to 90 days compared to the adult RBC life span of 120 days. Premature RBCs tend to be more fragile and have an even shorter lifespan [3]. Nucleated RBCs are not an uncommon finding, as shown in Figure 1.3.

Lymphocytes and Neutrophils

In newborns, in the first 24 hours, higher numbers of neutrophils circulate when compared to adults, quickly reaching adult levels by 72 hours of life. Mature segmented neutrophils are often seen by 4–6 days after birth. Similarly, granule numbers and maturation are also variable in newborns [4]. Neutrophils mature throughout gestation and therefore are at risk for defects if this maturation process or the pregnancy is impaired or shortened. Neutrophils circulate as the first responders against infections in a newborn. Even after birth, a balance between neutrophil maturation in the bone marrow, release into the circulation, and subsequent passage into the tissues is critical. While interpreting neutrophil numbers in newborns, it is important to take into account and correlate with their gestational age, birth weight, and ongoing comorbidities such as maternal medical history, infection, and drugs. Lymphocytes in a newborn ("baby lymphocytes") have an immature blastoid appearance with fine chromatin and clefted nuclei (Figure 1.4) and can be diagnostically challenging. Recognizing these features would be helpful when a differential diagnosis of lymphoblastic leukemia arises.

Platelets

In the fetus and newborn, platelets are mostly produced in the liver and spleen compared to bone marrow in adults. Platelet count depends on gestational age, but usually reach the adult range of 150,000–450,000/µL by 22 weeks

Table 1.1 Red blood cell and reticulocyte indices in neonatal and adult blood*

	Newborn (RBCs/ Reticulocytes)	Adult (RBCs/ Reticulocytes)
Red blood cells		
MCV (fL)	107.7/123	89.8/106
RDW (%)	22.1	11.6
CHCM (g/dL)	32.9/24.7	33.7/30.3
MCH (pg)	34.4/29.7	29.6/30.3
Life span	60–90 days	120 days
Reticulocytes		
	4.4%	1.2%

* Adapted from Nathan and Oski's *Hematology and Oncology of Infancy and Childhood*, 7th edition. The Neonatal Erythrocytes and Its Disorders, Chapter 2, 52–75.e8.

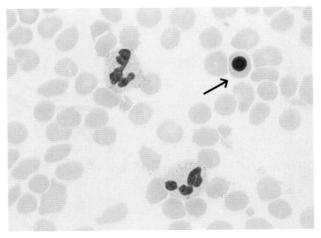

Figure 1.3 (Wright-Giemsa, 50x) Blood film from a healthy newborn showing a nucleated RBC (arrow).

of gestation. The platelet function is usually normal compared to adult platelets within a few days after a term birth. Several maternal and perinatal factors influence neonatal platelet dysfunction in at-risk infants, including maternal hypertension, medications, prematurity, birth weight, and infections, among others [5]. Many infections and systemic diseases can present with changes in the complete blood count and peripheral blood morphology. Next, we review general causes, and blood smears from infections and other causes are again discussed with pictures.

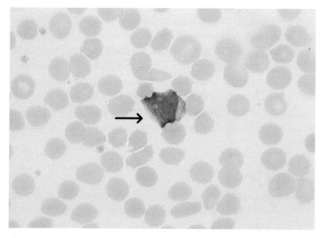

Figure 1.4 (Wright-Giemsa, 100x) Blast-like lymphocytes, often referred to as baby lymphocytes or pedi-lymphocytes, are seen in newborns.

Leukemoid Reaction

A leukemoid reaction is defined as a white blood cell (WBC) count greater than 50,000 cells/μL and is not secondary to a hematologic malignancy such as chronic myeloid leukemia. In most children, it is secondary to an acute infection, but other causes such as drugs – particularly steroids – solid organ cancers, and severe bleeding are possible. When a high WBC count is encountered, a thorough clinical history, physical examination, and blood smear review are essential for correct diagnosis. The blood smear in a leukemoid reaction is characterized by predominant neutrophilia and a left shift in maturation with many immature myeloid forms seen in the circulation (Figure 1.5a). Additionally, leukocyte alkaline phosphatase (LAP) can be markedly elevated (Figure 1.5b). LAP is predominantly found in neutrophils including immature forms, but not in lymphocytes or monocytes. In most cases, bone marrow examination is not required. When a bone marrow is performed, it is hypercellular with normal morphology and maturation of all cell lineages, along with normal immunophenotyping and cytogenetic studies [6].

Sepsis

Neutrophilia secondary to a bacterial infection is accompanied by toxic granulations in the neutrophils and precursors (Figure 1.6). Toxic granulations are blue-black or purplish granules distributed through the cytoplasm. Toxic granulation can also be seen in burns, drugs such as chemotherapy agents, and poisons. A higher proportion

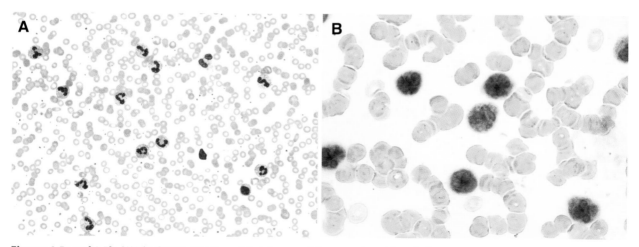

Figures 1.5a and 1.5b (Wright-Giemsa, 20x) Figure 1.5a is from a toddler presenting with viral infection resulting in a leukemoid reaction that shows neutrophilia and a left shift in myeloid maturation with toxic granulations. Figure 1.5b shows an elevated LAP score. For this test, naphthyl AS-B1 phosphate is hydrolyzed by alkaline phosphatase to diazonium salt, forming a blue dye within the cytoplasm of the WBCs, as shown in this picture.

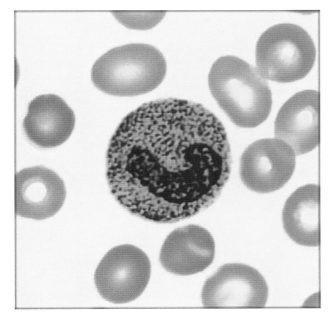

Figure 1.6 (Wright-Giemsa, 100x) Band with toxic granulations. Dark purple granules are in the cytoplasm of the band due to abnormal maturation of the primary granules.

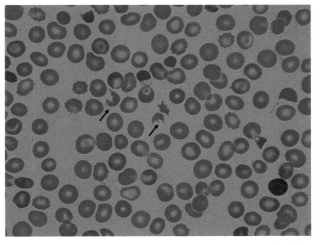

Figure 1.7 (Wright-Giemsa, 50x) Blood smear from a 2-year-old child presenting with drug-induced immune hemolytic anemia from ceftriaxone. The smear was taken a couple of days after presentation showing the presence of schistocytes (black arrows) and helmet cells (red arrows), along with paucity of platelets. This picture fits with drug-induced thrombotic microangiopathy.

of band forms (usually > 10%) is typically seen with sepsis. Alternatively, neutropenia can also be associated with infections, particularly viruses. It is important to note that there can be reduced number of erythrocytes with occasional clumping or even fragment cells, and platelet numbers can be either increased or decreased in severe cases [7].

Drugs

Drugs can induce quantitative and qualitative abnormalities of erythrocytes, platelets, and leukocytes to a variable degree. This can depend on the type of drug and the dose, and on the preexisting condition of the bone marrow. Review of clinical and medication history is crucial if findings on the blood smear are not within normal or expected range. Some of these conditions include drug-induced immune-hemolytic anemia, which may show schistocytes and thrombocytopenia (as shown in Figure 1.7 [8]), and drug-related eosinophilia (Figure 1.8). A common drug, recombinant granulocyte colony-stimulating factor, induces a marked leukocytosis with an increase in mature neutrophils, immature myeloid precursors, and monocytoid precursors [9].

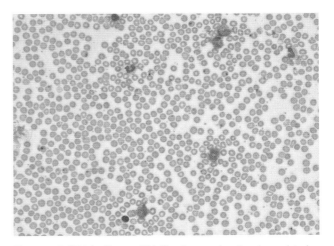

Figure 1.8 (Wright-Giemsa, 20x) Blood smear showing drug-related eosinophilia.

Stress Response

Bone marrow stress is a collective term used to identify the response of bone marrow or the general hematopoietic response to infection, inflammation, drugs, stem cell transplant, and so forth. This results in circulating nucleated red cells and polychromasia (reticulocytes) into the peripheral circulation prior to maturation. These enucleated polychromatic erythrocytes are larger and have higher levels of erythropoietin. Similarly, biological stress can result in leukocytosis and thrombocytosis.

SARS-CoV-2

COVID-19 caused by SARS-CoV-2 has brought about a global pandemic. The symptoms of COVID-19 range from mild flu-like symptoms to severe respiratory illness that can be fatal. Laboratory medicine plays an important role in diagnosis and prognosis in these patients. Recent studies have described hematology parameters such as lymphopenia, lymphocytosis, neutrophilia, and atypical coagulation. The peripheral blood smear findings seen in COVID-19–infected patients have been published and data continue to emerge. The morphology on peripheral blood smears seen in COVID-19 patients includes a spectrum of findings ranging from neutrophils with pseudo-Pelger-Huet anomalies (Figure 1.9), abnormal lobations (Figure 1.10), toxic granulations, atypical lymphocytes (Figure 1.11), plasmacytoid lymphocytes, vacuolated monocytes (Figure 1.12), platelet clumping, and RBCs with schistocytes and basophilic stippling. Pediatric patients who presented with multisystem inflammatory syndrome in children (MIS-C) showed RBC abnormalities significant for burr cells and increased schistocytes (Figures 1.13a and 1.13b) [10, 11, 12, 13].

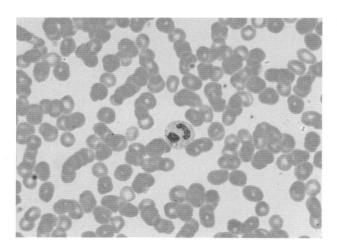

Figure 1.9 (Wright-Giemsa, 50x) Blood smear from a 16-year-old COVID-19 patient showing pseudo-Pelger-Huet anomaly.

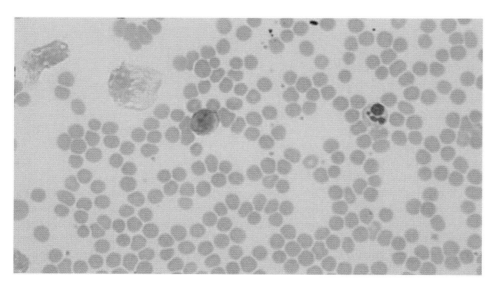

Figure 1.10 (Wright-Giemsa, 600x) Peripheral blood from a 10-year-old COVID-19 patient with neutrophil with abnormal lobation and an atypical lymphocyte.

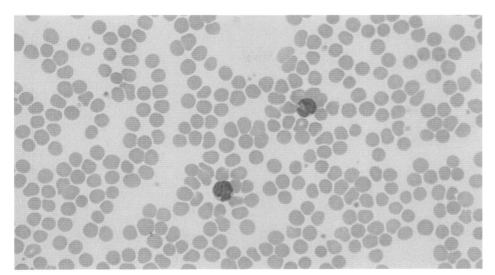

Figure 1.11 (Wright-Giemsa, 600x) Peripheral blood from a 12-year-old COVID-19 patient with atypical lymphocytes.

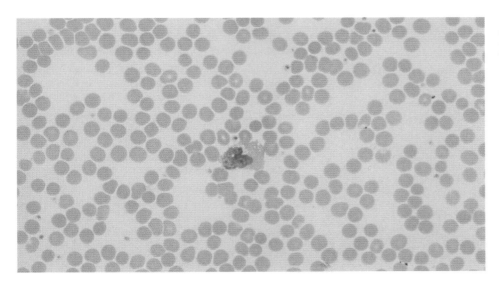

Figure 1.12 (Wright-Giemsa, 600x) Peripheral blood from a 8-year-old COVID-19 patient with vacuolated monocyte.

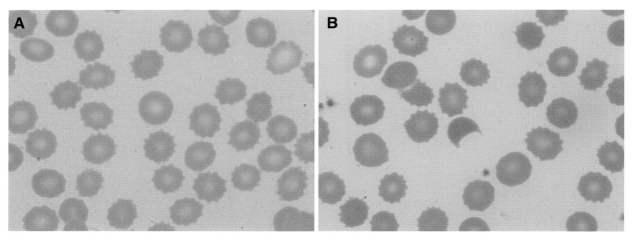

Figures 1.13a and 13b (Wright-Giemsa, 50x) Blood smear from a 10-year-old girl with COVID-19 and MIS-C with increased burr cells and schistocytes.

References

1. Gulati G, Song J, Florea AD, Gong J. Purpose and criteria for blood smear scan, blood smear examination, and blood smear review. Ann Lab Med. 2013; **33**(1): 1–7.

2. Bain BJ. Diagnosis from the blood smear. N Engl J Med. 2005; **353**: 498–507.

3. Steiner LA, Gallagher PG. Erythrocyte disorders in the perinatal period. Semin Perinatol. 2007; **31**(4): 254–61.

4. Lawrence SM, Corriden R, Nizet V. Age-appropriate functions and dysfunctions of the neonatal neutrophil. Front Pediatr. 2017; **5**: 23.

5. Kühne T, Imbach P. Neonatal platelet physiology and pathophysiology. Eur J Pediatr. 1998; **157**(2): 87–94.

6. Sakka V, Tsiodras S, Giamarellos-Bourboulis EJ, Giamarellou H. An update on the etiology and diagnostic evaluation of a leukemoid reaction. Eur J Intern Med. 2006; **17**(6): 394–8.

7. Aird WC. The hematologic system as a marker of organ dysfunction in sepsis. Mayo Clin Proc. 2003; **78**(7): 869–81.

8. Chonat S, Graciaa S, Shin HS, Newton JG, Quarmyne MO, Boudreaux J, et al. Eculizumab for complement mediated thrombotic microangiopathy in sickle cell disease. Haematologica. 2020. Dec 1; **105**(12): 2887–91.

9. Reykdal S, Sham R, Phatak P, Kouides P. Pseudoleukemia following the use of G-CSF. Am J Hematol. 1995; **49**(3): 258–9.

10. Nazarullah A, Liang C, Villarreal A, Higgins RA, Mais DD. Peripheral blood examination findings in SARS-Co-V-2 infection. AM J Clin Pathol. 2020; **154**(3): 319–29.

11. Berber I, Cagascar O, Sarici A, Berber NK, Aydogdu I, Ulutas O, et al. Peripheral blood smear findings of COVID-19 patients provide information about the severity of the disease and the duration of the hospital stay. Mediterr J Hematol Infect Dis. 2021; **13**(1): e2021009.

12. Diorio C, Henrickson SE, Vella LA, McNerney KO, Chase J, Burudpakdee C, et al. Multisystem inflammatory syndrome in children and COVID-19 are distinct presentations of SARS-CoV-2. J Clin Invest. 2020; **130**(11): 5967–75.

13. Merino A, Vlagea A, Molina A, Egri N, Laguna J, Barrera K, et al. Atypical lymphoid cells circulating in blood in COVID-19 infection: Morphology, immunophenotype and prognosis value. J Clin Pathol. 2020; **75**(2): 104–11.

Chapter 2

Red Blood Cell Disorders

Sara Graciaa, Michele E. Paessler, Satheesh Chonat

Congenital nonimmune hemolytic anemias are disorders of the red blood cells (RBCs) that occur infrequently in children and adults. These disorders can be divided into three categories: disorders affecting RBC metabolism, the RBC membrane, and hemoglobin synthesis. In this chapter, we briefly describe these conditions and the blood smear morphology. Increasing use of ektacytometry, flow cytometry, or the less sensitive osmotic fragility test can help in analyzing RBC membrane disorders. In addition to morphology of RBCs, RBC enzyme and/or genetic testing can be confirmatory for diagnosis.

Enzyme Deficiencies

Glucose-6-phosphate dehydrogenase (G6PD) deficiency: This is the most common RBC enzyme disorder worldwide. It is a genetic disorder characterized by a defect or deficiency in G6PD, which is involved in the hexose mono-phosphate pathway. It is required for the production of nicotinamide adenine dinucleotide phosphate (NADPH),

which protects RBCs from oxidative damage. Absence of the G6PD enzyme in RBCs results in the buildup of reactive oxidants, which causes hemoglobin to denature and precipitate, which in turn damages the structure and function of the RBC membrane [1]. Heinz bodies – particles of denatured hemoglobin – may be seen in supravital stained preparations. Figures 2.1a and 2.1b are examples of blister and bite cells that can be noted in patients with G6PD presenting with hemolytic crisis.

Pyruvate kinase (PK) deficiency: PK deficiency is the second most common RBC enzymopathy after G6PD deficiency, with an estimated incidence of 1 in 20,000 whites [2]. It is an autosomal recessive disorder characterized by a deficiency or complete absence of PK, which plays a vital role in the glycolytic pathway to produce pyruvate and adenosine triphosphate (ATP). Decreased ATP release shortens RBCs' life span due to membrane instability and results in a non-spherocytic hemolytic anemia, which can range from mild to a severe transfusion-dependent hemolytic anemia. Blood

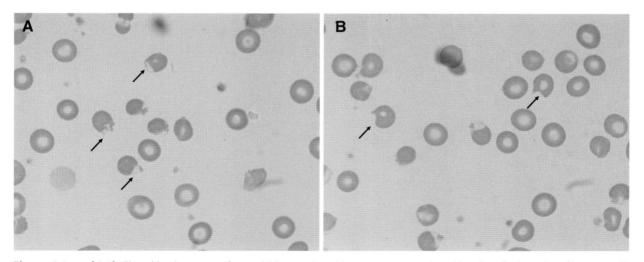

Figures 2.1a and 2.1b These blood smears are from a child presenting with acute severe anemia and jaundice after ingestion of large quantities of fava beans. The arrows in Figure 2.1a point to the blister cells with a thin rim of cytoplasm, including some cells that are in the process of rupturing. The black arrows in Figure 2.1b are the bite cells that form after the rupture of blister cells.

smear can show occasional echinocytes, which are increased after splenectomy (Figure 2.2).

Hexokinase (HK) deficiency: HK is required for the initial step of glycolysis and the pentose shunt. HK deficiency is rare with most patients belonging to Northern European ancestry. This is a heterogeneous disease characterized by mild bone marrow aplasia, and macrocytosis on blood smear. Notably, the deficiency also leads to decreased levels of 2,3-bisphosphoglyceric acid (BPG)

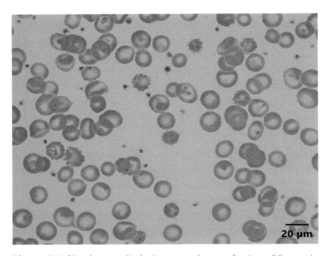

Figure 2.2 Blood smear displaying some degree of anisopoikilocytosis, characteristic echinocytes (densely staining spiculated cells with spicules of uniform size), among other polychromasia suggestive of reticulocytosis.

and a consequent leftward shift of the oxyhemoglobin dissociation curve.

Triosephosphate isomerase (TPI) deficiency: TPI deficiency is a rare glycolytic enzyme defect associated with congenital hemolytic anemia and progressive neurological dysfunction. It is an autosomal recessive multisystem disorder, affecting cardiac, neuromuscular, and immune function. Reduced TPI catalytic activity in erythrocytes leads to elevated levels of dihydroxyacetone phosphate (DHAP), which decomposes to methylglyoxal. Methylglyoxal is highly reactive and produces advanced glycation end products and consequential oxidative stress. Moreover, it is neurotoxic and may contribute to the associated neurodegeneration seen in TPI deficiency [3].

Glucose 6-phosphate isomerase (GPI) deficiency: GPI deficiency is an autosomal recessive disorder characterized by non-spherocytic hemolytic anemia. GPI deficiency primarily affects erythrocytes as it interferes with the second step of the Embden-Meyerhof glycolytic pathway and ATP production. It results in varying degrees of anemia and genotype does not easily dictate phenotype.

Red Blood Cell Membrane Disorder

Hereditary spherocytosis (HS): This is the most common RBC membranopathy. It is a genetic disorder caused by alteration in the vertical associations between the RBC lipid bilayer and inner membrane skeleton. The most commonly implicated proteins are α-spectrin, β-spectrin, ankyrin, band

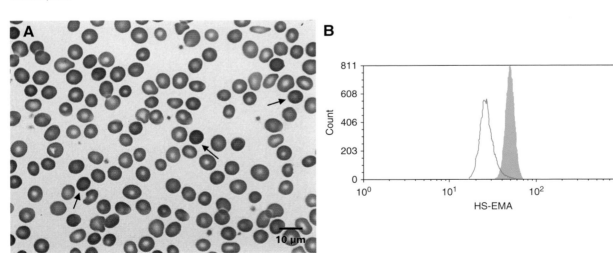

Figures 2.3a and 2.3b A. Peripheral blood film from a 12-year-old Caucasian female who was diagnosed with ankyrin deficiency-related hereditary spherocytosis (HS) at 3 weeks of life with no transfusion requirements. She presented with anemia and reticulocytosis of mild severity. Many of these RBCs have a spherical shape (spherocytes, black arrows). B. The eosin-5'-maleimide (EMA) binding assay is a flow-based assay measuring the amount of EMA binding to band 3 membrane protein. The mean fluorescence intensity of EMA-stained RBCs in this HS patient (shown by a thin orange line) is left shifted (lower) when compared with control RBCs (orange shaded), suggestive of reduced band 3 proteins seen in some HS patients.

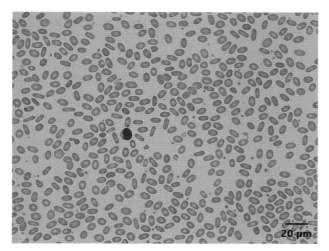

Figure 2.4 This smear is taken from a patient presenting with mild hemolytic anemia. RBCs are uniformly elliptical in shape, which is characteristic of HE.

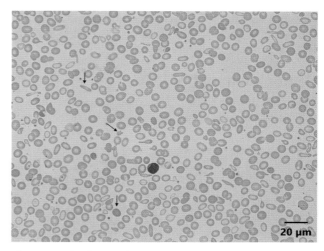

Figure 2.5 Blood smear demonstrates increased poikilocytosis, elliptocytes, and fragmented red blood cells.

3, and protein 4.1 [4]. As suggested by the name, peripheral smears in HS patients demonstrate hyperchromic, normocytic spherocytes, which lack central pallor. Certain subgroups of HS have more specific findings. For example, patients with band 3 deficiency can have pincer-like erythrocytes and those with β-spectrin deficiencies can have acanthocytic spherocytes on review of the smear.

Hereditary elliptocytosis (HE): HE is an inherited membranopathy characterized by the presence of elliptically shaped RBCs on the peripheral blood smear (Figure 2.4). Microspherocytes may be present as well, depending on the degree of hemolytic anemia. Defects in proteins linking the outer membrane and cytoskeleton result in reduced membrane stability and deformability. Similar to HS, defects in α-spectrin, β-spectrin, or protein 4.1 R cause HE.

Hereditary pyropoikilocytosis (HPP): HPP is an autosomal recessive disorder and, similar to HE, disease is caused by mutations in the *SPTA1* and *SPTB* genes, resulting in qualitative defects of α-spectrin and β-spectrin, respectively, and in the *EPB41* gene, leading to quantitative or qualitative defects of protein 4.1 R. The extent of the deficiency dictates the clinical severity. Affected individuals range from being asymptomatic to suffering from complications of severe anemia. Review of smear will reveal marked anisopoikilocytosis, red cell fragmentation (middle arrow), and microspherocytes (bottom arrow) (Figure 2.5).

Southeast Asian ovalocytosis (SAO): SAO is more common in individuals from Southeast Asia and the Pacific. It

is characterized by the presence of rigid, oval-shaped RBCs, often with a central slit (stoma) or transverse ridge. It stems from band 3 gene mutations that lead to rigidity of the RBC membrane. Clinically significant hemolysis is exclusive to the neonatal period. Otherwise, individuals with SAO are asymptomatic with normal hemoglobin and reticulocyte counts.

Stomatocytosis: Hereditary stomatocytosis can be split into two categories, overhydrated and dehydrated. Overhydrated stomatocytosis – also known as hydrocytosis caused by mutations in the *RHAG* gene – is a heterogeneous group of hemolytic anemias characterized by an elevated mean corpuscular volume, decreased mean corpuscular hemoglobin concentration (MCHC), and increased osmotic fragility of RBCs. A high percentage of stomatocytes will be evident on the peripheral smear. In contrast, dehydrated stomatocytosis or xerocytosis is caused from mutations of the *PIEZO or KCNN4* genes involving RBC membrane channels, characterized by an increased MCHC and decreased osmotic fragility. RBC dehydration produces stomatocytes, target cells, and xerocytes (dense, hyperchromic RBCs with hemoglobin puddled at the periphery), as shown in Figure 2.6.

Acanthocytosis: Acanthocytes are RBCs that are often contracted in size and hyperchromatic, with irregularly placed, short, pointed projections from the cell surface. They are characteristic of patients with abetalipoproteinemia and may be seen in smaller numbers in a variety of metabolic disorders such as severe chronic liver or renal disease, in the post-splenectomy state, and in small numbers in a variety of blood cell disorders affecting RBCs. This case is an example of spur cell anemia seen in chronic severe liver disease (Figure 2.7).

Hemoglobinopathy

Sickle cell disease (SCD): The common genetic types of SCD include homozygous hemoglobin (SS), heterozygous for hemoglobin S with either hemoglobin C or with thalassemia (Sβ+ or Sβ0 subtypes). Sickle hemoglobin (Hb S) is unstable and polymerizes under hypoxic conditions. The polymerization causes the RBCs to assume a sickle or crescent-like shape. The classic polymerization is only partially responsible for the clinical manifestations of SCD, namely hemolysis and vaso-occlusive pain. A number of pathophysiologic mechanisms have been implicated in the disease. See Figure 2.8 for blood smear findings seen in SCD. Capillary zone electrophoresis (CE) is commonly used to provide a fast and accurate diagnosis of hemoglobinopathies. See Figures 2.8b and 2.8c for the CE pattern for a person with normal hemoglobin (hemoglobin A [high peak] and A2 [small peak] and hemoglobin SC [hemoglobin A, S, A2, and C, from left to right]).

Thalassemia: Thalassemia syndromes derive from diminished or absent production of one or more globin chains. The altered production of these globin chains in thalassemia can lead to decreased hemoglobin, imbalanced accumulations of these chains, and, ultimately, hemolytic anemia. Thalassemia is better characterized as transfusion-dependent thalassemia (TDT) or nontransfusion-dependent thalassemia (NTDT). Alpha thalassemia is caused by decreased or absent production of alpha globin. Alpha globin is made by four genes, two on each strand of chromosome 16. The number of deletions/mutations generally determines the disease severity. On the other hand, beta globin is created by two genes. Point mutations abolish or decrease the production of beta

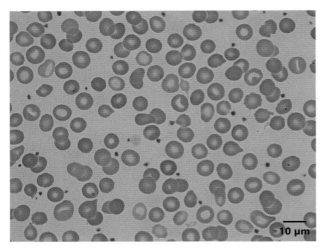

Figure 2.6 This picture is from a toddler who presented with mild hemolytic anemia, near normal hemoglobin, and increased MCHC. Blood smear shows moderate numbers of red cells with horizontal central clearing called stomatocytes, which result from the cation leak, leading to dysregulation of cellular volume and formation of abnormal-looking RBCs (stomatocytes) on the blood smear.

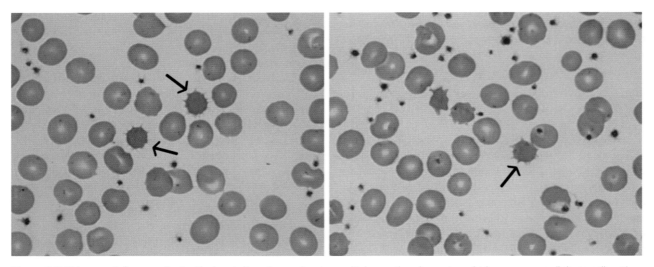

Figure 2.7 This smear is from a patient with chronic liver disease showing multiple acanthospherocytes, which appear as small dense cells with spicules of varying sizes (unlike in echinocytes where spicules are more uniform in size).

globin. Similar to the genetics of alpha thalassemia, the number of beta thalassemia alleles determines the severity of disease. See Figure 2.9.

Hemoglobin C: Hemoglobin C is a less soluble form of hemoglobin resulting from a beta globin mutation. It results when an individual inherits a substitution of lysine for the normal glutamic acid in the sixth amino acid position of the ß-globin chain on chromosome 11. Homozygous inheritance results in hemoglobin C disease and presents with mild anemia. See Figure 2.10 for characteristic findings seen in hemoglobin C disease.

Immune-Mediated Hemolytic Anemia

Autoimmune hemolytic anemia (AIHA) is caused by auto-antibody destruction of one's own RBCs. There are four types: warm, cold, paroxysmal cold hemoglobinuria (PCH), or mixed. Warm and cold are differentiated by the ideal temperature at which the autoantibodies bind the RBCs. These types can be further differentiated into primary or secondary, based on the presence or absence of an identifiable underlying disease. Primary or idiopathic AIHA occurs when patients have no identifiable underlying disease, whereas, in patients with an underlying diagnosis such as immune dysregulation, it is classified as secondary AIHA.

Warm autoimmune hemolytic anemia: Warm AIHA is the most common, with most cases in pediatrics being idiopathic or secondary to infection. In adults, it is often secondary to an underlying autoimmune disorder or malignancy. Warm AIHA is caused by antibodies that are maximally reactive with RBC antigens at 37°C, with most RBC destruction occurring in the reticulo-endothelial system. Figure 2.11 shows findings on blood smear of warm AIHA.

Cold agglutinin syndrome: CAS accounts for 10% of AIHA cases in pediatrics and is often secondary to infection by *Mycoplasma pneumoniae* or the Epstein-Barr virus. Cold autoantibodies are classically immunoglobulin M (IgM) and bind RBCs and recruit complement proteins. As the bound RBC travels centrally, blood warms and IgM falls off but the complement remains bound. This culminates in extravascular hemolysis by the spleen or intravascular hemolysis by the membrane attack complex. A blood smear should be made after warming the blood to ensure there is no RBC agglutination on the smear. The blood smear in CAS appears similar to paroxysmal cold hemoglobinuria (PCH), described next.

Paroxysmal cold hemoglobinuria: PCH is an acute, often self-limiting form of cold AIHA most commonly seen in younger children following a viral illness. The only confirmatory test is Donath-Landsteiner. This test involves incubating blood at 4°C to allow for antibody binding, followed by an additional incubation at 37°C to allow for complement activation and subsequent hemolysis. A direct agglutination test is usually immunoglobulin G (IgG) negative and C3d positive unless the test is performed at colder temperatures. The agglutination of RBCs seen in PCH, along with erythrophagocytosis, is shown in Figure 2.12.

Mixed autoimmune hemolytic anemia: Mixed AIHA is a rare entity defined by the coexistence of warm IgG autoantibodies and C3d in a direct antiglobulin test (DAT) and high-titer cold agglutinins. These patients tend to have an atypical presentation and a severe phenotype with very low hemoglobin (<6 g/dL), are refractory to standard treatment options (steroids, transfusion), and require other immune suppressants [6]. See Table 2.2 for serologic findings in DAT.

Secondary autoimmune hemolytic anemia: Secondary AIHA can result from various underlying disorders such as autoimmune disease, immune dysregulation, lymphoproliferative disorders, malignancy, infections, and medication (Table 2.1).

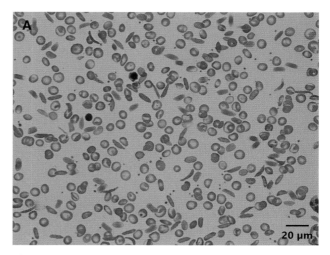

Figures 2.8a–2.8c A. The peripheral smear demonstrates the characteristic findings of SCD with "sickle-shaped" RBCs, along with target cells, polychromasia, and nucleated RBCs. B. The CE patterns for a person with normal adult hemoglobins (hemoglobin A and A2). C. The capillary electrophoresis pattern for a person with hemoglobin SC with extra peaks for hemoglobin S and C.

B

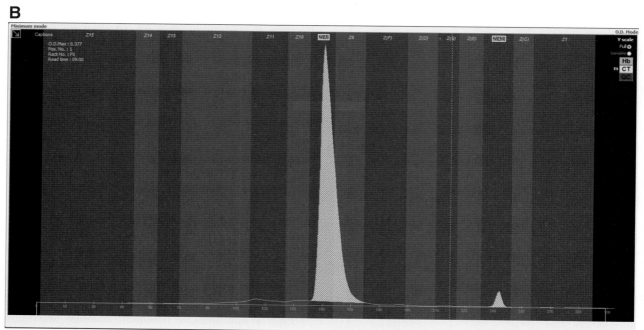

C

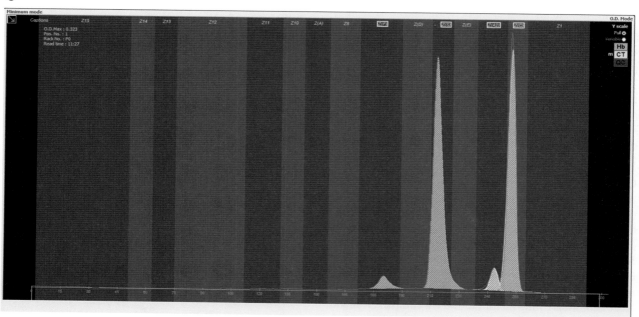

Figures 2.8a–2.8c (cont.)

Table 2.1 Conditions associated with autoimmune hemolytic anemia

Autoimmune Disorders	Infection
Evans syndrome	Epstein-Barr virus
Systemic lupus	Mycoplasma
Erythematosus	Parvovirus B19
Juvenile idiopathic arthritis	Cytomegalovirus
Graves' disease;	Varicella
Autoimmune thyroiditis	Hepatitis C
Autoimmune hepatitis	
Diabetes mellitus type I	
Crohn's disease	
Ulcerative colitis	

Immunodeficiency	Medications (most common)
Wiskott-Aldrich syndrome	Ceftriaxone
HIV/AIDS	Cefotetan
Combined	Piperacillin
immunodeficiency	
Common variable	
immunodeficiency	
Adenosine deaminase	
deficiency	

Malignancy	Lymphoproliferative
Acute leukemias	Disorders
(lymphocytic or myeloid)	Autoimmune
Lymphomas	lymphoproliferative disease

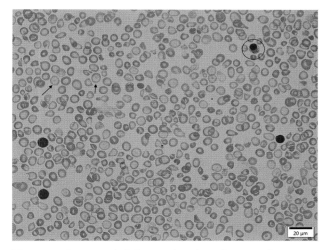

Figure 2.9 Patients with thalassemia have hypochromic and microcytic RBCs. The peripheral smear additionally will often reveal a large number of target cells (arrows), nucleated red blood cells (circles), and polychromasia.

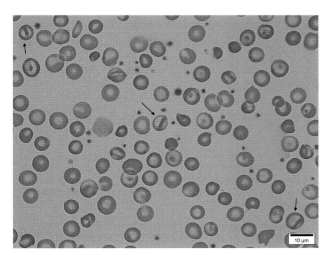

Figure 2.10 The RBCs are dehydrated, resulting in an increased MCHC. Target cells and hexagonal crystals (arrows) are classically seen on the smear.

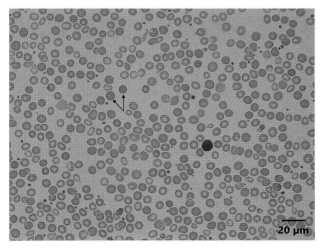

Figure 2.11 Blood smear from a patient with recently diagnosed systemic lupus erythematosus and warm immunoglobulin G (IgG) autoimmune hemolytic anemia. Microspherocytes (arrows) and occasional polychromasia suggestive of reticulocytes were present.

Table 2.2 Diagnostic table of autoimmune hemolytic anemia

	Warm Reactive	Cold Agglutinin Syndrome	Paroxysmal Cold Hemoglobinuria
Antisera	IgG or IgA	IgM	Biphasic IgG
Antibody reactivity	37°C	4°C	4°C
Direct antiglobulin test (Direct Coombs test)	IgG +/–C3d	C3d	C3d Perform Donath-Landsteiner test

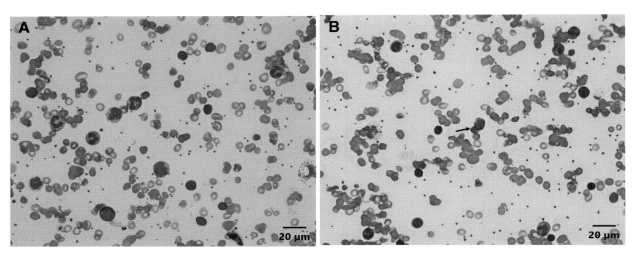

Figures 2.12a and 2.12b A 16-month-old boy presented with fever, respiratory symptoms, severe anemia of 3.9 g/dL, and absolute reticulocyte count of 141 x 10³/μL. DAT was C3d positive and IgG negative. Adjoining blood smears (50X) reveal agglutination of RBCs (Figures 2.12a and 2.12b); the arrow in Figure 2.12b depicts the process of neutrophil erythrophagocytosis. A positive Donath-Landsteiner test and mycoplasma IgM were confirmatory for Paroxysmal Cold Hemoglobinuria.

References

1. Beutler E. G6PD deficiency. Blood. 1994; **84**(11): 3613–36.

2. Beutler E, Gelbart T. Estimating the prevalence of pyruvate kinase deficiency from the gene frequency in the general white population. Blood. 2000; **95**(11): 3585–8.

3. Koralkova P, Van Solinge WW, Van Wijk R. Rare hereditary red blood cell enzymopathies associated with hemolytic anemia: Pathophysiology, clinical aspects, and laboratory diagnosis. Int J Lab Hematol. 2014; **36**(3): 388–97.

4. Risinger M, Kalfa TA. Red cell membrane disorders: Structure meets function. Blood. 2020; **136**(11): 1250–61.

5. Caruso C, Chonat S. Immune and nonimmune hemolytic anemia. In Kamat D, Frei-Jones M, eds. Benign hematologic disorders in children. Cham: Springer; 2021: 51–64. https://doi.org/10.1007/978-3-030-49980-8_4.

6. Berentsen S, Barcellini W. Autoimmune hemolytic anemias. N Engl J Med. 2021 Oct 7; **385**(15): 1407–19.

Neutrophil and Platelet Disorders

Satheesh Chonat, Silvia T Bunting, Kristian T. Schafernak, Michele E. Paessler

Neutrophils are known as the first responders at the sites of infection and injury, but their role in thrombosis is also being recognized. Platelets are known to be an important component in maintaining hemostasis and controlling the bleeding at the site of trauma, as well as in immune modulation [1]. Although some conditions are classified as neutrophilic disorders, they also show clinical manifestations associated with platelet dysfunction, or vice versa. For example, Chediak-Higachi disease is commonly known as neutrophil function disorder; however, it has bleeding history due to abnormal lysosome-like structures inside platelets. Similarly, MYH9-related disorders and Hemansky-Pudlak syndrome are associated with macrothrombocytopenia and storage pool defect but also characterized by neutropenia with recurrent infection and impaired cytotoxic activity.

Neutrophil Function Disorders

Chediak-Higashi syndrome: Chediak-Higashi syndrome is an autosomal recessive disease that is secondary to a mutation in the *LYST* gene, affecting vesicular trafficking and the formation of giant granules, mainly in melanocytes and leukocytes. These patients report moderate bleeding history, characteristic hypopigmentation of skin, and immune dysregulation [2]. These patients are at high risk for hemophagocytic lymphohistiocytosis (HLH) [3]. The peripheral blood smear features giant granules in neutrophil (see Figure 3.1), which, along with clinical manifestations, are diagnostic of this disease. It is important to note that these granules in the cytoplasm of the neutrophils are variably sized.

WHIM (warts, hypogammaglobulinemia, infections, and myelokathexis) syndrome: WHIM is an autosomal dominant-inherited immune-dysregulation disorder typified by heterozygous mutations in *CXCR4*, which codes for the chemokine receptor, also called CXCR4, which plays an important role in neutrophil and lymphocyte trafficking in the bone marrow [4]. Patients can present with hypogammaglobulinemia, warts, and

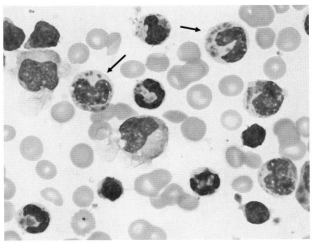

Figure 3.1 Blood smear showing giant granules in neutrophils from a patient with Chediak-Higashi disease. These granules can be of variable size, from large (left arrow) to giant (right arrow). These granules are characteristic of this disorder.

neutropenia and lymphocytopenia, leading to bacterial infections. Some of these patients develop bronchiectasis, anogenital dysplasia, or invasive cancer [5]. Rarely these patients present with Tetralogy of Fallot [6]. These patients are primarily managed with supportive care (antibiotics, granulocyte colony-stimulating factor). The CXCR4 antagonist plerixafor has shown some benefit in a recent clinical trial [7] (Figure 3.2).

May-Hegglin anomaly: This is part of a group of autosomal dominant disorders with mutations involving the *MYH9* gene [8]. This mutated gene encodes for the non-muscle myosin heavy chain II-A (NMMHC-IIA). These patients have macrothrombocytopenia and leucocyte inclusion bodies, resembling Döhle bodies [9]. Extra-hematology manifestations include deafness, nephropathy, and cataracts. As shown in the figure, Döhle bodies are large light blue-gray granules in the cytoplasm of neutrophils. The proposed

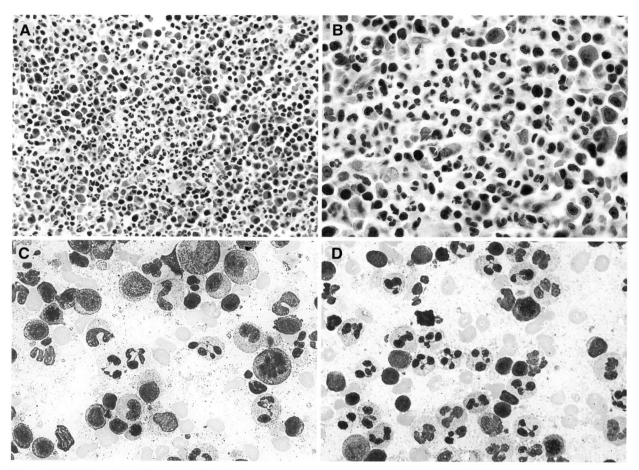

Figure 3.2 WHIM syndrome: This 6-year-old boy had a germline mutation in *CXCR4* and a history of infections, warts, neutropenia, and hypogammaglobulinemia. The core biopsy (A and B: H&E, 500x and 1,000x) shows a hypercellular marrow with granulocytic hyperplasia with increased proportion of segmented neutrophils. On the aspirate smear (C and D: Wright-Giemsa at 1,000x), many distinctive neutrophils (some containing cytoplasmic vacuoles) can be observed, with pyknotic nuclear segments attached by long, thin chromatin strands. The findings are indicative of myelokathexis, a Greek neologism meaning bone marrow (*myelo-*) retention (*-kathexis*) of neutrophils.

mechanism is that during periods of inflammation, remnants of rough endoplasmic reticulum remain in the cytoplasm as 1–3 μm Döhle bodies in the periphery of neutrophils, likely from augmented maturation of neutrophils. Figure 3.3 shows neutrophils with Döhle bodies in the periphery shown by arrows.

Barth syndrome: This is an X-linked cardioskeletal myopathy caused by mutations in the *TAZ* gene encoding tafazzin, a protein localized to the inner leaflet of the mitochondrial membrane, where it catalyzes the remodeling of cardiolipin [10, 11]. Cardiolipin plays important roles in the structure and function of mitochondria.

Due to its chemical composition, cardiolipin takes on a conical structure, allowing for membrane curvature in the form of cristae. It also is involved in energy production and intracellular protein transport. Many patients with Barth syndrome are at risk for recurring and sometimes serious bacterial infections because of neutropenia. Recent evidence suggests this is due to accelerated apoptosis of myeloid progenitors in the marrow, which have abnormal mitochondria with loss of cristae. In the original description of the disease, vacuoles were observed in nearly half of circulating neutrophils while the bone marrow showed a maturation arrest at the myelocyte stage (Figure 3.4).

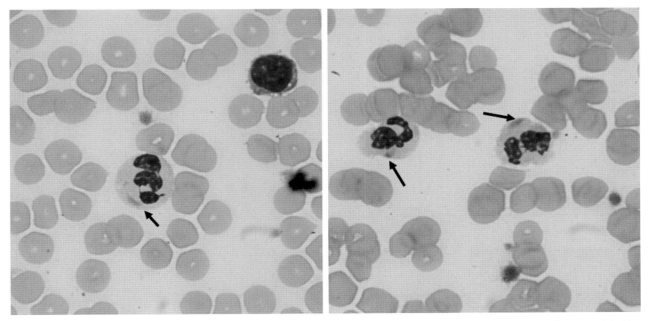

Figure 3.3 Blood smears from a patient with May-Hegglin disease showing a gray-blue neutrophil inclusion (black arrows) in the neutrophils. Also shown is a giant platelet in the picture on the right.

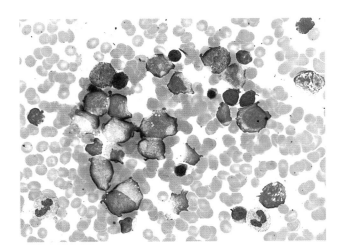

Figure 3.4 Barth syndrome. This bone marrow aspirate (Wright-Giemsa) from a child with Barth syndrome demonstrates a shift to immaturity and vacuoles in the neutrophil series.

Platelet Disorders

Platelet Glycoprotein Deficiency

Platelets have several glycoprotein (GP) complexes on their membrane, which serve as vital components for platelet aggregation through interaction with other cellular proteins, such as collagen in the exposed basement membrane, followed by shape change from smooth disks to spheres with pseudopodia, then release granular contents. The initial platelet aggregates can then "snowball" by adding platelets to form a "plug" to stop bleeding. Inherited defects related to these receptors result in abnormal hemostasis pathways and also, in some situations, lead to a characteristic change in platelet morphology on the blood smear [12]. Platelet aggregation testing (Figure 3.5) and flow cytometry analyses for surface glycoproteins are considered diagnostic tests.

Glanzmann's thrombasthenia results from a functional deficiency of GPIIb/IIIa receptors, leading to defective interaction with fibrinogen and von Willebrand factor (vWF). It is an autosomal recessive disorder. The blood smear shows normal platelet count and morphology. Patients with this rare autosomal recessive disorder exhibit symptoms related to mucocutaneous bleeding and rarely catastrophic bleeding [12]. Platelet aggregation study shows absent platelet aggregation with collagen/epinephrine and collagen/adenosine diphosphate (ADP), but these platelets have a normal agglutination curve with ristocetin (Figures 3.5 and 3.6).

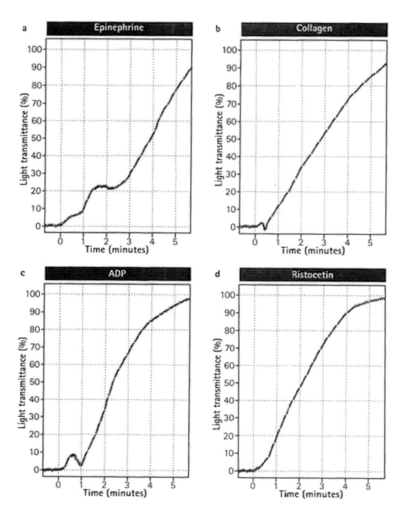

Figure 3.5 Platelet aggregation study using light transmission aggregometry is a diagnostic test for platelet dysfunction. Various agonists are added to the platelet-rich plasma and the percentage of light transmission is measured. If platelet aggregation occurs, the light transmission will increase as reaction occurs. If the platelets fail to aggregate, there will be no or low light transmission. This figure is an example of a normal platelet aggregation study. The light transmission increases as reaction takes place. The agonists used are epinephrine, collagen, ADP, and ristocetin.

Bernard-Soulier syndrome (BSS) is associated with quantitative or qualitative defects involving GPIb/IX/V complex, which is the receptor for vWF, thus affecting platelet adhesion to vascular endothelium. It is an autosomal recessive disorder. Blood smear displays thrombocytopenia and giant-sized platelets, often two or three times larger than normal-sized platelets (normal size 2–3 μm). While exact mechanisms are still unclear, functional deficiency of GPIb/X/V complex results in defective interaction between the platelet plasma membrane and its skeleton, leading to large-sized platelets. Affected individuals tend to have mucocutaneous bleeding, purpura, and prolonged bleeding after surgery. Platelet aggregation studies show normal aggregation for agonists such as ADP, collagen, epinephrine, and arachidonic acid, but reduced or absent ristocetin-induced platelet aggregation.

This pattern is opposite to what Glanzmann's thrombasthenia shows (not shown).

Platelet Storage Pool Deficiency

Normally, platelets contain two types of granules: alpha and delta granules (Figure 3.7). Release of granule contents upon activation is essential in the normal response to vascular damage. Alpha granules contain a plethora of proteins that comprise the bulk of the platelet secretome, including hemostatic factors such as Factor V, vWF, and fibrinogen; angiogenic factors such as angiogenin and VEGF; anti-angiogenic factors such as angiostatin and PF4; growth factors such as PDGF, bFGF, and SDF1α; proteases such as MMP2, MMP9; and necrotic factors such as TNFα, TNFβ, and other cytokines. Alpha granules are the bluish granules seen within the platelets on a Wright-Giemsa stain.

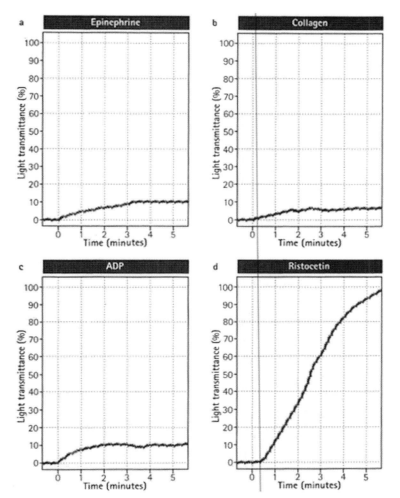

Figure 3.6 Light transmission aggregometry from a patient with Glanzmann's thrombasthenia. The patient has a functional deficiency of glycoprotein IIb/IIIa receptors, resulting in defective interaction with fibrinogen and vWF. The platelets fail to aggregate when epinephrine, collagen, and ADP are added. The antibiotic ristocetin causes vWF to bind the platelet receptor glycoprotein Ib (GpIb), which is intact in Glanzmann's thrombasthenia, thus ristocetin-induced platelet aggregation remains undamaged. For patients with Bernard-Soulier syndrome due to defect in glycoprotein Ib, the reverse happens – that is, normal aggregation with epinephrine, collagen, or ADP but abnormal aggregation with ristocetin.

Absence of alpha granules make the platelets appear gray or "ghostlike," hence the term *gray platelet syndrome*.

Delta granules are also known as dense bodies or dense granules. They are smaller than alpha granules. Dense granules are not visible in routine Wright-Giemsa stains but only on electronic microscope as electric dense elements. The dense granules of human platelets contain ADP, adenosine triphosphate (ATP), ionized calcium, and serotonin.

Gray Platelet Syndrome

Gray platelet syndrome is characterized by a deficiency in alpha granules of platelets. It results from biallelic mutations involving the *NBEAL2* gene, encoding for neurobeachin-like-2 protein [13]. This platelet defect manifests mild thrombocytopenia with moderate to severe bleeding phenotype. Clinical presentation could be similar to idiopathic thrombocytopenic purpura (ITP); however, review of the peripheral blood smear shows that the platelets are characteristically large and pale gray in color from lack of alpha granules in the platelets (Figure 3.8). Electron microscopy can also reveal these large pale gray platelets.

Hermansky-Pudlak syndrome (HPS): HPS is a platelet storage-pool deficiency disorder inherited as an autosomal recessive disease. It is characterized by oculocutaneous albinism with visual impairment and prolonged bleeding due to platelet dysfunction due to delta storage pool defect [14]. Some patients have pulmonary fibrosis, colitis, or abnormal storage of fatty-like substance. Diagnosis is usually suspected when a patient presents with hypopigmentation of skin and hair along with

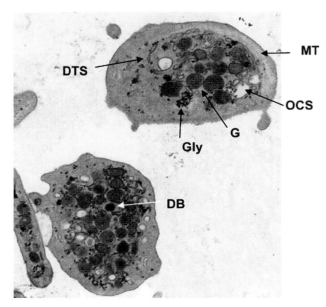

Figure 3.7 Electron microscopy (original magnification ×22,500) of platelets showing the dense tubular system (DTS), microtubules (MT), open canalicular system (OCS), alpha granules (G), glycogen (Gly), and the dense bodies (DB)

characteristic absent delta granules (dense bodies) on electron microscopy of platelets (see Figure 3.7 for dense granule morphology). Coagulation function testing reveals impaired secondary aggregation response to platelet aggregation and prolonged bleeding time. Many genes are associated with HPS (biallelic pathogenic variants in *AP3B1*, *AP3D1*, *BLOC1S3*, *BLOC1S6*, *DTNBP1*, *HPS1*, *HPS3*, *HPS4*, *HPS5*, or *HPS6*) [15].

Platelet Dysfunction Associated with Immune Disorder

Idiopathic thrombocytopenia purpura (ITP): ITP is the condition of having a low platelet count (thrombocytopenia) or no platelet function, of no known cause (idiopathic) [16]. Most causes appear to be related to antibodies against platelets. ITP is also known as immune thrombocytopenic purpura. The clinical presentation may be acute with severe bleeding or insidious with slow development with mild or no symptoms. Bone marrow biopsy is performed in refractory cases to rule out conditions such as familial platelet disorder with associated myeloid malignancy (*RUNX1*), congenital amegakaryocytic thrombocytopenia due to *MPL* (thrombopoietin receptor) mutation, Wiskott-Aldrich syndrome or its attenuated form (*WAS*), or

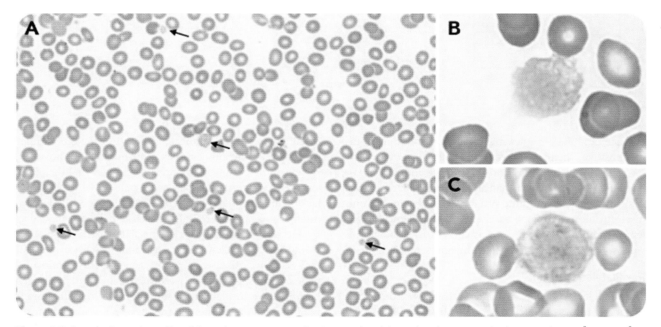

Figure 3.8 Gray platelet syndrome. Two siblings of a consanguineous family were referred due to thrombocytopenia (in the range of 30×10^3 to $80 \times 10^3/\mu L$), recurrent infections, and hepatosplenomegaly. In the blood smear, large and pale platelets were observed, compatible with the diagnosis of gray platelet syndrome (GPS) (panels A–C; arrows, abnormal platelets; original magnification ×500 [A] and ×1000 [B–C]; Wright-Giemsa stain).

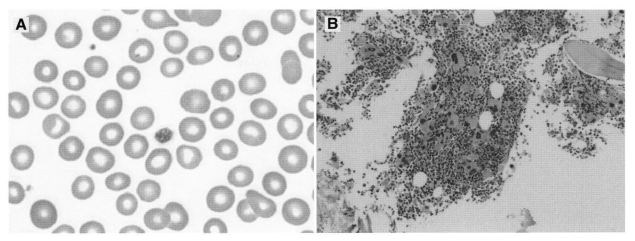

Figure 3.9 ITP. The peripheral blood showed marked thrombocytopenia with occasional giant platelets. (A, Wright-Giemsa stain). The marrow in ITP will demonstrate abundance of megakaryocytes at all stages of maturation and therefore vary widely in size (B: Wright-Giemsa, 100x; C: CD61 immunostain, 100x).

X-linked thrombocytopenia with *GATA1* mutation (Figure 3.9).

Wiskott-Aldrich syndrome (WAS): WAS is characterized by microthrombocytopenia, which is also dysfunctional [17]. WAS is an X-linked recessive disease involving the *WAS* gene, which produces WAS protein. This protein is believed to modulate cell motility through movements of actin filaments in the cytoskeleton. It is often seen in young children presenting with mild bleeding history, eczema of skin, and immune dysregulation (recurrent infections). Immune dysregulation is characterized by both T-cell and B-cell abnormality. Some of these patients can also have autoimmune manifestations. They are at higher risk of malignancies, especially leukemias and lymphomas. These patients are known to have small platelets (Figure 3.10).

Platelet Dysfunction Associated with a Defect in Enzymatic Activity (TTP)

Thrombotic thrombocytopenic purpura (TTP) is a rare blood disorder characterized by the pentad of fever, thrombocytopenia, hemolytic anemia, renal dysfunction, and neurologic dysfunction resulting from organ ischemia due to microvascular occlusion. This is a form of thrombotic microangiopathy (TMA), resulting from severe deficiency of ADAMTS13 (a disintegrin and metalloproteinase with thrombospondin motifs 13) activity [18].

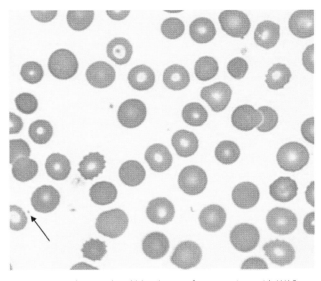

Figure 3.10 The peripheral blood smear from a patient with WAS shows small platelet (arrow).

Congenital TTP (cTTP) occurs from biallelic (homozygous or compound heterozygous) mutations involving ADAMTS13 in 5% of cases, or is acquired (immune-mediated [iTTP]) due to autoantibodies against ADAMTS13 in 95% of patients [19]. The ADAMTS13 deficiency results in the buildup of hyper-adhesive ultra-large von Willebrand multimers

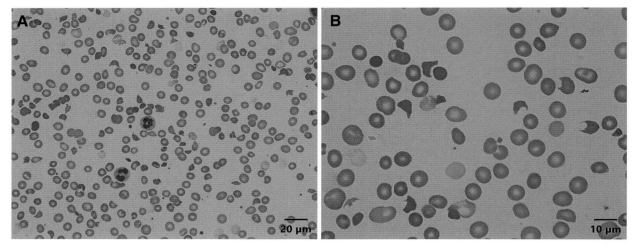

Figure 3.11 Blood smear from an adolescent female presenting with acute episodes of headaches, gum bleeding, fatigue, and dark urine. Laboratory work was remarkable for thrombocytopenia and microangiopathic hemolytic anemia with blood smear evident for schistocytes thought to be formed from the shearing of red blood cells by the micro-thrombi and paucity of platelets (A and B, Wright-Giemsa stain, 500x and 1,000x, respectively).

in the circulation leading to platelet adhesion and aggregation and subsequent formation of microvascular thrombi causing organ ischemia and damage. Blood smear in TTP is characteristic for thrombocytopenia and microangiopathic hemolytic anemia with schistocytes thought to be formed from the shearing of red blood cells by the micro-thrombi (Figure 3.11).

References

1. Lisman T. Platelet-neutrophil interactions as drivers of inflammatory and thrombotic disease. Cell Tissue Res. 2018; **371**(3): 567–76.
2. Kaplan J, De Domenico I, Ward DM. Chediak-Higashi syndrome. Curr Opin Hematol. 2008; **15**(1): 22–9.
3. Jessen B, Maul-Pavicic A, Ufheil H, Vraetz T, Enders A, Lehmberg K, et al. Subtle differences in CTL cytotoxicity determine susceptibility to hemophagocytic lymphohistiocytosis in mice and humans with Chediak-Higashi syndrome. Blood. 2011; **118**(17): 4620–9.
4. Liu Q, Pan C, Lopez L, Gao J, Velez D, Anaya-O'Brien S, et al. WHIM syndrome caused by Waldenström's macroglobulinemia-associated mutation CXCR4 (L329fs). J Clin Immunol. 2016; **36**(4): 397–405.
5. Badolato R, Donadieu J. How I treat warts, hypogammaglobulinemia, infections, and myelokathexis syndrome. Blood. 2017; **130**(23): 2491–8.
6. Badolato R, Dotta L, Tassone L, Amendola G, Porta F, Locatelli F, et al. Tetralogy of Fallot is an uncommon manifestation of warts, hypogammaglobulinemia, infections, and myelokathexis syndrome. J Pediatr. 2012; **161**(4): 763–5.
7. McDermott DH, Liu Q, Ulrick J, Kwatemaa N, Anaya-O'Brien S, Penzak SR, et al. The CXCR4 antagonist plerixafor corrects panleukopenia in patients with WHIM syndrome. Blood. 2011; **118**(18): 4957–62.
8. Kunishima S. [May-Hegglin anomaly: Past and present: MNovel diagnostic test and new concept of the disease]. Rinsho Byori. 2009; **57**(1): 54–9.
9. Barros Pinto MP, Marques G. MYH9 disorders (May-Hegglin anomaly): The role of the blood smear. J Pediatr Hematol Oncol. 2019; **41**(3): 228.
10. Clarke SL, Bowron A, Gonzalez IL, Groves SJ, Newbury-Ecob R, Clayton N, et al. Barth syndrome. Orphanet J Rare Dis. 2013; **8**: 23.
11. Ikon N, Ryan RO. Barth syndrome: Connecting cardiolipin to cardiomyopathy. Lipids. 2017; **52**(2): 99–108.
12. Diz-Kücükkaya R, López JA. Inherited disorders of platelets: Membrane glycoprotein disorders. Hematol Oncol Clin North Am. 2013; **27**(3): 613–27.
13. Gunay-Aygun M, Falik-Zaccai TC, Vilboux T, Zivony-Elboum Y, Gumruk F, Cetin M, et al. *NBEAL2* is mutated in gray platelet syndrome and is required for biogenesis of platelet α-granules. Nat Genet. 2011; **43**(8): 732–4.
14. De Jesus Rojas W, Young LR. Hermansky-Pudlak syndrome. Semin Respir Crit Care Med. 2020; **41**(2): 238–46.
15. Huizing M, Malicdan MCV, Wang JA, Pri-Chen H, Hess RA, Fischer R, et al. Hermansky-Pudlak syndrome: Mutation update. Hum Mutat. 2020; **41**(3):543–80.

16. LeVine DN, Brooks MB. Immune thrombocytopenia (ITP): Pathophysiology update and diagnostic dilemmas. Vet Clin Pathol. 2019; **48** Suppl 1: 17–28.

17. Massaad MJ, Ramesh N, Geha RS. Wiskott-Aldrich syndrome: A comprehensive review. Ann N Y Acad Sci. 2013; **1285**: 26–43.

18. Chiasakul T, Cuker A. Clinical and laboratory diagnosis of TTP: An integrated approach. Hematology Am Soc Hematol Educ Program. 2018; **2018**(1): 530–8.

19. George JN. Congenital TTP: Toward a turning point. Blood. 2019; **133**(15): 1615–17.

Infectious Diseases and Nutritional Deficiencies

Satheesh Chonat, Sara Graciaa, Silvia T Bunting

Infectious Diseases

The clinician often refers to the total and the differential leucocyte count when evaluating patients with fever or infection. Therefore, a complete blood count (CBC) and review of blood smear remain the most commonly ordered tests in these situations. In addition to the quantitative review of CBC, morphological analysis including inclusion bodies is often undertaken during this exercise. We review common infections and related characterized changes noted on their blood smear.

a. **Viral infections:** In general, viral infections are often typified by reactive or atypical lymphocytes, which are larger than a resting lymphocyte and feature a pleiomorphic shape, irregular nucleus, thin chromatin, and cytoplasm that can be pale or darker at the edges of the cell, where it is often indented by adjacent cells. Vacuoles or large azurophilic granules can be seen in the cytoplasm. These atypical cells are found in infectious mononucleosis, which can occur secondary to Epstein-Barr virus (EBV) or cytomegaloviral (CMV) infections (see Figures 4.1a and 4.1b). Blood smears from patients with EBV or CMV also show mild relative and absolute neutropenia and thrombocytopenia. These changes are also seen in patients with other viral infections, including rubella, hepatitis, toxoplasmosis, or human immunodeficiency virus.

b. **Malaria:** Thin and thick blood smears are a standard request in cases where malaria is suspected. While a thin smear helps identify the presence of a malarial parasite and the level of parasitemia, a thick smear can help identify the species of plasmodium parasite (Figure 4.2a) [1]. Four types of the plasmodium parasite (falciparum, vivax, ovale, and malariae) can affect humans. During blood smear evaluation, it is important to recognize the different forms of the parasite based on their life cycle: ring, trophozoite,

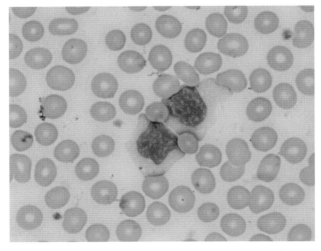

Figures 4.1a and 4.1b Blood film from a patient with EBV infection. These two smears show large lymphocytes with abundant cytoplasm and irregularly shaped nuclei. As shown in Figure 4.1b, the lymphocyte cell contour fits the outline of the surrounding red blood cells (RBCs).

schizont, and gametocyte [2]. Figures 4.2b and 4.2c show the ring and gametocyte stages of plasmodium falciparum, respectively.

c. **Yeast:** Occasionally, in patients who are immunocompromised, the presence of candidal elements or pseudohyphae can be found intracellularly in a neutrophil and extracellularly on a Giemsa stain, which can help early identification of a fungal infection (see Figure 4.3).

d. **Pertussis:** On fortuitous occasions, rare infections such as Bordetella can be diagnosed from a blood smear, where mature lymphocytes can be seen with a clefted nucleus, scant cytoplasm, and condensed chromatin (Figure 4.4) [3].

e. **Ehrlichiosis:** This can infect monocytes and neutrophils depending on the strain. A typical blood smear might reveal microcolonies of *Ehrlichiae*

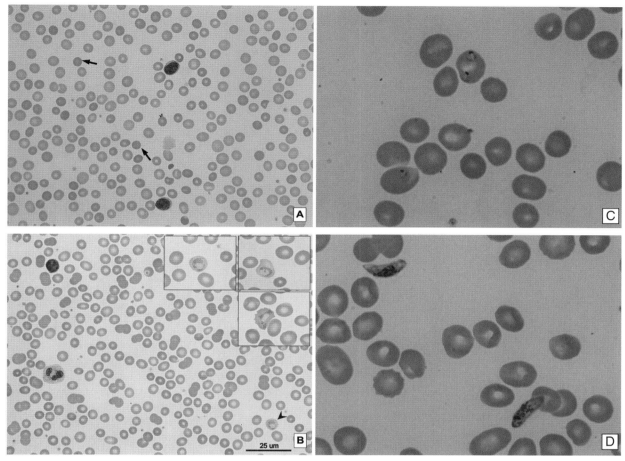

Figure 4.2 Blood smear showing microspherocytes (arrows, A), microcytic hypochromic RBCs and some erythrocytes with malarial parasitic inclusions (arrowhead and insets, B). Image taken from [1]. Figures 4.2b and 4.2c show the ring (first) and gametocyte (last) stages of the *Plasmodium falciparum* life cycle.

(Figure 4.5) in the cytoplasm of leucocytes, which look discrete and punctate a gray-blue color in the cytoplasm [4].

f. **Babesiosis:** Similar to other parasitic infections described earlier in this chapter, Babesia parasites can be found outside (Figure 4.6a) and within leucocytes or erythrocytes (Figure 4.6b) in varying shapes such as round, oval, and ring forms.

g. **Toxoplasmosis:** Though the confirmatory testing of this and many other infections is made using serological tests, diagnosis can be aided by direct observation of the parasite in tissue fluids, including blood (see Figure 4.7).

Nutritional Deficiencies

Nutritional deficiencies, especially iron deficiency, remain the leading causes of anemia globally. Review of a blood smear is not only vital but mostly confirmatory for diagnosis and treatment. Hence, a good understanding of the effect of these systemic nutritional disturbances on erythrocytes and other blood cells would come in handy for a naïve hematologist or pathologist in training.

h. **Iron deficiency** is one of the most common causes of anemia worldwide. Children are especially prone to iron deficiency when compared to adults, as they have increased requirement secondary to rapid growth and development. If unrecognized or not adequately

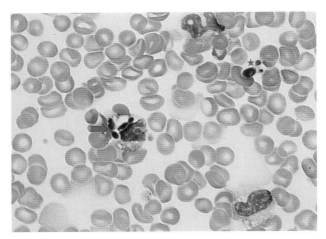

Figure 4.3 Blood smear shows yeasts inside a leukocyte (arrow) and extracellular (star) yeasts.

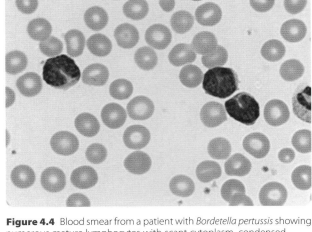

Figure 4.4 Blood smear from a patient with *Bordetella pertussis* showing numerous mature lymphocytes with scant cytoplasm, condensed chromatin, and clefted nuclei. Image taken from [3].

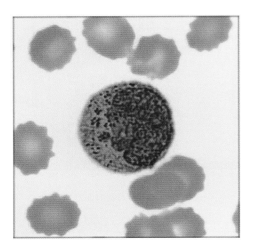

Figure 4.5 A characteristic blood smear showing discrete and punctate gray-blue colored microcolonies of *Ehrlichiae* within the cytoplasm of a monocyte, known as morulae.

treated, iron deficiency can lead to irreversible neurodevelopmental and cognitive sequelae. Iron deficiency can be caused by inadequate dietary intake, impaired absorption, or blood loss. Iron is required for hemoglobin synthesis and erythropoiesis and, in late stages of iron deficiency, anemia can develop. Patients with iron-deficiency anemia typically have a decreased RBC count, hemoglobin, hematocrit, and mean corpuscular volume. Platelet count may be elevated as erythropoietin stimulates platelet precursors in addition to erythroblasts (Figure 4.8).

i. **Folate/ Vitamin B12/ Copper deficiency.** Vitamin B12 (also known as cobalamin) and vitamin B9 (folate) are both required for hematopoiesis. When these vitamins are deficient due to poor dietary intake, decreased absorption, or an underlying genetic disorder, megaloblastic anemia can result. In cases of severe deficiencies, thrombocytopenia and neutropenia can be detected as well. In some cases, hyper-segmented neutrophils precede the development of macrocytic anemia (Figure 4.9). This underscores the importance of not solely relying on labs but also taking the crucial step of reviewing the peripheral blood smear, especially if the suspicion of the deficiency is high.

j. **Lead poisoning** should always be on the differential in a child presenting with microcytic anemia. Until the 1970s, lead was used in paint and children who live in older homes or in low-income countries therefore are more likely to be exposed. Young children are especially at risk due to numerous factors. First, young children have an incomplete blood-brain barrier and are more susceptible to the neurotoxic effects of lead. Moreover, children who are iron deficient have an increased absorption of lead through the gastrointestinal tract. As discussed earlier, iron deficiency is most prevalent in children under the age of 5, placing these children at even higher risk. Lead diffuses into soft tissues, including

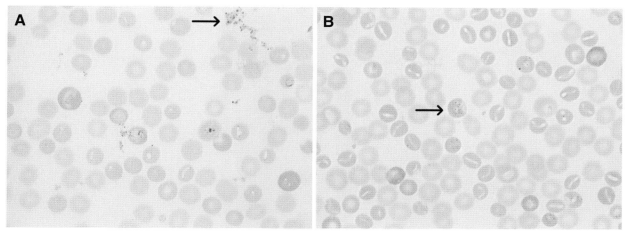

Figures 4.6a and 4.6b Babesia parasites are shown outside the leucocytes (a) on the blood film and inside the erythrocytes (b).

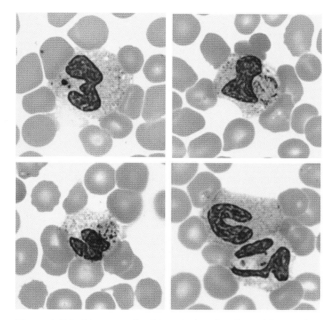

Figure 4.7 In this composite picture, tachyzoites, the rapidly growing stage of *Toxoplasma gondii*, are shown as inclusion bodies within infected neutrophils.

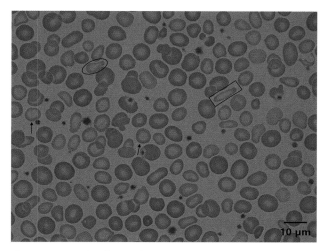

Figure 4.8 Peripheral smear from a toddler with an iron-deficient diet. The RBCs show hypochromasia and anisopoikilocytosis with teardrop-shaped RBCs (oval outline), "pencil" cells (rectangle outline), and hypochromic RBCs (arrow).

the kidneys, liver, brain, and bone marrow, and its toxicity interferes with enzymatic steps in the heme pathway, leading to decreased hemoglobin synthesis and a hypochromic, microcytic anemia. High lead levels (>70 μg/dL) lead to acute hemolysis. Lead poisoning alters ribosomes and causes aggregation, which ultimately leads to basophilic stippling of RBCs (Figures 4.10a and 4.10b) [5].

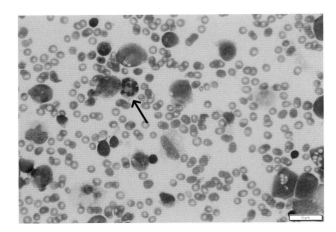

Figure 4.9 This smear was taken from an infant with pancytopenia secondary to severe vitamin B12 deficiency. On close examination, occasional hyper-segmented neutrophil can be seen (arrow).

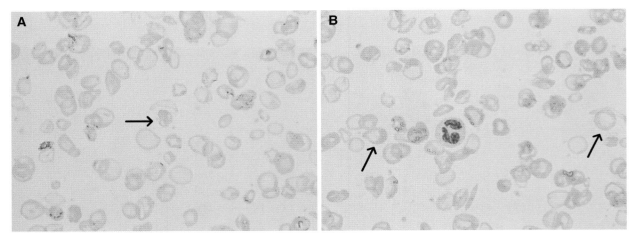

Figures 4.10a and 4.10b Blood smear in lead poisoning with hypochromic RBCs scattered around as shown in both pictures along with characteristic basophilic stippling (arrows in Figures 4.10A and 4.10B).

References

1. Graciaa S, Russell R, Chonat S. Complement mediated hemolytic anemia secondary to plasmodium ovale infection in a child. J Pediatr Hematol Oncol. 2019; **41**(7): 557–8.

2. Tsai MH, Yu SS, Chan YK, Jen CC. Blood smear image based malaria parasite and infected-erythrocyte detection and segmentation. J Med Syst. 2015; **39**(10): 118.

3. Pandey S, Cetin N. Peripheral smear clues for Bordetella pertussis. Blood. 2013; **122**(25): 4012.

4. Hamilton KS, Standaert SM, Kinney MC. Characteristic peripheral blood findings in human ehrlichiosis. Mod Pathol. 2004; **17**(5): 512–17.

5. Dapul H, Laraque D. Lead poisoning in children. Adv Pediatr. 2014; **61**(1): 313–33.

Chapter

5

Benign Non-neoplastic Noninfective Lymphadenopathy

Dehua Wang, Shunyou Gong

Lymphadenopathy (LAD) is a common presentation in the pediatric population. Cervical LAD with neck mass is the most common manifestation [1]. The etiology of LAD is diverse, including various benign nonspecific reactive conditions, infections, neoplasms, and immune disorders, among others. In spite of the initial concern of lymphoma or infectious conditions, most cases of LAD turn out to be benign and nonspecific reactive. The morphologic features of nonspecific reactive LAD can overlap with those of specific infective LAD or lymphoma. Although some features are more associated with certain etiologies, they are not pathognomonic. Clinical correlation would be essential on this ground. The goal of this chapter is to use case-based illustration to thoroughly demonstrate the morphological features of reactive lymph node and specific entities of non-neoplastic/ noninfective LAD.

The preserved nodal architecture with patent sinuses is the key feature for reactive lymph nodes. However, the nodal architecture may be variably or partially distorted depending on the degree of the involvement in some benign specific entities. Follicular hyperplasia (FH) (Figure 5.1), paracortical/interfollicular hyperplasia (PIH) (Figure 5.2), and sinus histiocytosis (Figure 5.3) are the most common morphological features seen in reactive LAD. Mixed pattern with a combination of more than one type of well-characterized lymphoid hyperplasia is also common. Not infrequently, focal immunoblast hyperplasia, mantle zone hyperplasia, marginal zone (monocytoid B-cell) hyperplasia, plasmacytoid dendritic cell (PDC) hyperplasia [2], or follicular lysis [3] (Figure 5.4) may be seen in a hyperplastic lymph node with certain specific entities or nonspecific reactive conditions. For instance, mantle zone hyperplasia is commonly seen in Castleman disease and progressive transformation of germinal centers (PTGC) (Figure 5.5). Florid FH (Figure 5.6) with disrupted large follicles, vague or loss polarization of germinal center, and scant to absent tangible macrophages should raise concern and prompt a workup for HIV infection, pediatric follicular lymphoma, or large cell

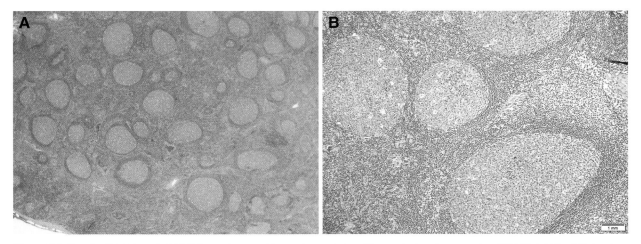

Figure 5.1 Reactive FH. A. Lymphoid follicles are increased in number and size with germinal center expansion (H&E, 20x). B. The follicles show preserved attenuated mantle zones, the polarization in light and dark zones, and numerous tangible body macrophages (H&E, 100x).

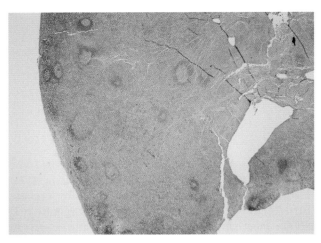

Figure 5.2 PIH. A lymph node biopsy shows marked expansion of the paracortical/interfollicular zone (H&E, 20x).

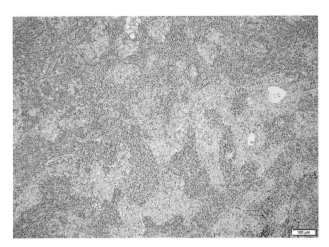

Figure 5.3 Sinus histocytosis. The lymph node sinuses are extended by pale, benign-appearing histiocytes/macrophages (H&E 100x).

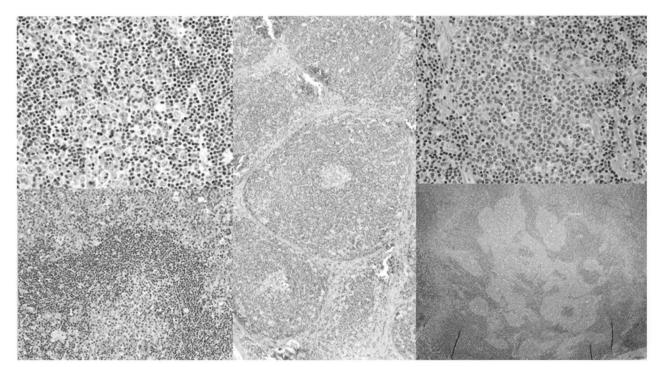

Figure 5.4 Hyperplastic lymph node with certain specific or nonspecific reactive conditions. Upper left: Immunoblastic hyperplasia, commonly seen in infectious mononucleosis, with the expansion of the paracortical zone, prominent increase in immunoblasts (large, transformed lymphocytes) with open chromatin, a single prominent nucleolus and small amount of cytoplasm. Lower left: Marginal zone hyperplasia/monocytoid B-cell hyperplasia. Focal marginal zone expansion forms a sheet of monocytoid B-cells with clear cytoplasm, small to intermediate, and round or indented nuclei (upper part of the image). Middle: Mantle zone hyperplasia. Commonly seen in Castleman disease. The mantle zone expands to an excessive thickness and is composed of small mature lymphocytes with a round nuclear contour and condensed chromatin. Upper right: PDC nodule/hyperplasia. Commonly seen in Castleman disease, Kikuchi-Fujimoto disease, and PTGC. A few small and pale distinct nodules in interfollicular areas, often near high endothelial venules. The nodule is composed of PDCs that are intermediate in size, slightly larger than small lymphocytes, and have round, oval, or indented nuclei, fine chromatin, inconspicuous nucleoli, pink cytoplasm, and well-defined cytoplasmic borders. Lower right: Follicular lysis. The germinal centers infiltrated by "tongues" of small lymphocytes, primarily T-cells admixed with a smaller number of mantle zone B-cells.

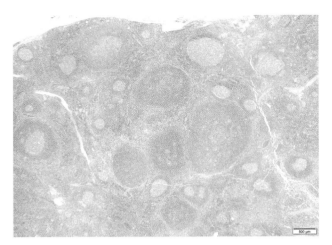

Figure 5.5 PTGC. A 15-year-old female developed an enlarged lymph node (2.7 × 3.8 cm) in the left neck. An excision of the lymph node was performed. The lymph node reveals a few enlarged follicles in the background of FH with intact, well-defined mantle zones (H&E, 20x). These enlarged follicles (PTGC) are more than two to three times larger than the surrounding hyperplastic follicles and are composed of predominant small lymphocytes migrated from the mantle zone, mixed with germinal center cells. PTGC can be associated with nodular lymphocytic predominant Hodgkin lymphoma.

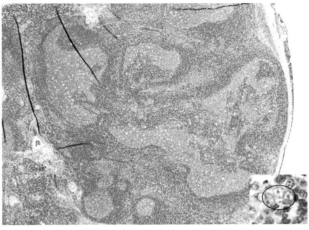

Figure 5.6 Florid FH. An 11-year-old female presented with left supraclavicular LAD for 2 weeks. The lymph node biopsy shows that some of the follicles are extremely large with prominent expanded germinal centers resembling "dumbbells" or having serpiginous appearances (H&E, 40x). The follicular dendritic cells in the light zone are characterized with cleared chromatin and small central nucleoli, which are often bilobed with flattening of the nuclear membranes called "kissing dendritic cells" (inset).

lymphoma. Nodular expansion of the paracortical/ interfollicular zone is commonly associated with dermatopathic LAD (Figure 5.7). Some neoplastic conditions involving the paracortical/interfollicular zone can also have nodular expansion. Although the etiology of necrotizing (Figure 5.8) and non-necrotizing (Figure 5.9) granulomatous LAD frequently results from infectious conditions and sarcoidosis, respectively, in young patients, sometimes infectious agents are not identified by microbiology study, molecular analysis, or serology study. Careful examination for the presence of neoplasm is prudent. Prominent granulomatous inflammation in the lymph node can be seen in Hodgkin lymphoma or peripheral T-cell lymphoma. The presence of marked polyclonal plasmacytic hyperplasia should alert doctors to the possibility of an autoimmune disease.

Castleman disease (CD) (Figures 5.10 and 5.11), Kikuchi-Fujimoto disease (KFD) (Figure 5.12), Kimura disease (Figure 5.13), Rosai-Dorfman disease (RDD) (Figure 5.14), and inflammatory myofibroblastic tumor (IMT) (Figure 5.15) of the lymph node are specific benign entities of LAD. The characteristic

features of morphology and clinical correlation are helpful for the diagnosis. The histologic features of lymph nodes in systemic lupus erythematous (SLE) can be heterogeneous, depending on the stage. The characteristic feature of SLE (Figure 5.16) mimics KFD when the hematoxylin body is not visible [4]. Other benign, noninfective situations may contribute to children's LAD – for instance, extramedullary hematopoiesis (EMH) (Figure 5.17), vascular transformation of lymph node sinuses (Figure 5.18), and a branchial cleft cyst in the lymph node (Figure 5.19).

Mucosa-associated organ and tissue with lymphoid hyperplasia (tonsil and Peyer's patches) can be seen in children. Extensive lymphoid hyperplasia can be atypical and mimic lymphoma. This entity was first presented in a case series by Attygalle and colleagues in 2004 [5]. The diagnosis of marginal zone lymphoma was immunoglobulin light chain restriction, usually by flow cytometry study, and aberrant CD43 expression by immunohistochemistry study. However, these cases lacked molecular evidence of clonality. Awareness of this entity will help to prevent the diagnostic pitfall.

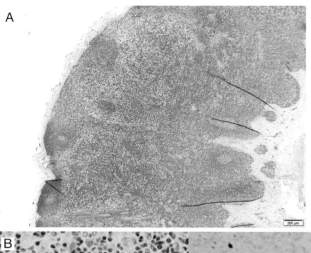

Figure 5.7 Dermatopathic LAD. A 13-year-old male presented with a right posterior neck LAD. A. The biopsy of the lymph node displays prominent nodular expansion in paracortical areas with proliferation of histiocytes, interdigitating dendritic cells, Langerhans cells, and reactive small lymphocytes imparting a mottled and pale appearance (H&E, 40x). B. Some histiocytes shows brown melanin pigment (left, H&E) with positivity by Fontana Masson stain (right). C. S-100 immunostain (left) demonstrates interdigitating dendritic cells and Langerhans cells. CD1a immunostain (right) highlights Langerhans cells.

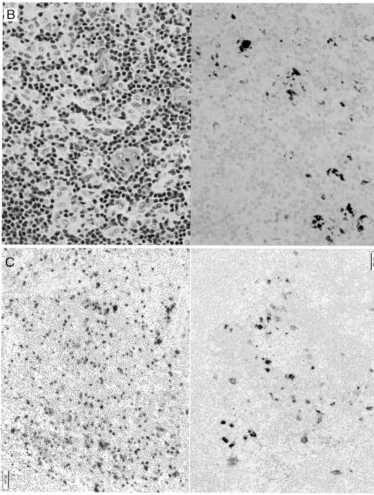

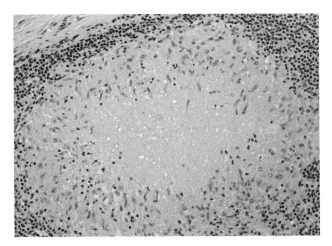

Figure 5.8 Necrotizing granulomatous lymphadenitis. A 6-year-old female presented with left elbow swelling for 4 weeks. A soft tissue mass was excised. The section of lymph node demonstrates architecture distortion by a few necrotizing granulomas. The granuloma in the image reveals central necrosis surrounded by palisading histiocytes mixed with lymphocytes (H&E, 200x). No microorganisms are identified (stains not shown).

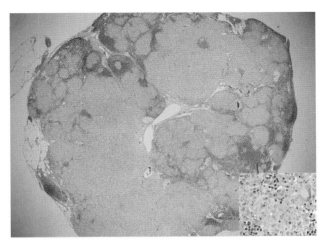

Figure 5.9 Noncaseating granulomatous lymphadenitis. A 17-year-old African American male presented with mediastinal LAD. Sarcoidosis was included in the differential diagnosis. The biopsy of a lymph node shows normal lymph node architecture replaced by confluent granulomas (H&E, 20x). The inset demonstrates granulomas composed of epithelioid histiocytes and multinucleated giant cells.

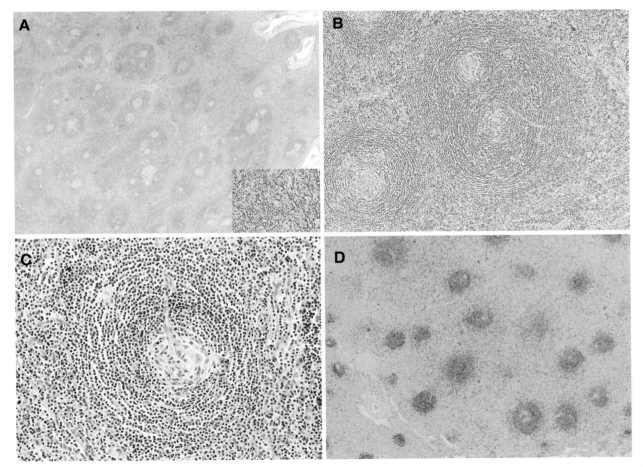

Figure 5.10 Unicentric CD-hyaline vascular variant. A 12-year-old male with right neck mass about 5 cm for 2 years; asymptomatic and doing well after neck mass excision. A. The lymph node shows increase in follicles throughout the node. The follicles are variably small in size (H&E, 20x). Interfollicular areas are expanded by prominent hyalinized vessels (inset). B. The characteristic features of follicles include more than one burned-out germinal center and mantle zone expansion arranged in multiple concentric layers ("onion skin" pattern) (H&E, 100x). C. A follicle crisscrossed by small vessels, giving the characteristic "lollipop" appearance (H&E, 200x). D. Follicular dendritic cell hyperplasia is highlighted by CD23 (Immunostain, 100x).

A

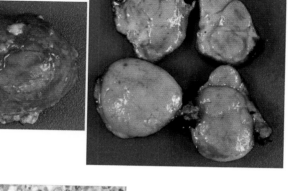

B

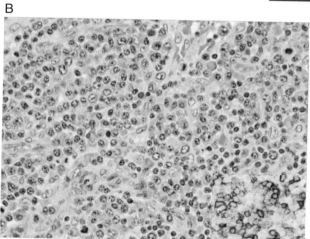

Figure 5.11 Multicentric CD-plasma cell variant. A 17-year-old male presented with multicentric LAD, constitutional symptoms, and increased serum IL6. The largest intra-abdominal mass was excised. A. The large mass measures 9.5 x 4.5 x 4 cm (left) with flesh nodular cut surface (right). B. Histological section of the mass shows lymph nodes with increase of follicles whose germinal centers are variable in size and some of them are atrophic(not shown). Interfollicular areas show sheets of plasma cells (H&E, 400x) with CD138 reactivity (immunostain, inset). Plasma cells were polytypic by in situ hybridization for kappa and lambda light chain stains (not shown). HHV-8 is not detected by immunostain (not shown).

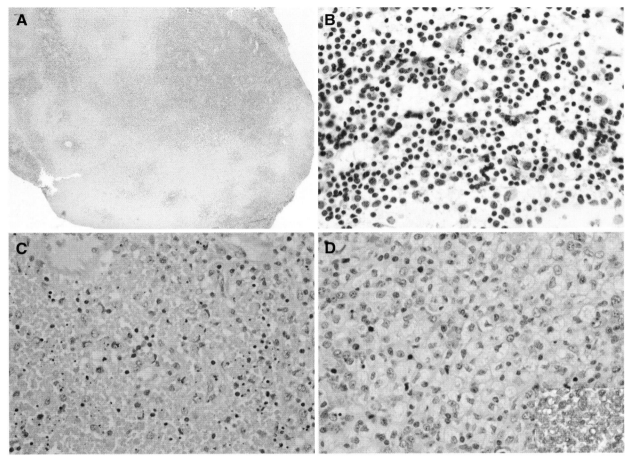

Figure 5.12 KFD. A 16-year-old male with a 1-month history of painful left cervical and right axillary LAD, leukopenia, anemia, intermittent fevers, weight loss, elevated LDH, CPK, CRP, and ferritin. A. Nodal architecture is effaced with extensive paracortex necrosis (H&E, 20x). B. A touch imprint reveals a number of macrophages with C-shaped nuclei and abundant cytoplasm filled with eosinophilic material (H&E, 400x). C. Some areas show features of the necrotic phase, which is composed of a number of atypical lymphocytes with vesicular chromatin and small distinct nuclei, histiocytes with C-shaped nuclei and eosinophilic material-filled cytoplasm, and necrotic cell debris (H&E, 400x). D. Other areas reveal characteristics of the xanthomatous phase with sheets of foamy histiocytes (H&E, 400x) that are positive for CD68 (inset).

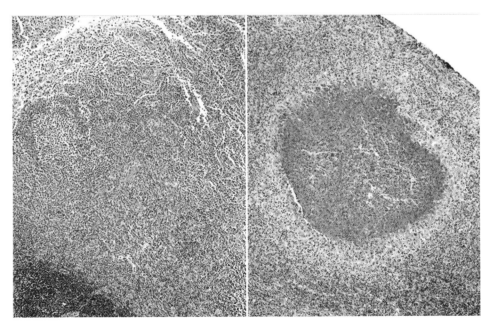

Figure 5.13 Kimura LAD. A 17-year-old male with an Asian ethnic background presented with left submandibular LAD for 2 months and marked eosinophilia. A left submandibular lymph node excision was performed. The lymph node shows a largely preserved nodal architecture and scattered reactive follicles with expansion of interfollicular area by eosinophilic infiltrate (H&E, left) and eosinophilic microabscess (right) in the paracortex, which is a typical feature of Kimura disease.

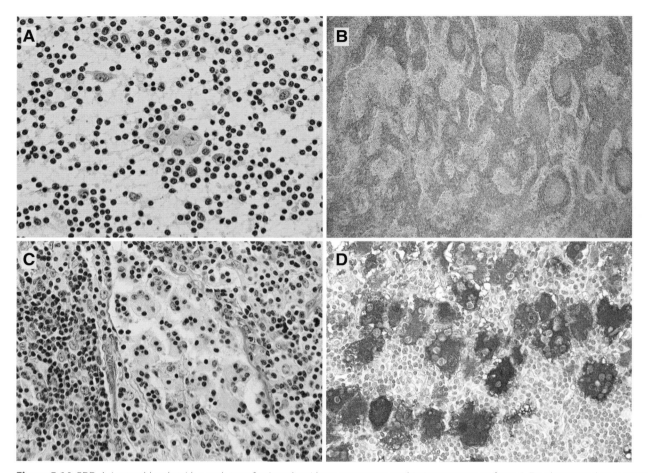

Figure 5.14 RDD. A 4-year-old male with a neck mass for 6 weeks without response to antibiotic treatment; no fever. A. Touch imprint demonstrates a large histiocyte in the center with emperipolesis characterized by intracytoplasmic mainly intact lymphocytes and/or rare plasma cells (H&E, 400x). B. Low-power view of the lymph node shows architecture distortion with pale areas for dilated sinus histiocytosis (H&E, 20x). C. At high magnification, dilated sinuses are filled with histiocytes showing emperipolesis (H&E, 400x). D. The histiocytes are positive for S-100, which highlights emperipolesis (immunostain, 400x).

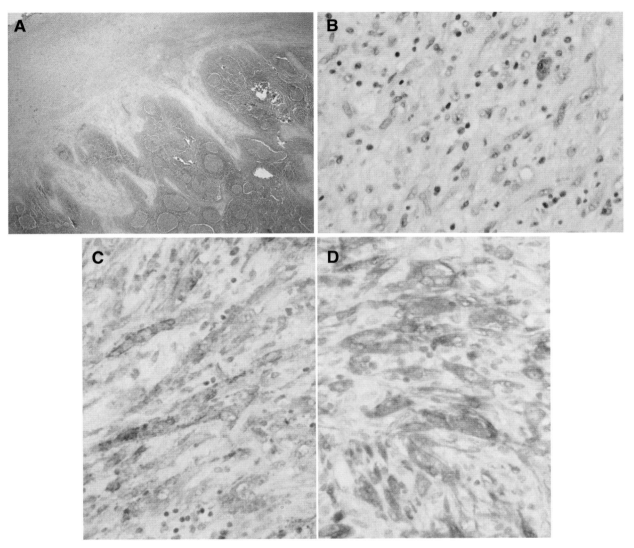

Figure 5.15 Inflammatory myofibroblastic tumor of the lymph node. A 13-year-old male with low-grade fever and isolated cervical LAD for 3 months and without response to antibiotics. A. The lymph node is largely replaced by a fibrotic lesion primarily involving the connective tissue framework and extending to the medulla/hilum, trabeculae, and capsule and a mixed inflammatory cell infiltrate (H&E, 20x). B. The lesion is composed of bland spindle cells (fibroblasts/myofibroblasts) mixed with inflammatory cells, including lymphocytes, plasma cells, and histiocytes in the background of variable collagen (H&E, 400x). C. The spindle cells are immunohistochemically positive for smooth muscle actin (SMA) and anaplastic lymphoma kinase 1 (ALK-1) (D) with a cytoplasmic staining pattern.

References

1. Deosthali A, Donches K, DelVecchio M, Aronoff S. Etiologies of pediatric cervical lymphadenopathy: A systematic review of 2687 subjects. Global Pediatric Health. 2019 Jul; **6**: 2333794X19865440.

2. Chang CC, Osipov V, Wheaton S, Tripp S, Perkins SL. Follicular hyperplasia, follicular lysis, and progressive transformation of germinal centers: A sequential spectrum of morphologic evolution in lymphoid hyperplasia. Am J Clin Pathol. 2003 Sep 1; **120**(3): 322–6.

3. Ioachim HL, Medeiros LJ. The normal lymph node. In Medeiros LJ, ed. Ioachim's lymph node pathology. 4th ed. Philadelphia, PA: Wolters Kluwer/Lippincott Williams & Wilkins; 2009:1–14.

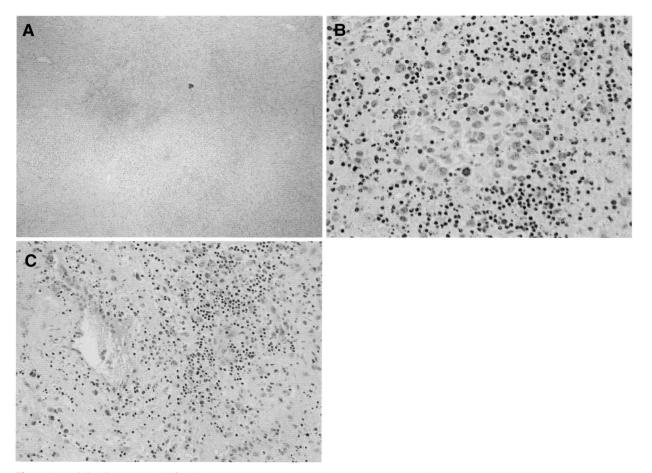

Figure 5.16 SLE LAD. A 14-year-old female presented with pleural effusion, abdominal pain, and retroperitoneal LAD. A biopsy of the retroperitoneal lymph node was performed. She was antinuclear antibody positive and diagnosed with SLE later. A. Lymph node biopsy shows extensive necrosis with residual lymphoid cells (H&E, 40x). B. The necrosis is surrounded by histiocytic proliferation, atypical lymphocytes, and karyorrhectic debris (H&E, 400x). Scant neutrophils and hematoxylin bodies can be seen, which are extracellular amorphous hematoxyphilic structures probably composed of degenerated nuclei that have reacted with antinuclear autoantibodies specific for SLE. C. Vasculitis is shown on the left. Scattered plasma cells are present on the right part of the image (H&E, 200x).

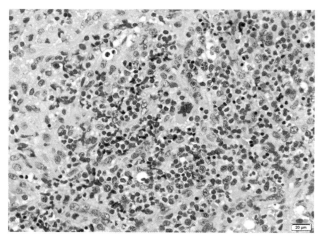

Figure 5.17 EMH of the lymph node. A 2-year-old female with hypoplastic left heart syndrome, status post multiple procedures and extracorporeal membrane oxygenation (ECMO), and on anticoagulation presented with thrombosis, fever, and enlarged right axillary lymph nodes. A biopsy of the lymph node was performed. The lymph node shows normal architecture with extramedullary hematopoietic elements observed in sinusoids and paracortical regions. EMH appears commonly in clusters mixed with lymphocytes. Megakaryocytes and nucleated red blood cells are demonstrated in this image (H&E, 400x).

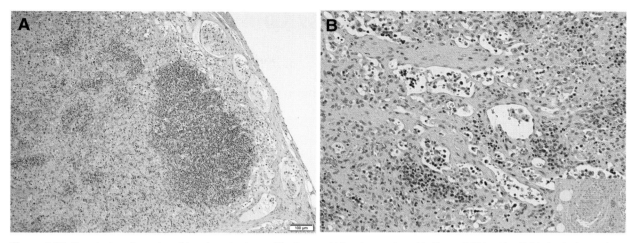

Figure 5.18 Vascular transformation of lymph node sinuses. The 2-year-old female mentioned in Figure 5.17, besides EMH, also had vascular transformation of sinuses in her lymph node biopsy. A. The lymph node shows dilated vascular channels in the sinuses located in the subcapsular area and small vascular proliferation in interfollicular areas (H&E, 100x). B. High magnification reveals endothelium-lined vascular channels in the medulla (H&E, 200x). The vascular channels are dilated with variably round, cleft, or anastomosing networks. The lymphocytes are markedly depleted. Thrombosis and fibrosis are commonly present (inset).

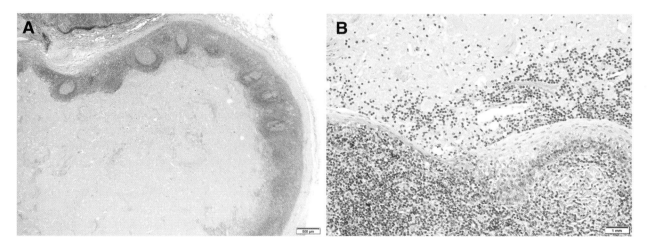

Figure 5.19 Branchial cleft cyst of the lymph node. A 13-year-old female with autism spectrum disorder, failure to thrive, and right cervical LAD. A. A biopsy of the lymph node shows a cyst filled with pink material and residual lymphoid follicles pushed to the peripheral rim (H&E, 20x). B. The cyst is lined by undulating squamous epithelium with focally dense intraepithelial lymphocytic infiltrate shown at the lower part of the image. The cyst, filled with cellular debris of squamous epithelial cells, lymphocytes, and cholesterol clefts, is shown in the upper part of the image (H&E, 400x).

4. Shrestha D, Dhakal AK, KC SR, Shakya A, Shah SC, Shakya H. Systemic lupus erythematosus and granulomatous lymphadenopathy. BMC Pediatrics. 2013 Dec; **13**(1): 1–6.

5. Attygalle AD, Liu H, Shirali S et al. Atypical marginal zone hyperplasia of mucosa-associated lymphoid tissue: A reactive condition of childhood showing immunoglobulin lambda light-chain restriction. Blood. 2004; **104**(10): 3343–8.

Chapter 6

Normal Bone Marrow Components in Pediatric Patients

Karen M. Chisholm, Gerald Wertheim

Bone marrow studies may be requested to evaluate for hematopoietic or solid neoplasms, or to help elucidate the etiology of abnormalities in the peripheral blood or lesions identified by imaging studies. These bone marrow specimens may include aspirate smears, clot sections, particle preparations, core touch preparations, and core biopsies. These specimens (preferably aspirates) can also be used for ancillary studies such as flow cytometry, cytogenetics, and molecular analysis to supplement the morphologic picture.

The bone marrow is composed of trilineage hematopoiesis (Figures 6.1 and 6.2), mainly myeloid cells, erythrocytes, and megakaryocytes (Figure 6.3), as well as background lymphoid cells, macrophages, fewer plasma cells, mast cells, and stromal cells (Figures 6.4 and 6.5). Maturing granulocytic lineage cells comprise the majority of the marrow (Figure 6.6), with maturing erythroid precursors representing a lesser percentage (Figure 6.7). The one exception is within the first 24 hours after birth, when erythroid cells can represent up to 40% of the marrow cellularity. In most other circumstances, the myeloid:erythroid ratio is approximately 2.5–3:1 but can be higher in younger children (Figure 6.8). Stromal cells include vessels, adipocytes, fibroblasts, and reticulin. Osteoblasts and osteoclasts can also be identified in pediatric marrows, especially in close relationship to bone (Figure 6.9).

The maturation spectrum and histologic features of the hematopoietic cells in the marrow are the same between pediatric and adult marrows. However, the overall cellularity (percentage of hematopoietic tissue to fat) of the marrow does change with age. Bone marrow cellularity is best determined using H&E-stained core biopsies. Newborns (age < 1 week) have essentially 100% marrow cellularity, which then declines with increasing age, with relative increases in the amount of adipose tissue in the marrow (Figure 6.10). *Hypocellular* and *hypercellular* are terms employed when the marrow has less or more cellularity than typical for age, respectively.

Pediatric bone marrows also often have increased B-lymphocyte precursors called hematogones. Such cells are most prominent in young children with amounts that decrease with age [7]. Hematogone percentages up to 72% have been reported [8]. Hematogones morphologically are mildly larger than mature lymphocytes with homogenous condensed chromatin, inconspicuous nucleoli, and scant amounts of basophilic agranular cytoplasm. These cells have a stereotypic or progressive pattern of antigen expression that aids in their recognition and discrimination from neoplastic lymphoid processes such as B-lymphoblastic leukemia/lymphoma [7]–[9]. Flow cytometric analysis is the best way to identify hematogones and to differentiate them from a neoplastic lymphoblastic population, especially in minimal residual disease (Figure 6.11).

Age range	Cellularity	Myeloids	Erythroids	M:E ratio	Lymphocytes (including hematogones)
Birth–3 months	80–100%	40–60%	5–40%	3–5:1	10–60%
3 months–4 years	70–90%	50–60%	10–25%	2.5–3.5:1	20–50%
4–10 years	60–80%	50–70%	15–25%	2.5–3:1	10–30%
10–15 years	50–75%	50–70%	15–25%	2.5–3:1	10–20%
15–20 years	45–70%	50–70%	15–25%	2.5–3:1	10–20%

Adapted from [1] to [6].

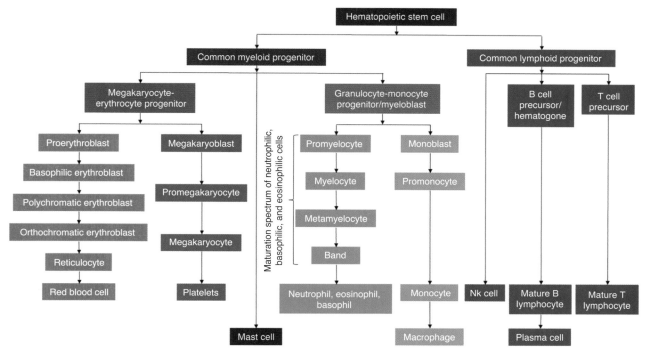

Figure 6.1 Development of hematopoietic stem cells to mature cells present in the bone marrow.

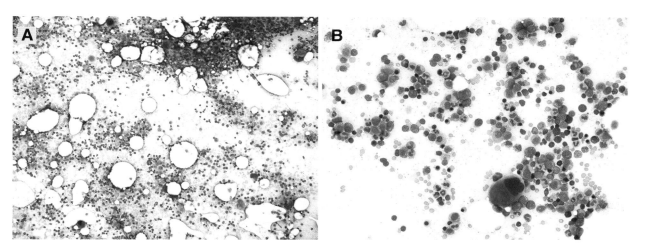

Figure 6.2 Bone marrow aspirate smears. A–B. Wright-Giemsa-stained aspirate smears in healthy children demonstrate trilineage hematopoiesis. Darkly stained cellular particles contain hematopoiesis as well as stromal cells, shown at the top right of the image (A, 100X), with more dispersed trilineage hematopoiesis adjacent to the particle. Further from particles, more distinct cells can be appreciated, including maturing myeloid cells, erythroid cells, lymphocytes, and a megakaryocyte (B, 200X).

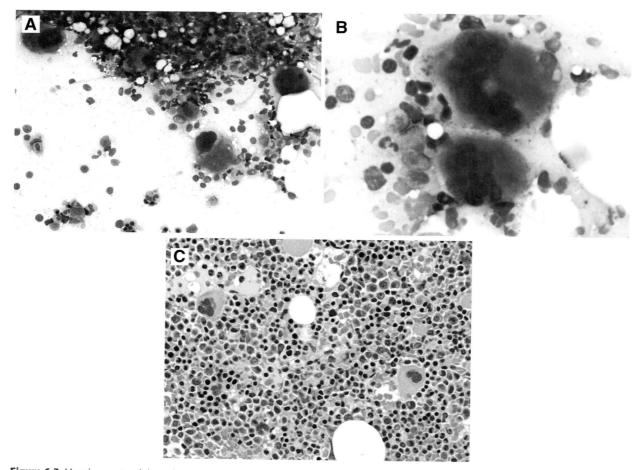

Figure 6.3 Megakaryocytes. A. In aspirate smears, megakaryocytes are often concentrated within and around bone marrow particles (Wright-Giemsa aspirate smear, 200X). B. Megakaryocytes usually have multilobated nuclei (Wright-Giemsa aspirate smear, 1,000X). C. In core biopsies, megakaryocytes are scattered throughout the marrow, though often identified adjacent to capillary sinuses (C, H&E, 400X).

Iron stores can also be evaluated in the bone marrow. In children less than 1 year old, iron is usually absent; starting at 4 years, the iron stores increase until they reach adult levels, usually by age 5 or 6 [10]. Thus, it is important not to overdiagnose iron deficiency in young children. Iron is usually in the form of hemosiderin within macrophages identified in the aspirate smears, but can also be identified in erythroid precursors (Figure 6.12). While large amounts of hemosiderin can be identified by usual Wright-Giemsa staining of the aspirate or H&E of the core biopsy, Perl's/Prussian blue stains may further highlight iron deposits. Notably, decalcification of the core biopsy may decrease the amount of iron identified [11].

Bone marrow core biopsies in pediatrics also have similar histologic features to those in adults, but with increased cellularity. Immature myeloid cells are located along the bony trabeculae, usually one to three cells thick. Erythroid cells form small clusters or erythroid islands, and megakaryocytes are scattered throughout the marrow. Hematogones are interstitial and do not form aggregates. Within the sampled bone, the subcortical region in

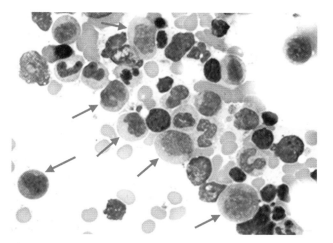

Figure 6.4 Wright-Giemsa-stained aspirate smear demonstrating multiple variably mature monocytes (highlighted by red arrows) (1,000X).

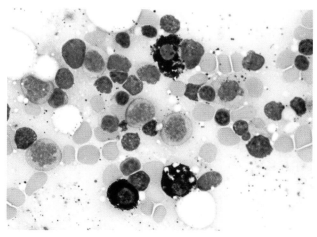

Figure 6.5 Wright-Giemsa-stained aspirate smear depicting three mast cells characterized as round to elongate/oval cells with round nuclei and abundant purple granules that can overlap the nucleus (1,000X).

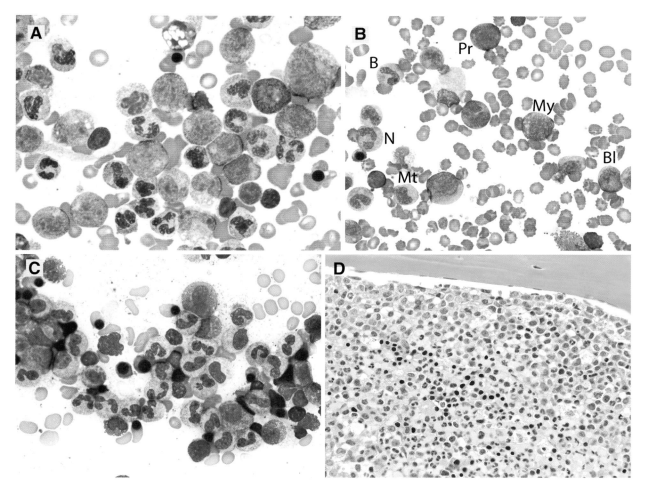

Figure 6.6 Myeloid maturation. A–D. Myeloid precursors mature in the bone marrow. A. Wright-Giemsa aspirate smear (1,000X). B. From least mature to mature, myeloid precursors are blasts (Bl), cells with high nuclear:cytoplasmic ratios, fine chromatin, and variably prominent nucleoli; promyelocytes (Pr), cells with perinuclear hof and azurophilic granules; myelocytes (My), cells with round nucleus, more condensed chromatin, and numerous granules; metamyelocytes (Mt), cells with slightly elongate, indented nucleus and many cytoplasmic granules; bands (B), cells with more elongated nucleus, sometimes horseshoe-shaped, and cytoplasmic granules; and neutrophils (N), cells with multilobated/segmented nuclei and condensed chromatin (Wright-Giemsa aspirate smear, 1,000X). C. In some foci, one can find more abundant band and neutrophil forms (Wright-Giemsa aspirate smear, 1,000X). D. In core biopsies, myeloids mature as they get farther away from the trabecular bone. The most immature myeloids are present paratrabecularly and neutrophils are furthest from the bone (H&E, 400X).

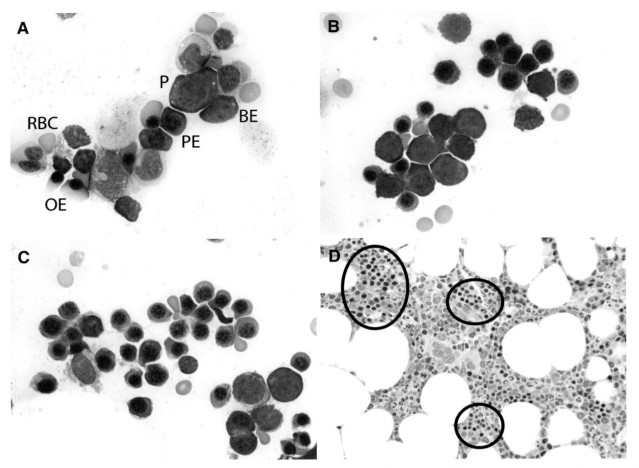

Figure 6.7 Erythroid maturation. A. As the erythroid precursors mature from proerythroblasts (P) to red blood cells (RBC), the nucleus becomes smaller with more condensed chromatin while the cytoplasm changes from deeply basophilic to more pink with increased hemoglobin production (basophilic erythroblast [BE] and polychromatic erythroblast [PE]). Between orthochromatic erythroblast (OE) and reticulocyte (R) stages, the nucleus is extruded (Wright-Giemsa aspirate smear, 1,000X). B. In some marrows, there may be clusters of erythroid cells; here basophilic erythroblasts in the lower left and more polychromatic erythroblasts in the upper right (Wright-Giemsa aspirate smear, 1,000X). C. Other areas might show many polychromatic and some orthochromatic erythroblasts. Some basophilic erythroblasts are also identified (Wright-Giemsa aspirate smear 1,000X). D. In core biopsies, erythroid cells often appear as cells with dark round nuclei and are often present in islands, or clusters, shown by black circles (H&E, 400X).

children younger than 10 years of age is typically hypercellular relative to more central areas, and then progressively becomes hypocellular with age (Figure 6.13) [3]. Thus, an adequate core biopsy is essential, especially when cellularity is an important parameter, for example, in a diagnosis of aplastic anemia.

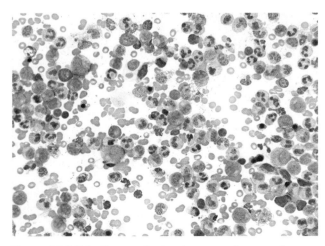

Figure 6.8 Wright-Giemsa-stained aspirate smear demonstrating an increased myeloid:erythroid cell ratio (400X).

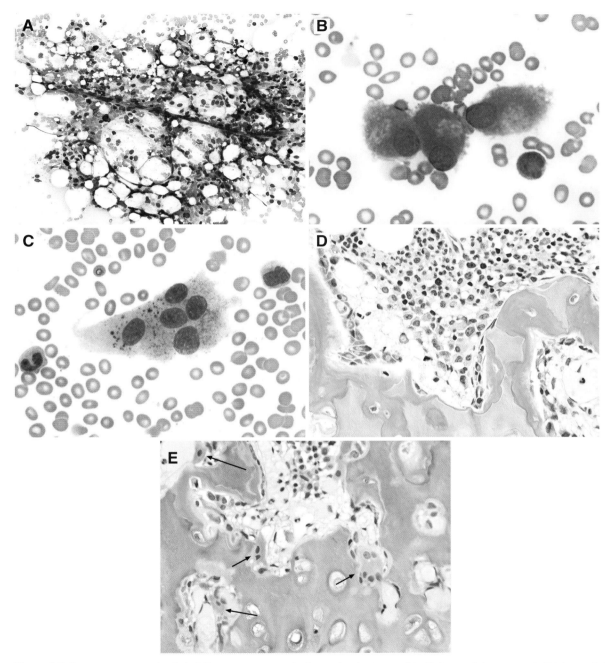

Figure 6.9 Bone marrow stromal cells. A–E. Bone marrow stromal cells are often best appreciated in hypocellular marrows. In this hypocellular particle, vessels, adipocytes (fat cells), and fibroblasts are identified, along with scattered lymphocytes, histiocytes, and mast cells (A, Wright-Giemsa aspirate smear, 100X). Osteoblasts and osteoclasts may also be identified in bone marrow aspirates, especially from children. Osteoblasts are characterized as large cells with single round and extremely eccentric nuclei with bluish cytoplasm. A cytoplasmic gray/light blue hof is present that is not adjacent to the nucleus (B, Wright-Giemsa aspirate smear, 1,000X). Osteoclasts have multiple round nuclei and coarse "bone sand" in their cytoplasm" (C, Wright-Giemsa aspirate smear, 1,000X). In pediatric bone marrow core biopsies, osteoblasts may sometimes be identified rimming the bony trabeculae. These osteoblasts have a prominent cytoplasmic hof and should not be confused with plasma cells (D, H&E, 400X). Bone formation in pediatrics may not only have rimming osteoblasts but also scattered osteoclasts as highlighted by the arrows (E, H&E, 400X).

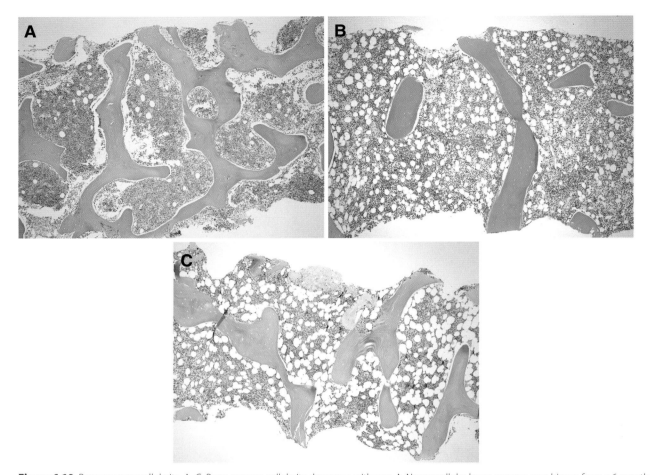

Figure 6.10 Bone marrow cellularity. A–C. Bone marrow cellularity decreases with age. A. Normocellular bone marrow core biopsy from a 6-month-old boy without hematologic pathology. Cellularity is approximately 90–95%. Some bony trabeculae are with incomplete ossification, a common finding in pediatric marrow studies (H&E stain, 40x). B. Normocellular bone marrow core biopsy from a 2-year-old girl without hematologic pathology. Cellularity is approximately 80% (H&E stain, 40x). C. Normocellular bone marrow core biopsy from a 12-year-old boy without hematologic pathology. Cellularity is approximately 60% (C, H&E stain, 40x).

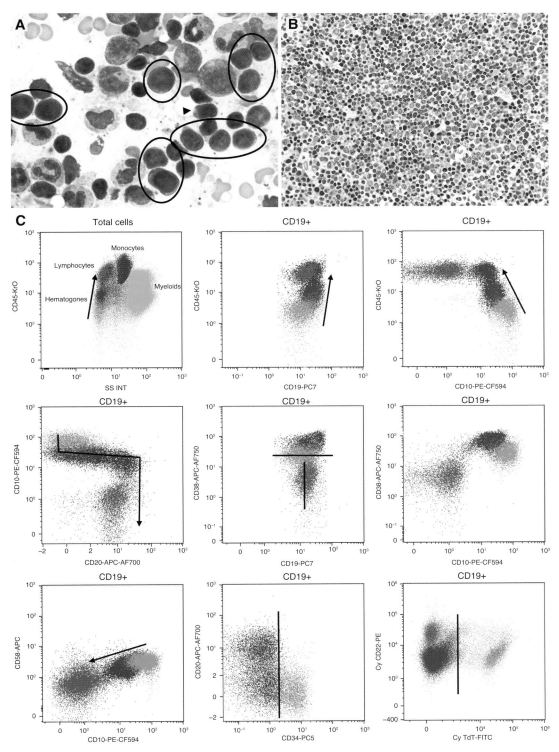

Figure 6.11 Hematogones. A. Hematogones can be increased in young children. In comparison to mature lymphocytes (arrowhead), hematogones are larger in size with round to mildly irregular nuclear contours, homogenous condensed chromatin, inconspicuous nucleoli, and scant amounts of basophilic agranular cytoplasm. All stages of hematogones are increased in this 3-month-old boy (Wright-Giemsa aspirate smear, 1,000X). B. In core biopsies, hematogones are present interstitially. In this 9-month-old girl, there is a markedly increased hematogone population. The admixture of

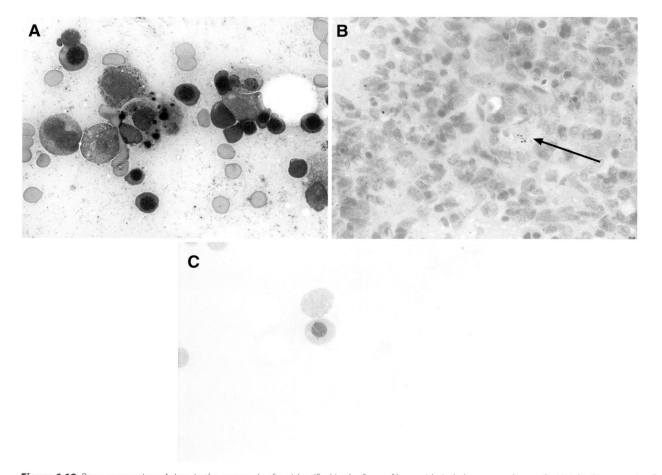

Figure 6.12 Bone marrow iron. A. Iron in the marrow is often identified in the form of hemosiderin-laden macrophages. On Wright-Giemsa stain of aspirate smears, the hemosiderin is a deep green/blue hue (Wright-Giemsa, 1,000X). B. Prussian blue stain on bone marrow aspirates highlight ferric iron as a bright blue color. Iron is stored within macrophages (arrow highlights such a hemosiderin-laden macrophage, 400X). C. Iron may also be identified in red blood cell precursors (sideroblastic iron) (Prussian blue stain, 1,000X).

Caption for Figure 6.11 (cont.)

immature and mature lymphoid cells is indicative of physiologic hematogones rather than a lymphoid neoplasm (H&E, 400X). C. By flow cytometry, the three stages of hematogones can be identified, from the least mature (stage I [teal], stage II [purple], stage III [blue]), to mature B lymphocytes (green). On the CD45 versus side scatter (SS) plot, the hematogones have low side scatter with progressively increasing CD45 intensity as they progress to maturation. When just gating on CD19+ cells, on the CD45 versus CD19 and CD45 versus CD10 dot plots, the hematogones show progressively increasing CD45 and decreasing CD10 expression from stage I to stage III. On the CD10 versus CD20 dot plot, the stage I hematogones are CD10 bright but negative for CD20; the stage II hematogones are slightly dimmer for CD10 and show progressively increasing CD20 expression as they become stage III hematogones, at which point they lose CD10 expression and mature to lymphocytes. On the CD38 versus CD19 dot plot, the hematogones (all three stages) tend to show fairly stable CD38 expression (as a straight horizontal line), while the mature lymphocytes show variable but dimmer CD38 expression, forming a "T" shape. On the CD58 versus CD10 plot, the hematogones can be seen with decreasing levels of CD58 expression, which is a useful tool in differentiation from lymphoblasts, which typically show overexpression of CD58. Only stage I hematogones are positive for CD34 and TDT while stage II and III hematogones are negative for both markers.

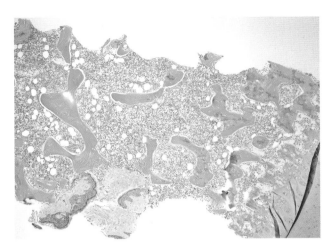

Figure 6.13 Bone marrow core biopsy from a 20-month-old boy demonstrating hypercellularity in the subcortical region. The subcortical marrow can remain hypercellular until up to 10 years of age, but then progressively becomes hypocellular. Also note the fragments of superficial skin, which are a procedural artifact that can be seen (H&E stain, 40x).

References

1. Greer JP, Arber DA, Glader B, List AF, Means RT, Paraskevas F, et al. Wintrobe's clinical hematology. 13th ed. Philadelphia, PA: Lippincott Williams & Wilkins; 2014.

2. Bain BJ, Clark DM, Lampert IA, Wilkins BS. Bone marrow pathology. 3rd ed. Oxford: Blackwell Science; 2001.

3. Foucar K, Reichard K, Czuchlewski D. Bone marrow pathology. 4th ed. Hong Kong: American Society for Clinical Pathology Press; 2020.

4. Foucar K, Viswanatha DS, Wilson CS. Non-neoplastic disorders of bone marrow. Atlas of nontumor pathology. Washington, DC: American Registry of Pathology; 2008.

5. Friebert SE, Shepardson LB, Shurin SB, Rosenthal GE, Rosenthal NS. Pediatric bone marrow cellularity: Are we expecting too much? J Pediatr Hematol Oncol. 1998; **20**(5): 439–43.

6. Hartsock RJ, Smith EB, Petty CS. Normal variations with aging of the amount of hematopoietic tissue in bone marrow from the Anterior Iliac Crest: A study made from 177 cases of sudden death examined by necropsy. Am J Clin Pathol. 1965; **43**: 326–31.

7. McKenna RW, Washington LT, Aquino DB, Picker LJ, Kroft SH. Immunophenotypic analysis of hematogones (B-lymphocyte precursors) in 662 consecutive bone marrow specimens by 4-color flow cytometry. Blood. 2001; **98**(8): 2498–507.

8. Rimsza LM, Larson RS, Winter SS, Foucar K, Chong YY, Garner KW, et al. Benign hematogone-rich lymphoid proliferations can be distinguished from B-lineage acute lymphoblastic leukemia by integration of morphology, immunophenotype, adhesion molecule expression, and architectural features. Am J Clin Pathol. 2000; **114**(1): 66–75.

9. McKenna RW, Asplund SL, Kroft SH. Immunophenotypic analysis of hematogones (B-lymphocyte precursors) and neoplastic lymphoblasts by 4-color flow cytometry. Leuk Lymphoma. 2004; **45**(2): 277–85.

10. Penchansky L. Pediatric bone marrow. Berlin: Springer; 2004.

11. Stuart-Smith SE, Hughes DA, Bain BJ. Are routine iron stains on bone marrow trephine biopsy specimens necessary? J Clin Pathol. 2005; **58**(3): 269–72.

Infectious Diseases

Shunyou Gong, Dehua Wang, Kristian T. Schafernak

Introduction

Lymphadenopathy (LAD) refers to the enlargement and/or abnormal consistency of lymph nodes and may be localized or diffuse. It reflects the results of immune responses to different insulants such as infection, autoimmunity, or malignancy [1]. Children with LAD are much more likely to have benign etiologies than adults, and most commonly present with a cervical mass [2]. While most benign LADs in children have no identifiable cause and are defined as nonspecific reactive LAD, some cases are found to be of infectious origin, including bacteria, yeast, parasite, or virus, often referred to as lymphadenitis [3].

Occasionally, infections may not present as LAD but more occultly or as fever of unknown origin (FUO). In these cases, the differential diagnosis includes infection, inflammatory disorders, and hematologic malignancy. A bone marrow biopsy may render a definitive diagnosis. Systemic infections may be diagnosed in the bone marrow. Morphologic findings can be nonspecific and include necrosis or granulomata, or the identification of an infectious organism.

Cat scratch disease (CSD) is caused by *Bartonella henselae*, a Gram-negative, facultative intracellular bacillus acquired from exposure to cats or cat fleas. After infection, the patient generally develops erythema, then a papular and vesicular lesion oozing fluid at the inoculation site, followed by swelling of the regional draining lymph node(s), which often adhere to the surrounding soft tissue and skin. Some patients may develop low-grade fever, malaise, and bone or joint pain [4]. If the history of cat exposure is not evident or revealed, the lymph node may be biopsied to rule out lymphoma. CSD lymphadenitis is usually a self-limiting disease in an immunocompetent child but may manifest as a life-threatening systemic, multi-organ disease in patients with an underlying immunodeficiency such as HIV/AIDS [4]. When typical features are not present in the lymph node removed from early-phase and recovering-phase patients, serological tests for immunoglobulin G (IgG) and immunoglobulin M (IgM) antibodies to *Bartonella henselae* may be required to reach a diagnosis (Figure 7.1).

Syphilis is a sexually transmitted disease caused by infection of *Treponema pallidum*, a spirochete bacterium. The natural history of syphilis is characterized by three clinical stages of disease, with the secondary phase likely demonstrating diffuse LAD with cervical LAD most noticeable [5]. The primary stage of syphilis usually presents with ulcerated painless lesions on the genitalia called chancre, but this history is often not disclosed, resulting in a lymph node biopsy. Serological assays including rapid plasma reagin (RPR) and venereal disease research laboratory (VDRL) tests identify the heterophile antibodies in syphilis patients and are commonly used for screening; positive reactions are confirmed by specific *Treponema pallidum* antibody tests (Figure 7.2) [5].

Mycobacterial lymphadenitis may be caused by *Mycobacterium tuberculosis* (TB), the pathogen once considered one of the most severe human diseases prior to the era of antibiotics, or a variety of other atypical (nontuberculous) mycobacteria that usually infect immunocompromised hosts. In the United States, the incidence of TB has decreased and TB lymphadenitis is uncommon in children. Most pediatric mycobacterial lymphadenitis cases seen in Western countries are caused by nontuberculous mycobacteria, particularly *Mycobacterium avium-intracellulare* (MAI) complex [6]. Mycobacteria are gram-positive bacilli with thick, lipid-rich cell walls that make them resistant to decolorization with acidified organic solvents, and thus called "acid-fast bacilli." *M. tuberculosis* is highly pathogenic and transmissible among humans via droplets or aerosol. MAI is present in the normal environment (soil and water) and less pathogenic to the general population, although increasing numbers of immunocompetent children with MAI lymphadenitis cases have been reported in recent years [7]. Immunocompromised children, particularly those affected by HIV/AIDS, are the most vulnerable population to nontuberculous mycobacterial infection [8].

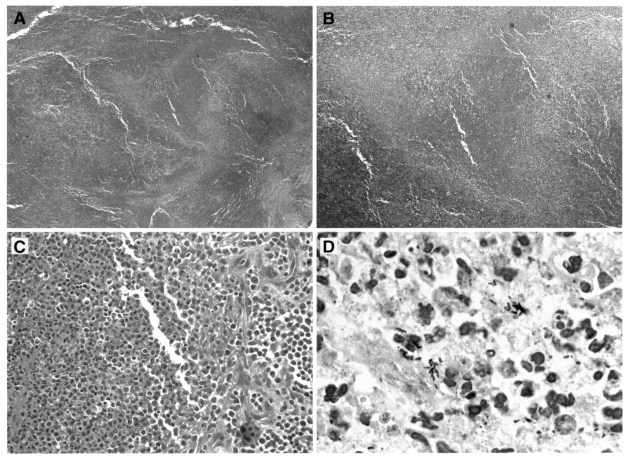

Figure 7.1 A 7-year-old boy presented with right axillary LAD, measuring 2.5 cm, which is nonmovable, tender to touch, with swelling and redness on the overlying skin. He has a cat at home; however, he did not remember a cat bite or scratch. The excisional biopsy showed the classic morphology. A. Stellate necrotizing granuloma (H&E, original magnification x 20). B. The necrotic center contains abundant neutrophils forming microabscesses (H&E, original magnification x 40). C. High-power view showed a peripheral rim of epithelioid histiocytes around the abscess (H&E, original magnification x 200). D. The diagnosis of CSD was confirmed by Warthin-Starry stain, which showed many histiocytes containing clusters of rod-shaped microorganisms (original magnification x 1,000); serologic tests were positive for IgM antibody to *Bartonella henselae*.

The histopathology of TB or MAI lymphadenitis may be very similar if not indistinguishable; therefore culture and molecular methods such as polymerase chain reaction (PCR) are required for definitive diagnosis (Figure 7.3).

Histoplasmosis infection may be pulmonary or extra-pulmonary (disseminated), with isolated cervical LAD rarely reported [9]. *Histoplasma capsulatum* (*H. capsulatum*) is a dimorphic fungus and grows as an intracellular yeast form at human body temperature. It is endemic in the river valleys of the Midwestern and South Central United States and causes opportunistic infections called histoplasmosis in immunocompromised individuals. The patients acquire the infection through inhaling the spores of *H. capsulatum*, which contaminate the soil through the excreta of chickens, birds, and bats (Figure 7.4).

Human toxoplasmosis may present with disseminated disease in immunocompromised individuals, but it commonly causes localized LAD in immunocompetent hosts [10, 11]. *Toxoplasma gondii* (*T. gondii*) is a proto-zoal parasite of the intestine of cats and with other animals serve as its intermediate hosts. Humans may be infected by ingestion of the oocytes of toxoplasma from food or water contained in cat feces, eating undercooked meat from infected livestock animals, or maternal-fetal transmission across the placenta [10]. While toxoplasma trophozoites in macrophages are very difficult to observe

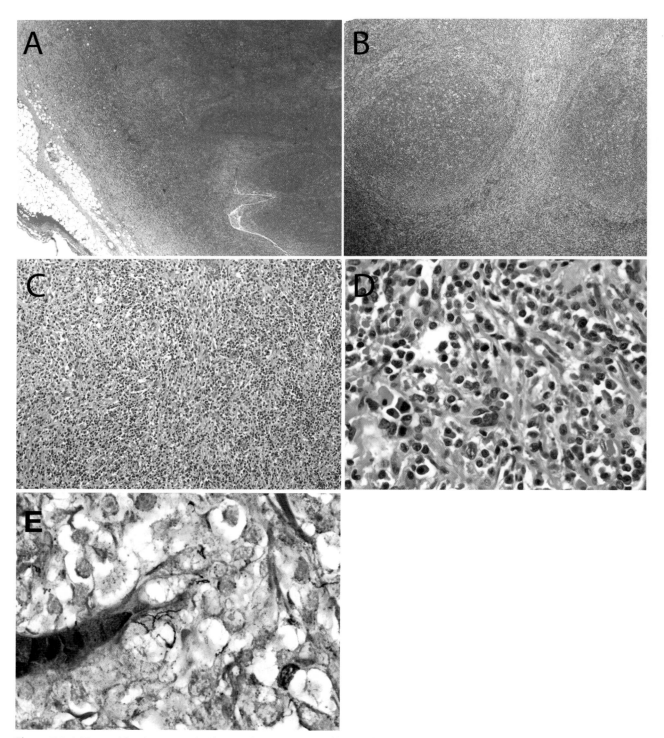

Figure 7.2 A 17-year-old male presented with cervical LAD. An excisional biopsy showed characteristic morphologic features. A. Thickened capsule with fibrosis and hyperplastic follicles (H&E, original magnification x 40). B. The follicles demonstrated polarized germinal centers and diminished mantle zones, with delicate fibrosis in the paracortex (H&E, original magnification x 100). C. Marked perivascular lymphoplasmacytic infiltrate was noted. D. High-power view showed numerous mature plasma cells mixed with small lymphocytes, histiocytes, and frequent fibroblasts (H&E, original magnification x 200). E. The diagnosis of syphilitic lymphadenitis was confirmed by Warthin-Starry stain, which showed many corkscrew-like spirochetes (original magnification x 1,000); serologic studies showed a positive IgM antibody to *Treponema pallidum*.

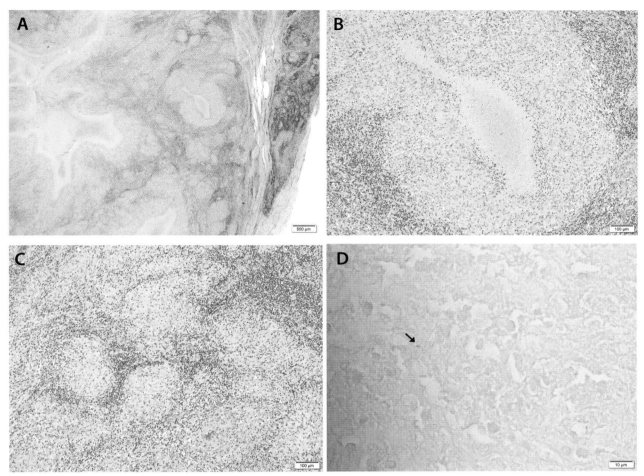

Figure 7.3 A 10-month-old male infant presented with oral ranula and right cervical LAD. A. Excisional biopsy showed an enlarged lymph node containing numerous necrotizing and non-necrotizing granulomas (H&E, original magnification x 20). B. One necrotizing granuloma shows caseous necrosis in the center and surrounding concentric layers of epithelioid histiocytes and an outer rim of lymphocytes (H&E, original magnification x 100). C. Several non-necrotizing granulomas are composed of non-palisading epithelioid histiocytes, with one granuloma containing multinucleated giant cells of Langerhans cell type (H&E, original magnification x 100). D. Fite's acid-fast stain revealed a bacillus (original magnification x 1,000), which was later identified as MAI complex by culture.

in infected lymph nodes, immunohistochemical stains for *T. gondii* help confirm the diagnosis (Figure 7.5).

Infectious mononucleosis (IM) is caused by the primary infection of Epstein-Barr virus (EBV) in adolescents or young adults. EBV is a member of the human herpesvirus family and infects around 95% of the population in the United States. In immunocompetent individuals, IM is usually self-limiting [12]. Patients commonly have cervical LAD, which is rarely biopsied. If IM is not diagnosed clinically and the LAD is prolonged, a biopsy may be performed to rule out malignancy [13]. The involved lymph node typically shows partially preserved architecture with marked

expansion of the paracortex by numerous immunoblasts, sometimes with patchy necrosis, mimicking diffuse large B-cell lymphoma. The infected cells are positive for Epstein-Barr virus encoded RNA (EBER), but negative or only a small subset are positive for LMP-1. A diagnosis of acute EBV lymphadenitis can be confirmed by EBV serologic tests, which typically reveal high-titer IgM antibody and negative or low-titer IgG antibody (Figure 7.6).

Cytomegalovirus (CMV) may cause LAD because of primary infection or viral reactivation, and a lymph node biopsy may be performed to rule out malignancy [14]. CMV is also a member of the humanherpes virus family

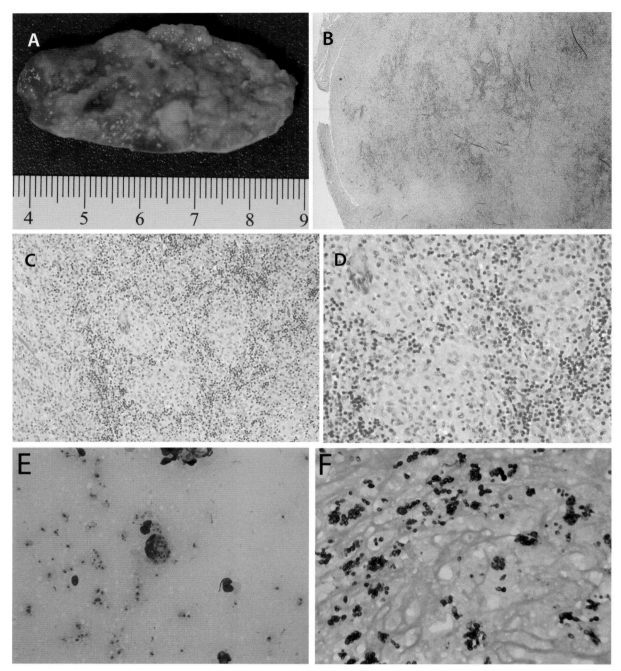

Figure 7.4 A 9-year-old girl with a history of kidney transplant presented with fever, cough, and cervical LAD. A. Excisional biopsy showed an enlarged lymph node measuring 5 cm in greatest dimension with cut surface revealing mostly gray, soft, caseous areas intermixed with minimal normal nodal texture. B. Low-power view demonstrated predominantly sheets of histiocytes and minimal normal residual lymph node architecture (H&E, original magnification x 20). C. Many non-necrotizing granulomas were present (H&E, original magnification x 40). D. Frequent multinucleated cells were noted (H&E, original magnification x 200). E. Touch imprints of the lymph node showed numerous intracellular microorganisms in histiocytes (Papanicolaou stain, original magnification x 1,000). F. A Grocott-Gomori methenamine silver (GMS) stain highlighted the yeasts on tissue sections, with occasional narrow-based budding noted (original magnification x 1,000). The diagnosis of histoplasmosis lymphadenitis was confirmed by positive urine antigen test for *H. capsulatum*.

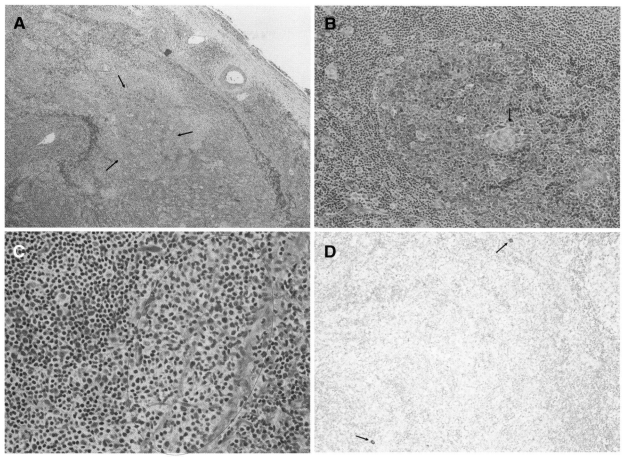

Figure 7.5 Lymph nodes with toxoplasmosis commonly show the triad of follicular hyperplasia, monocytoid B-cells, and clusters of epithelioid histiocytes encroaching on the germinal center. A 9-year-old boy presented with low-grade fever and cervical LAD. He has a cat at home. A. Excisional biopsy showed thickened capsule, preserved nodal architecture and numerous small epithelioid granulomas imposing a mottled appearance. A large follicle with attenuated mantle zone and hyperplastic germinal center (arrows) was shown (H&E, original magnification x 100). B. A small epithelioid granuloma encroaching on reactive follicle is shown (H&E, original magnification x 100). C. Sheets of monocytoid cells were noted focally (H&E, original magnification x 200). D. The diagnosis of toxoplasma lymphadenitis was confirmed by immunohistochemical stain for *T. gondii*, which showed two large histiocytes positive for the stain (original magnification x 100).

and transmitted by blood transfusion, person-to-person contact through saliva and respiratory secretions, as well as maternal-fetal passage through the placenta. CMV causes a flu-like illness in immunocompetent people but, like EBV, conversion to permanent latent infection is common [15]. CMV is a major pathogen in immunocompromised hosts, who may reactivate latent CMV and develop life-threatening disseminated infection (Figure 7.7).

Human immunodeficiency virus (HIV) lymphadenitis is occasionally diagnosed in adolescents and young adults in the United States, where around 21% of documented new infections occur in patients aged 12 to 24 years [16]. HIV-1 is an enveloped double-stranded RNA virus belonging to the lentivirus subfamily of retroviruses. HIV-1 infects CD4+ T-cells through the interaction of the viral envelop protein gp120 and CD4 receptor on T-cells and monocytes [17]. Acute HIV infection causes a nonspecific flu-like syndrome that may include low-grade fever, weight loss, fatigue, skin ash, and LAD [18]. Enlarged lymph nodes may be biopsied to exclude malignancy. In practice, a diagnosis of HIV lymphadenitis is often delayed because the histomorphologic findings in the early phase are nonspecific and may resemble other

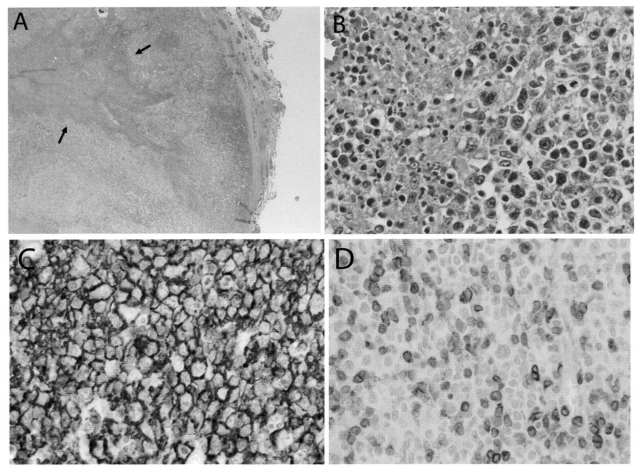

Figure 7.6 A 17-year-old previously healthy female presented with persistent low-grade fever for 3 weeks and cervical LAD. A. Excisional biopsy showed partially preserved architecture with patchy necrosis (arrows) (H&E, original magnification x 40). B. The paracortex was expanded by numerous large lymphoid cells with prominent central nucleoli and many apoptotic bodies (H&E, original magnification x 400). IHC stains showed that the large cells were positive for CD20 (C, original magnification x 400). CD3 (D, original magnification x 400) highlighted scattered small T-cells. The large cells are positive for CD30 (E, original magnification x 400), but negative for CD15 (F, original magnification x 400), consistent with immunoblasts. CD15 outlined a few neutrophils. G. The infected cells are positive for EBER (Original magnification x 100). H. IHC stain for LMP-1 was largely negative (original magnification x 100). The patient later underwent serology tests for antibodies to EBV nucleocapsid protein. The results were positive for IgM and negative for IgG, consistent with EBV lymphadenitis.

types of viral lymphadenitis, and social risk factors may not be known. Advanced HIV lymphadenitis show involution of germinal centers and proliferation of blood vessels (subacute), which slowly progresses to Castleman-like morphology, including totally "burned-out" fibrotic follicles and penetrating hyalinized blood vessels (chronic). The diagnosis of HIV lymphadenitis may be confirmed by serologic and/or HIV-RNA tests (Figure 7.8).

Several infectious diseases predominantly involve extranodal tissue and LAD may not be their initial presentation. However, they are sometimes confused with other noninfectious benign or malignant entities and thus are briefly described here.

Aspergillosis is a fungal infection that generally affects severely immunocompromised individuals. If the infection can disseminate into bone marrow, the patient may present with marked cytopenia and systemic symptoms such as fever, septic shock, and even death. Diagnosis relies on recognition of the necrosis associated with fungal infection and highlighting the characteristic hyphae through a GMS stain (Figure 7.9).

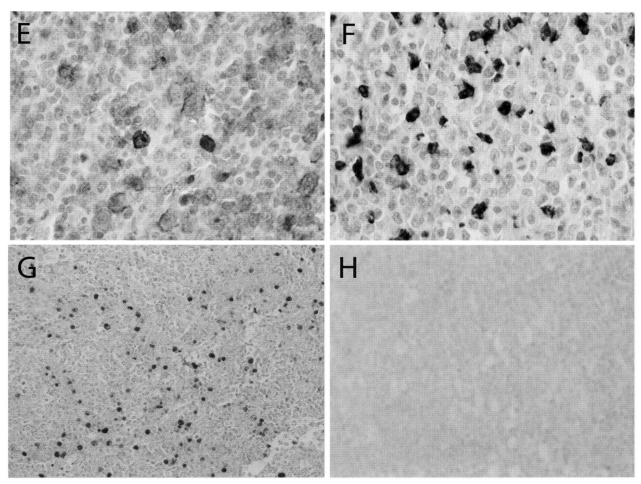

Figure 7.6 (cont.)

Coccidioidomycosis is caused by inhalation of the arthroconidia of *Coccidioides immitis* or *C. posadasii*, found in desert soil, and patients commonly present with a respiratory disease known as valley fever. Extrapulmonary dissemination occurs in only about 0.5% of infections in the general population, but immunodeficient patients are at much higher risk of disseminated disease (Figure 7.10).

Parvovirus B19 is a single-stranded DNA virus that causes asymptomatic infections in most individuals, but in the presence of an underlying red cell survival defect or immune suppression, transient aplastic crisis can lead to a serious anemia (Figure 7.11).

Leishmaniasis is a parasitic disease caused by infection with Leishmania parasites. Disseminated leishmaniasis is rare in the United States but may be seen in patients who have recently traveled to areas where this disease is endemic. Recognition of the morphologic features of this parasite on bone marrow aspirate and biopsy is crucial for timely diagnosis and proper treatment (Figure 7.12).

In summary, infectious diseases may share clinical features of lymphoid or myeloid malignancies. Pathologists must carefully examine the tissue morphologically and sometimes perform ancillary studies to render a correct diagnosis.

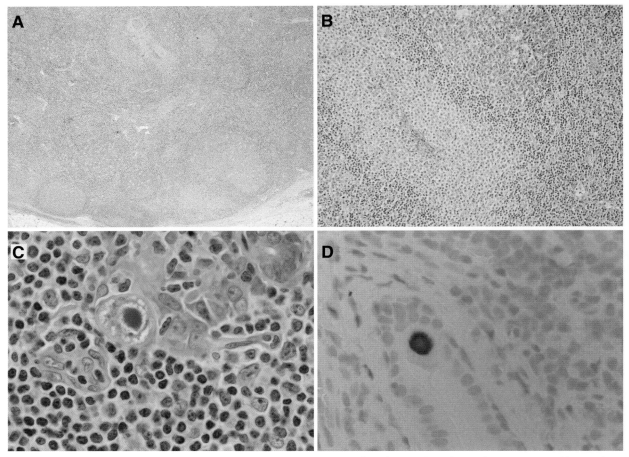

Figure 7.7 A 13-year-old boy with a history of asthma presented with low-grade fever for 2 weeks and cervical LAD. A. Excisional biopsy showed preserved architecture with follicular hyperplasia (H&E, original magnification x 40). B. Aggregates of monocytoid cells and large immunoblasts were commonly seen in the expanded paracortex (H&E, original magnification x 100). C. An enlarged CMV-infected cell with prominent eosinophilic nuclear inclusion surrounded by a clear halo – so-called Owl's eye – was seen in the background of many immunoblasts (H&E, original magnification x 400, image from another case, courtesy of Dr. Michele Paessler). D. A diagnosis of CMV lymphadenitis was confirmed by a CMV IHC stain, which showed dense nuclear stain in an infected cell (original magnification x 400, image from another case, courtesy of Dr. Michele Paessler).

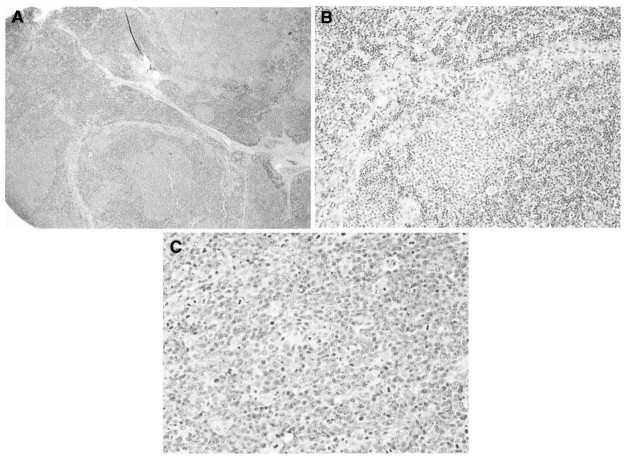

Figure 7.8 A 16-year-old boy presented with mediastinal mass and cervical LAD. He was suspected to have lymphoma and a cervical lymph node was excised. A. At low-power view, the lymph node demonstrates florid follicular hyperplasia with irregular-shaped reactive germinal centers with a diminished mantle zone (naked germinal center) (H&E, original magnification x 20). B. Aggregates of monocytoid cells with abundant pale cytoplasm are commonly found near blood vessels or sinuses (H&E, original magnification x 100). C. The germinal centers show numerous apoptotic bodies and mitotic figures, suggesting robust immune response (H&E, original magnification x 400). The diagnosis of HIV lymphadenitis was confirmed by peripheral blood PCR, which revealed >140,000 HIV RNA/mL.

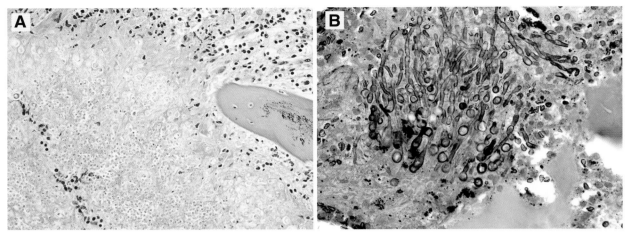

Figure 7.9 A 9-year-old girl with persistent B-lymphoblastic leukemia s/p chemotherapy died during the pretransplant phase and an autopsy was performed. A. At low magnification, the area of interest might resemble necrosis, but abundant fungal elements are identified (H&E, original magnification x 200). B. Septate hyphae with dichotomous branching were demonstrated with GMS stain (original magnification x 400).

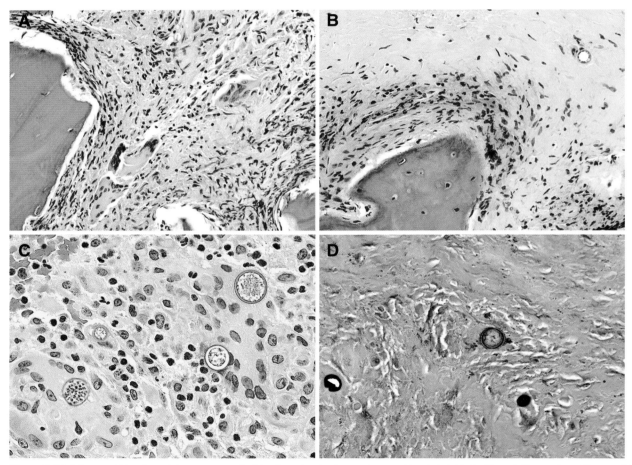

Figure 7.10 A 9-year-old boy from Arizona presented with a frontal scalp abscess that was biopsied. A. Marked bone inflammation with necrotizing granuloma (H&E, original magnification x 200). Variously sized spherules containing endospores were noted (H&E) B. Original magnification x 200. C. Original magnification x 400. D. The spherules were highlighted by GMS stain (original magnification x 400).

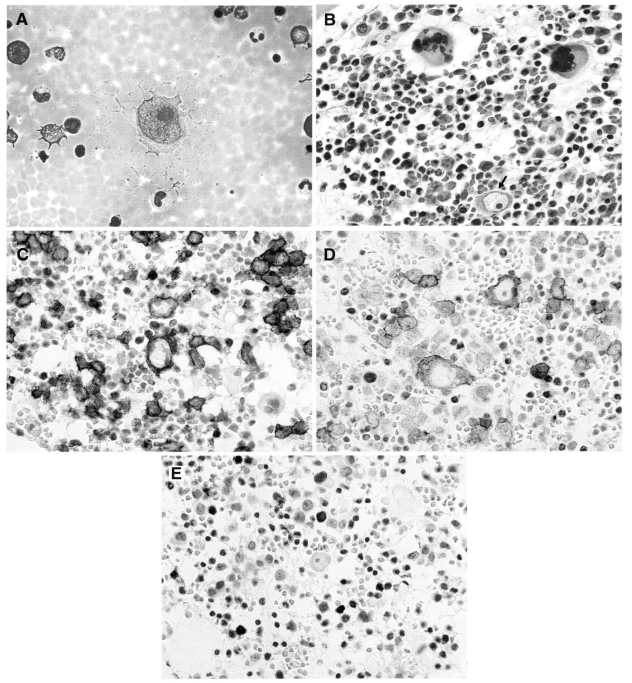

Figure 7.11 An 11-year-old girl who underwent bone marrow examination for anemia and thrombocytopenia. Rare scattered giant proerythroblasts with granular chromatin and a prominent nucleolus were noted in the bone marrow aspirate (A. Wright-Giemsa, original magnification x 400) and core biopsy (B. H&E, original magnification x 400; the cell of interest is in the center of the bottom of the image with the arrow and two megakaryocytes are provided at the top of the image for a size comparison). The giant proerythroblasts are positive for CD71 (C, original magnification x 400) and CD117 (D, original magnification x 400). Note that the parvovirus immunostain does not stain the giant proerythroblasts (E, original magnification x 400) but still stains smaller erythroid precursors.

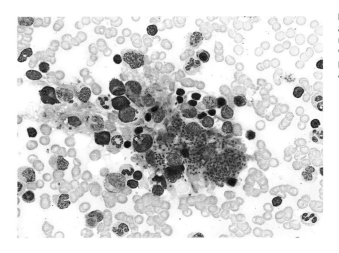

Figure 7.12 A 2-year-old Albanian child presented with fever and anemia. This bone marrow aspirate smear (Wright-Giemsa, original magnification x 400) showed numerous Leishmania infantum amastigotes within disrupted macrophage cytoplasm. Their size is similar to that of platelets; therefore, it is important to verify that the amastigotes have both a nucleus and a smaller kinetoplast.

References

1. Oguz A, Karadeniz C, Temel EA, Citak EC, Okur FV. Evaluation of peripheral lymphadenopathy in children. Pediatr Hematol Oncol. 2006; 23(7): 549–61.

2. Rajasekaran K, Krakovitz P. Enlarged neck lymph nodes in children. Pediatr Clin North Am. 2013; 60(4): 923–36.

3. Deosthali A, Donches K, DelVecchio M, Aronoff S. Etiologies of pediatric cervical lymphadenopathy: A systematic review of 2687 subjects. Glob Pediatr Health. 2019; 6: 2333794X19865440.

4. Chen Y, Fu YB, Xu XF, Pan Y, Lu CY, Zhu XL, et al. Lymphadenitis associated with cat-scratch disease simulating a neoplasm: Imaging findings with histopathological associations. Oncol Lett. 2018; 15(1): 195–204.

5. Yuan Y, Zhang X, Xu N, Wang L, Li F, Zhang P, et al. Clinical and pathologic diagnosis and different diagnosis of syphilis cervical lymphadenitis. Int J Clin Exp Pathol. 2015; 8(10): 13635–8.

6. Cruz AT, Ong LT, Starke JR. Mycobacterial infections in Texas children: A 5-year case series. Pediatr Infect Dis J. 2010; 29(8): 772–4.

7. Reuss AM, Wiese-Posselt M, Weissmann B, Siedler A, Zuschneid I, An der Heiden M, et al. Incidence rate of nontuberculous mycobacterial disease in immunocompetent children: A prospective nationwide surveillance study in Germany. Pediatr Infect Dis J. 2009; 28(7): 642–4.

8. Lewis LL, Butler KM, Husson RN, Mueller BU, Fowler CL, Steinberg SM, et al. Defining the population of human immunodeficiency virus-infected children at risk for Mycobacterium avium-intracellulare infection. J Pediatr. 1992; 121 (5 Pt 1): 677–83.

9. Mishra DP, Ramamurthy S, Behera SK. Histoplasmosis presenting as isolated cervical lymphadenopathy: A rare presentation. J Cytol. 2015; 32(3): 188–90.

10. Li B, Zou J, Wang WY, Liu SX. Toxoplasmosis presented as a submental mass: A common disease, uncommon presentation. Int J Clin Exp Pathol. 2015; 8(3): 3308–11.

11. Saxena S, Kumar S, Kharbanda J. Toxoplasmosis submandibular lymphadenitis: Report of an unusual case with a brief review. J Oral Maxillofac Pathol. 2018; 22(1): 116–20.

12. Pittaluga S. Viral-associated lymphoid proliferations. Semin Diagn Pathol. 2013; 30(2): 130–6.

13. Childs CC, Parham DM, Berard CW. Infectious mononucleosis: The spectrum of morphologic changes simulating lymphoma in lymph nodes and tonsils. Am J Surg Pathol. 1987; 11(2): 122–32.

14. Lum EL, Schaenman JM, DeNicola M, Reddy UG, Shen JI, Pullarkat ST. A case report of CMV lymphadenitis in an adult kidney transplant recipient. Transplant Proc. 2015; 47(1): 141–5.

15. Staras SA, Dollard SC, Radford KW, Flanders WD, Pass RF, Cannon MJ. Seroprevalence of cytomegalovirus infection in the United States, 1988–1994. Clin Infect Dis. 2006; 43(9): 1143–51.

16. Yusuf H, Fields E, Arrington-Sanders R, Griffith D, Agwu AL. HIV preexposure prophylaxis among adolescents in the US: A review. JAMA Pediatr. 2020; 174(11): 1102–8.

17. Posner MR, Cavacini LA, Emes CL, Power J, Byrn R. Neutralization of HIV-1 by F105, a human monoclonal antibody to the CD4 binding site of gp120. J Acquir Immune Defic Syndr (1988). 1993; 6(1): 7–14.

18. Henn A, Flateau C, Gallien S. Primary HIV infection: Clinical presentation, testing, and treatment. Curr Infect Dis Rep. 2017; 19(10): 37.

Chapter

8

Mature B-Cell Non-Hodgkin Lymphoma

Xiayuan Liang, Billie Carstens

Non-Hodgkin lymphomas (NHLs) comprise about 10% of all childhood cancers [1]. They include a diverse collection of malignant neoplasms that arise from mature and immature lymphoid cells of B-cell and T-cell origin [1]. Adult and pediatric NHLs have a number of differences, including subtypes, tumor locations, and biologic behaviors, which are summarized in Table 8.1 [1]. Morphologic evaluation of adequate tissue, immunophenotyping, and cytogenetic and molecular analysis are essential approaches in the diagnosis of NHLs. This chapter focuses on mature B-cell NHLs in children. Mature T-cell NHLs and immature lymphoid neoplasms are discussed in Chapters 9 and 13.

Burkitt Lymphoma

Burkitt lymphoma (BL) is defined by the World Health Organization (WHO) classification as a highly aggressive lymphoid neoplasm, often presenting at extranodal sites or as an acute leukemia (Figure 8.1). This tumor comprises approximately 40–50% of NHLs in children [1]. Three clinical variants are summarized in Table 8.2 [1, 2].

Approximately 80% of cases have t(8;14)(q24;q32)/ *MYC-IGH* rearrangement. The remaining cases have either t(2;8)(p12;q24)/*MYC-IgK* (about 15%) or t(8;22) (q24;q11)/*MYC-Ig* λ (5% of cases) [1, 2]. Intensive chemotherapy results in a good prognosis.

Burkitt-Like Lymphoma with 11q Aberration

In the 2016 WHO classification, Burkitt-like lymphoma with 11q aberration (BLL, 11q) is recognized as a new entity in the category of mature B-cell lymphoma [3]. It is

Table 8.1 Major differences of Non-Hodgkin lymphoma between children and adults

	Pediatric NHLs	Adult NHLs
Subtypes	Limited	Broad
Grade	Intermediate to high grade	>2/3 low grade
Clinical behavior	Aggressive in most cases	Indolent and nonaggressive in low-grade tumors
Mature versus immature	More precursor lymphomas	More mature lymphomas
Lineage	Even split of B-cell and T-cell tumors	Most B-cell tumors
Tumor location	More extranodal disease	More nodal disease
Stage	More high-stage disease	Less high-stage disease

Table 8.2 Features of clinical variants of Burkitt lymphoma

	Age	Geographic Location	Site	EBV Status
Endemic BL	Young children	Malaria belt of equatorial Africa	Extranodal (jaw, facial bones, and orbit common)	+
Sporadic BL	Children, young adults	Throughout the world	Gastrointestinal tract (ileocecal region common)	<30%+
Immunodeficiency-associated BL		HIV-infected or other immunocompromised individuals		+

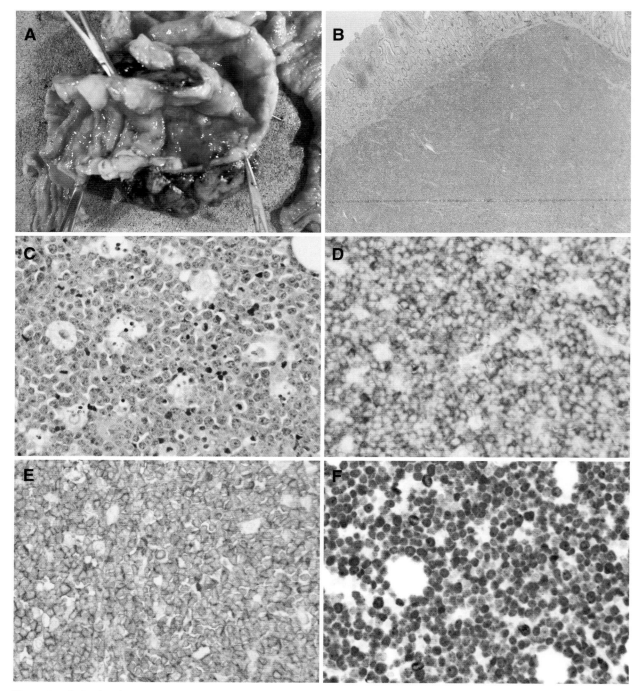

Figure 8.1 Burkitt lymphoma.

a. A small bowel resection: The right shows normal intestinal wall; the left shows abnormal thickened intestinal wall.

b. The intestinal wall is infiltrated by a diffuse tumor cell proliferation (H&E, 20x).

c. There is a starry-sky pattern. Tumor cells are homogenous and intermediate in size with square-off border of retracted cytoplasm, round nuclei, finely clumped and dispersed chromatin, and multiple basophilic medium-sized, paracentrally situated nucleoli (H&E, 400x).

d. Tumor cells are CD10 positive (CD10 immunostain, 400x).

e. Tumor cells are CD20 positive (CD20 immunostain, 400x).

f. Mib-1 demonstrates >99% proliferation activity (Mib-1 immunostain, 400x).

g. Tumor cells in peritoneal fluid show deeply basophilic cytoplasm (left: Wright-Gimesa, 1,000x) containing vacuoles due to lipid droplets (right: Oil Red O, 1,000x).

h. Cytogenetics. The upper panel is a FISH interphase study. *MYC* is labeled red. *IGH* is labeled green. Chromosome 8 centromere is labeled light blue. The upper left shows a normal cell with two red and two green signals. The upper middle shows that two interphase tumor cells have *MYC-IGH* rearrangement with red-green fusion signals. The upper right is the schematic representation. The lower image shows chromosome analysis with 46,XY,t(8;14)(q24;q32).

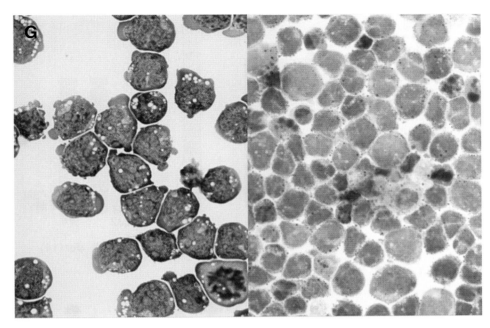

Figure 8.1 (cont.)

a subset of high-grade B-cell lymphomas resembling BL morphologically (Figure 8.2), phenotypically, and genetically through analysis by microRNAs and gene expression profile, but that lack *MYC* rearrangements [3]. Instead, this tumor carries a chromosome 11q alteration characterized by proximal gains and telomeric losses: specifically, interstitial gains in 11q23.2-23.3 and losses of 11q24.1-ter [4]. BLL, 11q usually has more complex karyotypes and more cytological pleomorphisms than typical BL. Patients often have a nodal presentation with a predilection for the head and neck, and a biologic behavior similar to that of BL. However, the 11q-gain/loss is not exclusively specific for BLL, 11q. While chromosomal analysis can be used to detect 11q Burkitt, SNP array, NGS copy number, or FISH are more accurate.

Diffuse Large B-Cell Lymphoma

Diffuse large B-cell lymphoma (DLBCL) is defined by the WHO as a neoplasm of large B lymphoid cells with nuclear size equal to or exceeding normal macrophage nuclei or more than twice the size of a normal lymphocytes, and that have a diffuse growth pattern [5]. DLBCL makes up approximately 15% of pediatric NHLs. Patients are usually >10 years of age. Clinically, patients often present with a rapidly enlarging tumor mass at single or multiple nodal and/or extranodal sites (skin, bone, gastrointestinal tract, genital tract, and central nervous system) [1]. DLBCL may display a variety of morphologic appearances (Figure 8.3). Morphologic variants of DLBCL are considered to be of similar clinical aggressiveness [1, 5].

There are various subtypes of DLBCL. However, in pediatric patients, only a few subtypes (Figure 8.4) are seen in practice. As with adult patients, the DLBCL, NOS is further divided into germinal center B-cell type (GCB type) and activated B-cell type (ABC type) based on cell origin, genetic signature, and prognostic significance [5]. GCB DLBCL expresses BCL-6, CD10, and cyclin H. GCET1, a germinal center marker, is highly correlated with GCB type. ABC DLBCL arises from post-germinal center B-cells that are arrested during plasmacytic differentiation and expresses MUM1, CD138, PAK1, CD44, and BCL-2 [5].

No specific, highly recurrent characteristic cytogenetic abnormalities are associated with DLBCL in children and adolescents [6]. The *cMYC* translocations, such as t(8;14) are seen in 20–40% of cases [1, 6]. Complex karyotypes occur in most cases of pediatric DLBCL [1, 6]. Clonally rearranged *IG*-heavy and light chain genes are detectable in all cases [5].

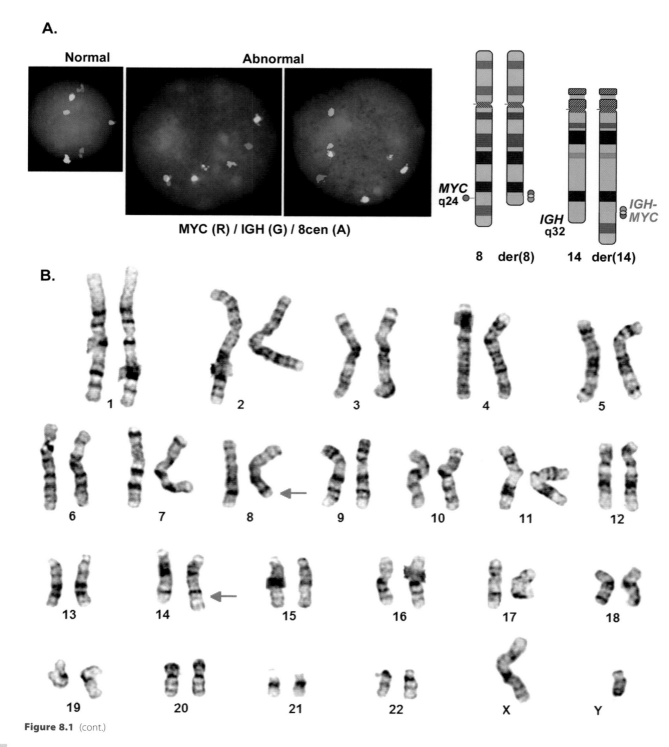

A.

Normal | Abnormal

MYC (R) / IGH (G) / 8cen (A)

MYC
q24

IGH
q32

IGH-MYC

8   der(8)   14   der(14)

B.

1   2   3   4   5

6   7   8   9   10   11   12

13   14   15   16   17   18

19   20   21   22   X   Y

Figure 8.1 (cont.)

High-Grade B-Cell Lymphoma with *MYC* and *BCL-2* and/or *BCL-6* Rearrangement

High-grade B-cell lymphoma with *MYC* and *BCL-2* and/ or *BCL-6* rearrangement is rarely seen in pediatric patients; DLBCL with coexpression of MYC and BCL2 protein (double-expressers) is more frequent in the ABC subtype [5].

Primary Mediastinal Large B-Cell Lymphoma

Primary mediastinal (thymic) large B-cell lymphoma (PMLBCL) is a mature and aggressive large B-cell lymphoma arising in the anterior mediastinum from putative thymic B-cell origin. It accounts for about 2–3% of NHLs [7]. It occurs predominantly in older adolescents. Patients often present with symptoms related to the bulk of anterior mediastinal tumor mass including dyspnea, cough, chest discomfort, or superior vena cava syndrome. Image studies often reveal a large mass in the anterior mediastinum. It can involve the lymph nodes, kidneys, adrenal glands, liver, or central nervous system. Bone marrow involvement is uncommon [7].

The tumor cells are usually uniform and medium to large in size with moderate to abundant pink/clear cytoplasm, round to oval, irregular, or multilobated nuclei, open chromatin, and one to several nucleoli. Association with fibrosis is common, ranging from delicate collagen fibers surrounding individual cell or groups of lymphoid tumor cells (compartmentalizing alveolar fibrosis) to broad septa of dense collagen (Figure 8.5).

Immunophenotypically, tumor cells express B-cell markers (CD19, CD20, CD22, CD79a, PAX-5, BOB.1, OCT-2, and PU1) with absence of surface immunoglobulins [7, 8]. CD30 expression is seen in 80% of cases, weaker than in classical Hodgkin lymphoma (cHL). Epstein-Barr virus is absent. Expression of BCL-2 and BCL6 is variable [7].

PMLBCL lacks *BCL2*, *BCL6*, and *cMYC* translocations [7]. Gene expression profiling studies of PMLBCL are distinct from those of other DLBCLs but significantly overlap with those of cHL [8, 9]. PMLBCL often shows gains in chromosome 2p16.1 where candidate gene *REL* and *BCL11A* are amplified, leading to a frequent nuclear accumulation of their proteins, which distinguishes PMLBCL from other subtypes of DLBCL [9]. PMLBCL is associated with a more favorable outcome than conventional DLBCL [7].

Pediatric-Type Follicular Lymphoma

Follicular lymphoma (FL) is defined as a neoplasm composed of follicle center (germinal center) B-cells (both centrocytes and centroblasts) that usually has at least a partially follicular pattern [10]. Pediatric- type FL (PTFL) is a nodal disease that occurs primarily in children and young adults with a male-to-female ratio of ≥10:1 [1, 11]. The differences between PTFL and adult-type FL are summarized in Table 8.3 [1, 10, 11].

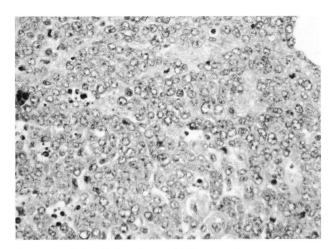

Figure 8.2 Burkitt-like lymphoma with 11q aberration. The tumor cells are more pleomorphic than classic Burkitt lymphoma and are intermedium to large in size, have open chromatin, and have high mitotic figures (H&E, 400x).

Table 8.3 Comparison of pediatric-type follicular lymphoma and adult-type follicular lymphoma

	Pediatric-type FL	Adult-type FL
Incidence	<5% pediatric lymphomas	20% of all lymphomas
Locations	Head and neck lymph nodes, tonsils	Lymph nodes, spleen, bone marrow, GI tract, skin
Clinical presentation	More localized disease	Less localized disease
Histology	Grade 3 common	Grades 1–3
BCL-2 protein	−	+
BCL-2 translocation	−	+

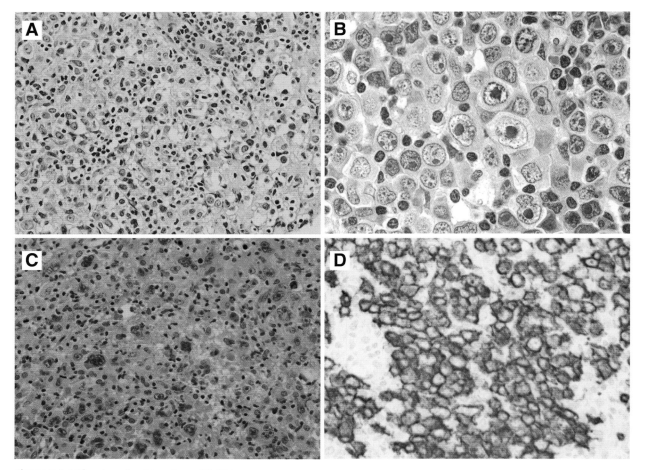

Figure 8.3 Diffuse large B-cell lymphoma (DLBCL).

a. Centroblast morphology demonstrates large neoplastic lymphoid cells with moderate amount of cytoplasm, oval to indented nuclei, vesicular chromatin, and two to four nuclear membrane-bound nucleoli. Mitosis and apoptotic cells are also present (H&E, 400x).

b. Immunoblastic morphology shows large neoplastic lymphoid cells with moderately abundant eosinophilc cytoplasm and very prominent, centrally placed eosinophilic nucleoli (H&E, 1,000x).

c. Anaplastic variant displays very large neoplastic cells with bizarre pleomorphic nuclei resembling Reed-Sternberg/Hodgkin cells or neoplastic cells in anaplastic large cell lymphoma (H&E, 400x).

d. Lymphoma cells demonstrate CD20 reactivity (CD20 immunostain, 400x).

e. Germinal center B-cell type shows BCL-6 positivity (BCL-6 immunostain, 400x).

f. Germinal center B-cell type shows CD10 positivity (CD10 immunostain, 400x).

g. Activated B-cell type shows MUM1 reactivity (MUM1 immunostain, 400x).

h. Flow cytometry demonstrates a monoclonal B-cell population with kappa light chain restriction.

Morphologically, FL is characterized by nodal effacement by a nodular proliferation of densely packed abnormal follicles containing a mixture of centrocytes and centroblasts [10]. The neoplastic follicles lack an intact mantle zone and loss of germinal center polarization, creating a back-to-back nodular pattern (Figure 8.6). The WHO classification recommends using a three-grade system (grade 1: 0–5 centroblasts/40x field; grade 2: 6–15 centroblasts/40x field; grade 3: >15 centroblasts/40x field) [10, 11]. Grade 3 can be further divided into grade 3A and grade 3B (grade 3A: has >15 centroblasts per high-power field but also contains centrocytes within the neoplastic follicle; grade 3B has solid sheets of centroblasts within the

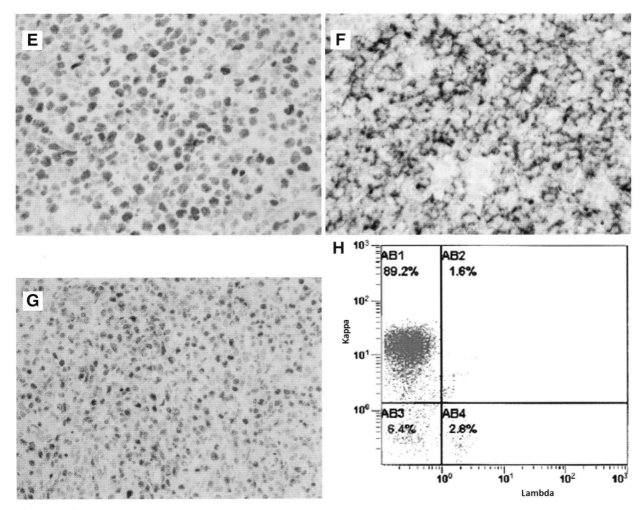

Figure 8.3 (cont.)

neoplastic follicle) [10]. Immunophenotype reveals CD19+, CD20+, CD79a+, PAX-5+, BCL6+, CD10+, CD5−, CD23−, CD25−, CD11c−, and CD43−. BCL-2 is usually positive in adult-type FL, but usually negative in PTFL [1, 10, 12].

Immunoglobulin-heavy or light chain rearrangement can be detected. Adult-type FL is characterized by carrying t(14;18) (q32; q21) and *BCL-2* gene rearrangements, resulting in overexpression of BCL-2 protein.

PTFL cases are much less likely to have *BCL-2* rearrangements or overexpression of BCL-2 protein, suggesting an alternative mechanism of lymphomagenesis in children, adolescents, and young adults [1, 10, 11].

The main differential diagnosis for PTFL is reactive follicular hyperplasia (Table 8.4). PTFL is usually indolent. Treatment includes excision, chemotherapy, or radiotherapy. Patients usually achieve durable remission [1, 10–12].

Pediatric Marginal Zone Lymphoma

Nodal marginal zone lymphoma (NMZL) and extranodal marginal zone lymphoma (EMZL) can be seen in children with much lower frequency than in adults [1, 13]. Pediatric patients with NMZL are predominantly male and usually present with asymptomatic and localized disease, mainly in the head and neck lymph nodes (Figure 8.7) [13]. Among the reported pediatric EMZL

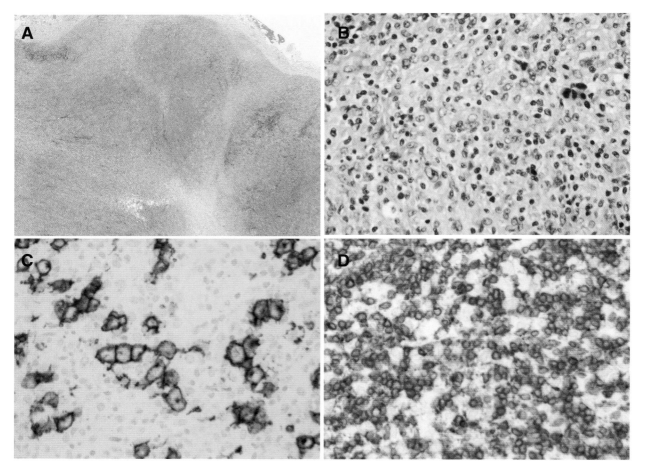

Figure 8.4 T-cell/histiocyte-rich large B-cell lymphoma characterized by a limited number of scattered, large B-cells embedded in a background of predominant T-cells and histiocytes.

a. A biopsy shows effacement of normal lymph node architecture (H&E, 20x).
b. Scattered large atypical lymphoid cells are identified in the background of small lymphocytes (H&E, 400x).
c. CD20 is positive in large neoplastic cells (CD20 immunostain, 400x).
d. Small lymphocytes in the background are CD3-positive (CD3 immunostain, 400x).

cases, about half arise in patients with immunodeficiency, most commonly secondary to HIV infection. The typical locations of EMZL include the stomach, orbit and ocular adnexa (Figure 8.8), tonsils, adenoids, submandibular gland, nasal sinus, skin, and lips [1, 14, 15]. Many mucosa-associated lymphoid tissue (MALT) lymphoma cases have a history of a chronic inflammatory disorder causing accumulation of extranodal lymphoid tissue. The chronic inflammation may be the result of infection, autoimmune disorders, or idiopathic stimuli. The patient age range in the pediatric group is 1–18 years with approximately equal numbers of males and females [1].

Histologically and immunophenotypically, pediatric NMZL and EMZL are similar to adult cases, except that there are often large follicles with extension of mantle zone B-cells into the germinal centers, resembling progressive transformation of germinal centers in NMZL cases. The neoplastic cells surrounding reactive follicles show proliferation and expansion. Cytologically, the neoplastic lymphoid cells are characterized by cells that are small to medium in size with a moderate amount of cytoplasm, and irregular nuclear contours that resemble small lymphocytes, centrocyte-like cells, large centroblasts, monocytoid B-cells, and monotypic plasma cells. Some cases have more numerous large transformed cells

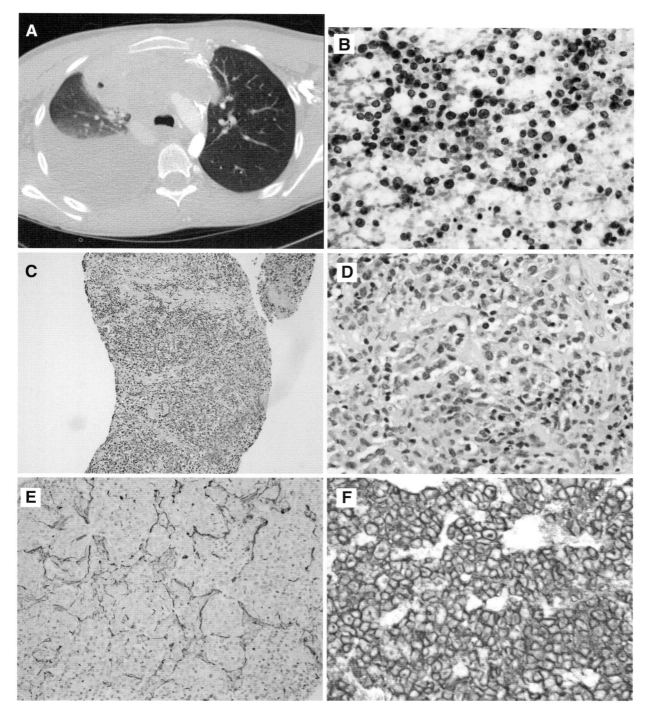

Figure 8.5 Primary mediastinal large B-cell lymphoma.

a. CT image shows a large anterior mediastinal mass.
b. Touch imprint shows a number of medium to large-sized neoplastic lymphocytes with vesicular chromatin and small nucleoli (H&E, 400x).
c. A needle core biopsy reveals diffuse infiltrate by neoplastic lymphocytes (H&E, 100x).
d. Medium to large-sized neoplastic lymphocytes show clear cytoplasm, round to irregular nuclei, open chromatin, and inconspicuous nucleoli (H&E, 400x).
e. Reticulin stain shows compartment fibrosis (Reticulin stain, 200x).
f. Neoplastic cells are CD20 strongly positive (CD20 immunostain, 400x).

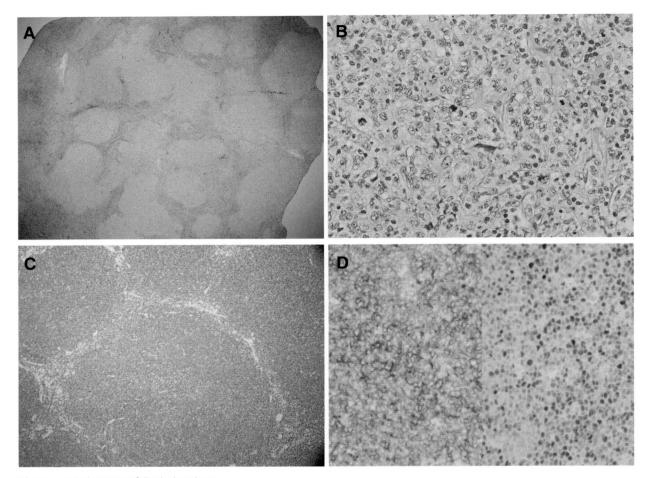

Figure 8.6 Pediatric-type follicular lymphoma.

a. Lymph node shows nodular growth pattern with back-to-back lymphoid follicles (H&E, 20x).
b. Neoplastic follicles contain predominantly large centroblasts with round or oval nuclei, vesicular chromatin, one to three peripheral nucleoli, a small to moderate amount of cytoplasm, and rare mitotic figures (H&E, 400x).
c. Tumor cells are positive for CD20 (CD20 immunostain, 20x).
d. Tumor cells are positive for CD10 (left: CD10 immunostain, 400x) and BCL-6 (right: BCL-6 immunostain, 400x).

(sometimes >20%). Plasma cell differentiation is present to varying degrees. Follicular colonization (the neoplastic cells infiltrate into surrounding reactive follicles) and prominent eosinophilia may be present. In EMZL, the neoplastic lymphoid cells can infiltrate mucosal epithelium to form lymphoepithelial lesions. NMZL and EMZL express pan-B-cell markers (CD19, CD20, CD22, CD79a, and PAX-5), often with CD43 coexpression [13]. There is usually no CD5, CD10, CD23, or cyclin D1 expression. Light chain restriction can be detected by flow cytometry, immunohistochemical staining, or in situ hybridization.

Polymerase chain reaction analysis can detect the presence of both heavy and light chain immunoglobulin rearrangements in almost all cases. Chromosomal translocations associated with MALT lymphomas include t(11;18) (q21; q21), t(1;14) (p22; q32), t(14;18) (q32; q21) and t(3;14) (p14.1; q32), resulting in the production of a chimeric protein (BIRC3-MALT1) and in transcriptional deregulation of BCL10, MALT1, and FOXP1, respectively. Trisomy 18 may occur in 20% of cases, rarely trisomy 3. Treatment for NMZL and EMZL is variable ranging from conservative to more aggressive approaches. The prognosis is excellent due to the indolent natural course of this tumor [1, 13].

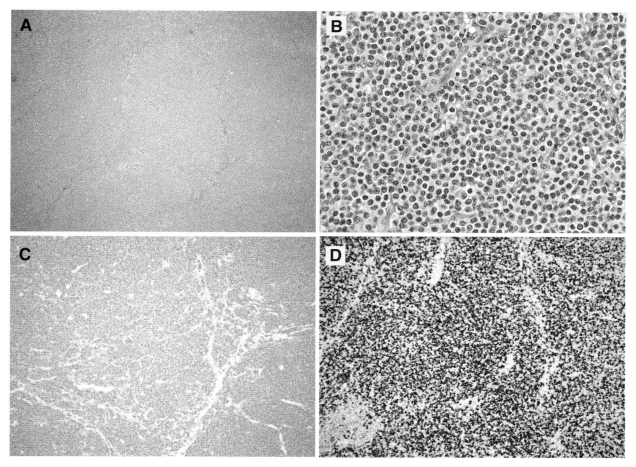

Figure 8.7 Pediatric nodal marginal zone lymphoma (images courtesy Dr. Karen Marie Chisholm).

a. A lymph node reveals vague nodule formation composed of paler-staining cells in a lymph node biopsy (H&E, 40x).

b. High power demonstrates neoplastic cells with mildly enlarged size, oval to slightly irregular nuclei, moderately abundant pale cytoplasm, and small nucleolus. Rare reactive small lymphocytes are intermixed with neoplastic lymphocytes (H&E, 400x).

c. Neoplastic cells are positive for CD20 (CD20 immunostain, 100x).

d. Neoplastic cells are positive for myeloid cell nuclear differentiation antigen (MNDA) by immunohistochemical stain (100x).

References

1. Perkins SL. Pediatric mature B-cell non-Hodgkin lymphomas. In Proytcheva, MA, ed. Diagnostic pediatric hematopathology. Cambridge: Cambridge University Press; 2011:395–428.

2. Leoncini L, Campo E, Stein H, Harris NL, Jeffe ES, Kluin PM. Burkitt lymphoma. In Swerdlow SH, Campo E, Harris NL, et al., eds. WHO classification of tumours of haematopoietic and lymphoid tissue. Revised 4th ed. Lyon: IARC Press; 2017:330–4.

3. Leoncini L, Campo E, Stein H, Harris NL, Jeffe ES, Kluin PM. Burkitt-like lymphoma with 11q aberration. In Swerdlow SH, Campo E, Harris NL, et al., eds. WHO classification of tumours of haematopoietic and lymphoid tissue. Revised 4th ed. Lyon: IARC Press; 2017:334.

4. Salaverria I, Martin-Guerrero I, Wagener R, Kreuz M, Kohler CW, Richter J, et al. A recurrent 11q aberration pattern characterizes a subset of MYC-negative high-grade B-cell lymphomas resembling Burkitt lymphoma. Blood. 2014 Feb 20; **123**(8): 1187–98.

5. Gascoyne RD, Campo E, Jaffe ES, Chan WC, Chan JKC, Rosenwald A, et al. Diffuse large B-cell Lymphoma, NOS. In Swerdlow SH, Campo E, Harris NL, et al., eds. WHO classification of tumours of haematopoietic and lymphoid tissue. Revised 4th ed. Lyon: IARC Press; 2017:291–7.

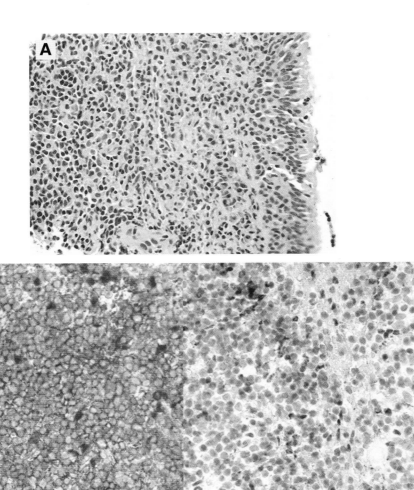

Figure 8.8 Pediatric extranodal marginal zone lymphoma.

a. A right posterior lacrimal sac lesion shows underlying mucosal atypical lymphoid proliferation (small lymphoid cells and plasma cells) with neoplastic lymphocytes infiltrating mucosal epithelium (H&E, 400x).

b. Neoplastic cells are positive for kappa light chain (left: Kappa immunostain, 400x) and negative for lambda light chain (right: Lambda immunostain, 400x).

6. Poirel HA, Cairo MS, Heerema NA, Swansbury J, Auperin A, Launay E, et al. Specific cytogenetic abnormalities are associated with a significantly inferior outcome in children and adolescents with mature B-cell non-Hodgkin's lymphoma: Results of the FAB/LMB 96 international study. Leukemia. 2009 Feb; **23**(2): 323–31.

7. Gaulard P, Harris NL, Pileri SA, Stein H, Kovrigina AM, Jeffe ES, et al. Primary mediastinal (thymic) large B-cell lymphoma. In Swerdlow SH, Campo E, Harris NL, et al. WHO classification of tumours of haematopoietic and lymphoid tissues. Revised 4th ed. Lyon: IARC Press; 2017:314–16.

8. Savage KJ, Monti S, Kutok JL, Cattoretti G, Neuberg D, De Leval L, et al. The molecular signature of mediastinal large B-cell lymphoma differs from that of other diffuse large B-cell lymphomas and shares features with classical Hodgkin lymphoma. Blood. 2003 Dec 1; **102**(12): 3871–9.

Table 8.4 Pathologic features of follicular lymphoma versus reactive follicular hyperplasia

		Follicular Lymphoma	Follicular Hyperplasia
Architectural features	Architecture pattern	Effaced Back-to-back follicular pattern	Preserved Intervening lymphoid tissue between follicles
	Lymphoid follicles	Slight to moderate variation in size and shape	Marked variation in size and shape
	Capsular infiltration	Yes	No
	Density of follicles	High	Low
	Follicle polarization	Absent mantle zone and polarization	Definite mantle zone and polarization
Cytologic features	Germinal center cells	Monomorphic	Polymorphic
	Mitotic activity	Relatively low	Moderate to high
	Tingible body macrophages	Absent	Prominent
	Interfollicular areas	Tumor cells present	Reactive lymphoid cells
Mib-1		Evenly distributed across the follicle	Highlight polarization of the follicle
B-cell clonality		Monoclonal	Polyclonal
Genetics	Polymerase chain reaction	Monoclonal	Polyclonal
	Cytogenetics	t(14;18)(q32;q21) in adult-type not in pediatric-type	Normal

9. Weniger MA, Gesk S, Ehrlich S, Martin-Subero JI, Dyer MJ, Siebert R, et al. Gains of REL in primary mediastinal B-cell lymphoma coincide with nuclear accumulation of REL protein. Genes Chromosomes Cancer. 2007 Apr; **46** (4): 406–15.

10. Jaffe ES, Harris NL, Swerdlow SH, Ott G, Nathwani BN, De Jong D, et al. Follicular lymphoma. In Swerdlow SH, Campo E, Harris NL, et al., eds. WHO classification of tumours of haematopoietic and lymphoid tissue. Revised 4th ed. Lyon: IARC Press; 2017:266–73.

11. Jaffe ES, Harris NL, Siebert R. Pediatric-type follicular lymphoma. In Swerdlow SH, Campo E, Harris NL, et al., eds. WHO classification of tumours of haematopoietic and lymphoid tissue. Revised 4th ed. Lyon: IARC Press; 2017: 278–9.

12. Liu Q, Salaverria I, Pittaluga S, Jegalian AG, Xi L, Siebert R, et al. Follicular lymphomas in children and young adults: A comparison of the pediatric variant with usual follicular lymphoma. Am J Surg Pathol. 2013 Mar; **37**(3): 333–43.

13. Campo E, Pileri SA, Jaffe ES, Nathwani BN, Stein H, Muller-Hermelink, HK. Nodal marginal zone lymphoma. In Swerdlow SH, Campo E, Harris NL, et al., eds. WHO classification of tumours of haematopoietic and lymphoid tissue. Revised 4th ed. Lyon: IARC Press; 2017:263–5.

14. Swerdlow SH. Pediatric follicular lymphomas, marginal zone lymphomas, and marginal zone hyperplasia. Pathol Patterns Rev. 2004 Dec 1; **122**(suppl 1): S98–S109.

15. Quintanilla-Martinez L, Sander B, Chan JK, Xerri L, Ott G, Campo E, Swerdlow SH. Indolent lymphomas in the pediatric population: Follicular lymphoma, IRF4/MUM1+ lymphoma, nodal marginal zone lymphoma and chronic lymphocytic leukemia. Virchows Archiv. 2016 Feb 1; **468**(2): 141–57.

Mature T-Cell and NK-Cell Non-Hodgkin Lymphomas

Xiayuan Liang, Billie Carstens

Mature T-cell non-Hodgkin lymphomas (NHLs) in the pediatric population comprise about 10–15% of the NHLs. Natural killer (NK) cell neoplasms in this age group are even rarer. Both groups of lymphomas tend to present with a broad spectrum of clinical manifestations, including nodal, extranodal, and leukemic diseases, and are frequently associated with paraneoplastic phenomena such as hemophagocytosis, fevers, or rashes [1].

Anaplastic Large-Cell Lymphoma, ALK-Positive

The WHO classification defines anaplastic large-cell lymphoma, ALK positive (ALCL, ALK+) as a systemic T-cell lymphoma composed of large pleomorphic cells with abundant cytoplasm, often horseshoe-shaped nuclei with a translocation involving the *ALK* gene and expression of ALK protein, and expression of CD30 [2]. ALCL, ALK+ is the most common subtype of mature T-cell lymphoma in the pediatric population with a male predominance (M:F ratio 1.5:1) [1, 2].

Most patients present with advanced-stage (stage III or IV) diseases. Clinically, ALCL, ALK+ has a variety of presentations, including nodal and extranodal disease. There is a high propensity for involving extranodal tissue (skin, bone, soft tissues, lungs, and liver) either as the only sites of disease or, more commonly, in association with nodal disease. The bone marrow involvement is approximately 10% [2]. Rare cases may present with leukemic blood involvement, which is associated with an extremely poor prognosis. Secondary skin involvement must be distinguished from primary cutaneous ALCL. Patients often have B symptoms, especially high fever [1, 2].

ALCL, ALK+ shows a broad morphologic spectrum (Figures 9.1a–e). All of the morphologic subtypes contain a variable proportion of the hallmark cells. The pathologic features of morphologic variants are summarized in Table 9.1 [2].

The tumor cells of all subtypes are positive for CD30 (Figure 9.1f) on the cell membrane and in the Golgi region. CD45 expression is variable. ALCLs may or may not demonstrate staining with T-cell markers (Figure 9.1g). CD3 is negative in >75% of cases and CD8 is usually negative [2]. Most tumors express CD4, CD5, and/or CD2 [2]. Expression of cytotoxic antigens (TIA-1 or granzyme-B) is commonly seen. Most ALK+ ALCL are positive for epithelial membrane antigen (EMA). Expression of CD56 is seen in some cases and appears to be associated with a poor prognosis.

ALK antibodies detect the fusion protein generated by translocations. In the majority of the cases that have the t(2;5)/*NPM* (nucleophosmin)-*ALK* translocation (Figure 9.1j), ALK staining of tumor cells is nuclear with or without cytoplasmic staining pattern (Figure 9.1h). A small percentage of ALCL, ALK+ cases exhibit cytoplasmic or membrane ALK staining pattern (Figure 9.1i), and these cases show a good correlation with variant ALK gene translocations involving partner genes other than *NPM* [1, 2].

The long-term survival rate of this disease is high, approaching 80% [2]. Poor prognostic factors include organ involvement, mediastinal disease, extensive skin disease, leukemic phase, systemic symptoms, small-cell variant, CD56 expression, and concurrent *MYC* rearrangement [1-3]. Children with refractory or relapsed ALCL are often treated with allogeneic bone marrow transplant.

Anaplastic Large-Cell Lymphoma, ALK-Negative

Anaplastic large-cell lymphoma, ALK-negative (ALCL, ALK−) is classified as a distinct entity in the 2016 WHO classification [4]. It is defined as a CD30+ T-cell neoplasm that is not reproducibly distinguishable on morphological grounds from ALCL, ALK+, but lacks ALK protein expression [4, 5].

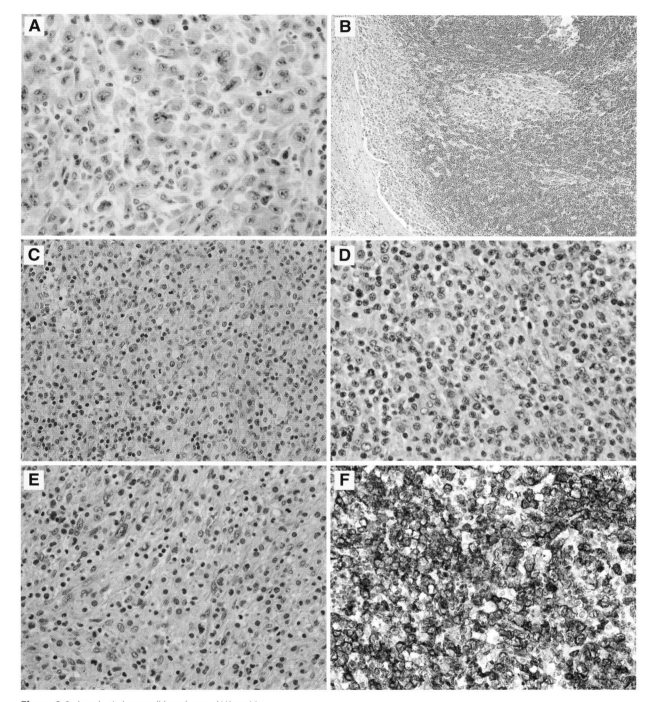

Figure 9.1 Anaplastic large-cell lymphoma, ALK-positive.

a and b. Anaplastic/common variant.

a. Hallmark cells show large-sized, abundant basophilic cytoplasm with eosinophilia near the nucleus, eccentric horseshoe-shaped or kidney-shaped nuclei, and prominent nucleoli (H&E, 400x).

b. Sinusoidal invasion by anaplastic large cells, a common pattern in systemic ACLC (H&E, 100x)

c. Lymphohistiocytic variant. A number of histiocytes are admixed with large neoplastic cells (H&E, 400x).

d. Small-cell variant. Tumor cells are predominantly small but are atypical with irregular nuclei. Hallmark cells are not prominent in this case (H&E, 400x).

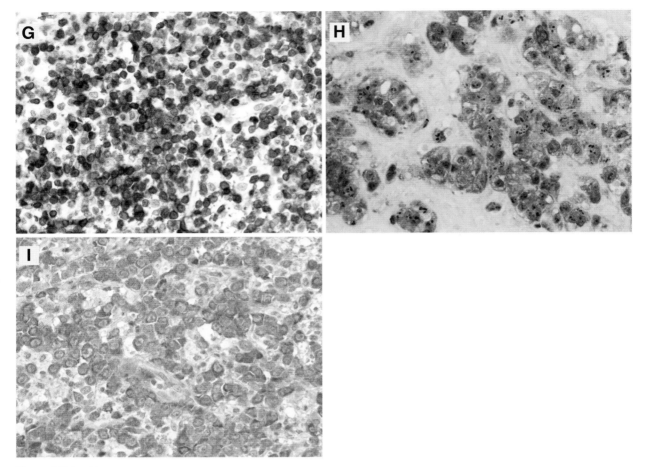

Figure 9.1 (cont.)

e. Composite variant. This variant shows more than one pattern seen in a single lymph node biopsy. There are a number of spindle-shaped neoplastic cells with pink cytoplasm and pleomorphic nuclei and hallmark cells with kidney-shaped nuclei, and monomorphid tumor cells with round nuclei in this lymph node biopsy (H&E, 400x).

f. Neoplastic cells are positive for CD30 (CD30 immunostain, 400x).

g. Neoplastic cells are positive for CD3 (CD3 immunostain, 400x).

h. Neoplastic cells are positive for ALK-1 with both nuclear and cytoplasmic staining pattern indicating t(2;5) translocation (ALK-1 immunostain, 400x).

i. Neoplastic cells are positive for ALK-1 with cytoplasmic staining pattern indicating non-t(2;5), variant *ALK* translocation (ALK-1 immunostain, 400x).

j. Cytogenetics. The upper panel shows interphase FISH break apart assay for *ALK*. 3'*ALK* is labeled red and 5'*ALK* is labeled green. The upper left shows a normal cell pattern with un-rearranged fusion (red-green) signals. The upper middle shows two interphase cells with an *ALK* rearrangement (separate red and green signals). The upper right is the schematic representation. The lower panel is chromosomal analysis revealing t(2;5)(p23;q35).

Among all systemic ALCLs, those that are ALK-negative constitute 15–50% of cases. It primarily affects adults (40–65 years), although cases can occur at any age [4–6]. There is a slight predominance in males [4, 6]. It usually involves lymph nodes at diagnosis and, less frequently, extranodal sites [4–6]. Two-third of patients present with advanced stage of disease and B symptoms [6].

ALCL, ALK– demonstrate a similar cytological spectrum to ALCL, ALK+ (Figure 9.2a), although a "small-cell variant" is not recognized [4–6]. In addition to homogenous CD30 expression (Figure 9.2b), more than 50% of cases are positive for one or more T-cell markers. CD2 and CD3 are more often expressed than CD5. CD43 (Figure 9.2c) is almost always positive [4]. CD4 (Figure 9.2d)

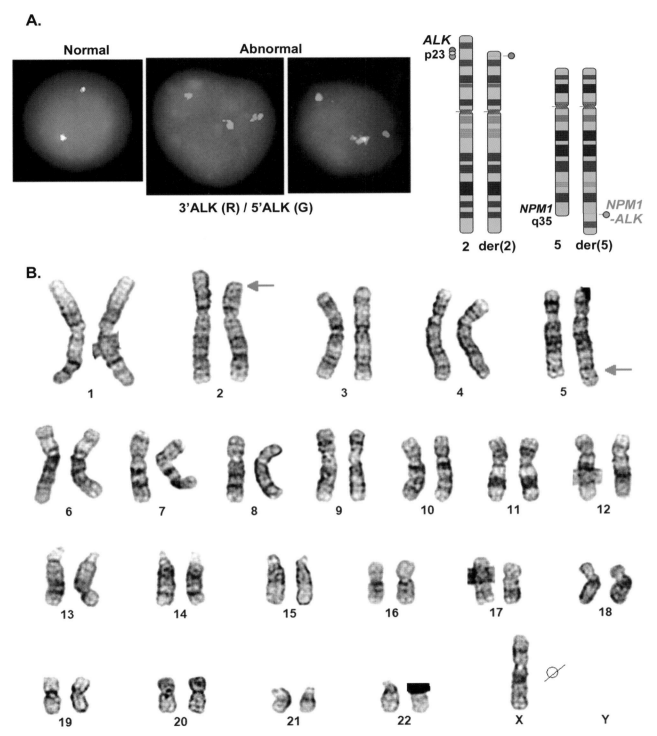

Figure 9.1 (cont.)

Table 9.1 Pathologic features of morphologic variants of ALCL, ALK+

	Frequency	Morphologic Features	Other Features
Anaplastic/common variant	60%	Anaplastic large cells and hallmark cells showing a sinusoidal to diffuse infiltration	
Lymphohistiocytic variant	10%	Neoplastic cells admixed with a large number of reactive histiocytes	More rarely seen in children
Small-cell variant	5–10%	– Predominance of small to medium- sized neoplastic cells with irregular nuclei and only scattered hallmark cells – Diffuse effacement of lymph node architecture – Hallmark cells tend to cluster along vascular structures	– Often misdiagnosed as peripheral T-cell lymphoma, NOS – More commonly associated with high-stage disease – More aggressive behavior
Hodgkin-like variant	3%	Difficult to distinguish from classical Hodgkin lymphoma, nodular sclerosis subtype	
Composite variant	15%	More than one pattern may be seen in a single lymph node biopsy	
Monomorphic variant	Rare	Neoplastic cells with rounded nuclei	
Sarcomatoid variant	Rare	Spindle-shaped neoplastic cells	

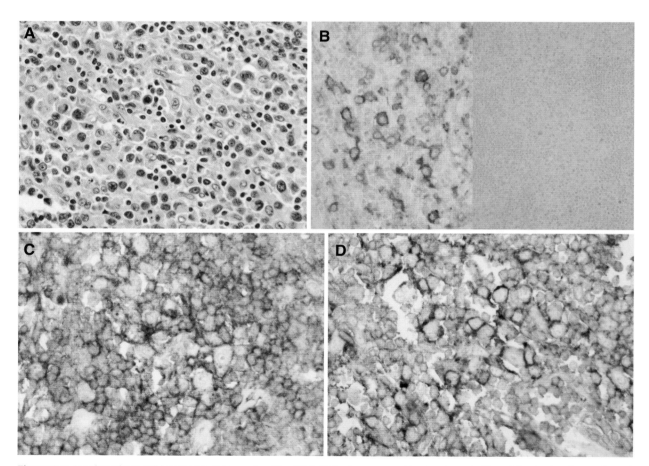

Figure 9.2 Anaplastic large-cell lymphoma, ALK-negative. Like ACLC, ALK+, the organ architecture is eroded by solid, cohesive sheets of neoplastic cells. In the lymph node, sinuses show lymphoma cell proliferation. However, the neoplastic cells are large and more pleomorphic in most cases of ALCL, ALK– than those seen in ALCL, ALK+.

a. Neoplastic cells are large and show abundant pink cytoplasm, pleomorphic and anaplastic nuclei, and prominent nucleoli (H&E, 400x).
b. The left panel shows neoplastic cells positive for CD30 staining. The right panel shows neoplastic cells negative for ALK-1 staining.
c. Neoplastic cells show CD43 reactivity (CD43 immunostain, 40x).
d. Neoplastic cells show CD4 positivity (CD4 immunostain, 40x).

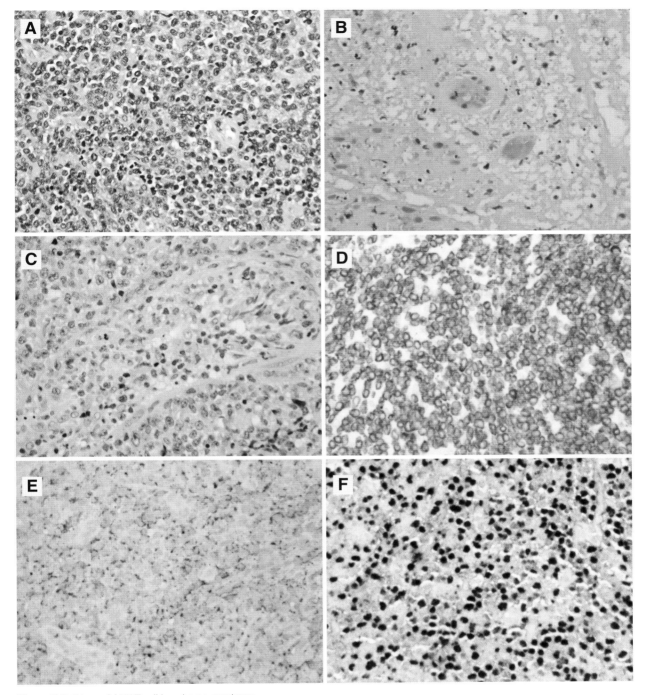

Figure 9.3 Extranodal NK/T-cell lymphoma, nasal type.

a. The lymphomatous infiltrate is diffuse and permeative. The neoplastic lymphoid cells are medium-sized to large and show irregular nuclear contours and granular to vesicular chromatin with inconspicuous nucleoli. The cytoplasm is moderate in amount. Mitotic figures are easily found (H&E, 400x).
b. Coagulative necrosis is present surrounding the blood vessel. The blood vessel shows fibrinoid changes (H&E, 400x).
c. A blood vessel shows angiocentric and angioinvasive features (H&E, 400x).
d. Tumor cells are positive for CD3 (CD3 immunostain, 400x).
e. Tumor cells are positive for cytotoxic molecule, Granzyme B (Granzyme B immunostain, 400x).
f. Epstein-Barr virus (EBV) signals (EBER+) are detected in tumor cells (EBER in situ hybridization, 400x).

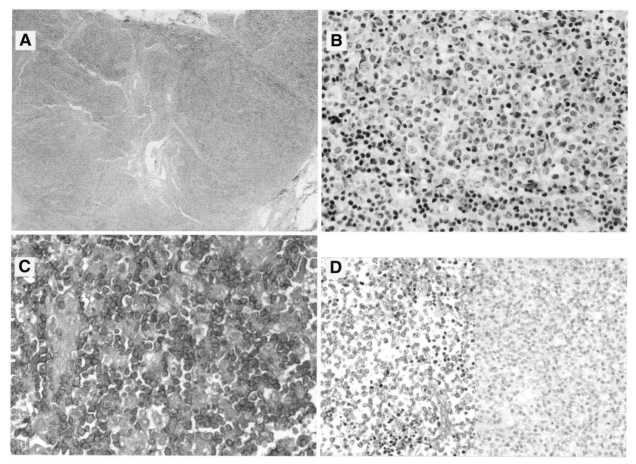

Figure 9.4 Peripheral T-cell lymphoma, NOS.

a. A lymph node biopsy shows an effacement of normal architecture by a diffuse (sometimes a paracortical) lymphoid proliferation (H&E, 20x).

b. High-power shows moderate pleomorphism of the moderate to large-sized tumor cells with moderate to abundant clear to basophilic cytoplasm, variably irregular nuclear configuration, vesicular chromatin, variably prominent nucleoli, and mitosis. The background is composed of small lymphocytes, rare eosinophils, and plasm cells. Clusters of benign epithelioid histiocytes may be seen occasionally, but not in this case (H&E, 400x).

c. The neoplastic cells express CD3 (CD3 immunostain, 400x).

d. The neoplastic cells are negative for CD30 (left: CD30 immunostain, 400x) and ALK-1 (right: ALK-1 immunostain, 400x).

is expressed in a significant proportion of cases, whereas CD8+ cases are rare [4]. Cytotoxic markers (TIA1, granzyme B, and/or perforin) are positive in many cases [4].

Differential diagnosis includes ALCL, ALK+, primary cutaneous ALCL (C-ALCL) when tumor involves skin, peripheral T-cell lymphoma, not otherwise specified (PTCL, NOS), classical Hodgkin lymphoma (cHL). The clinicopathologic comparison of these entities are summarized in Table 9.2 [1, 4, 6].

Genetically, T-cell receptor genes are clonally rearranged in most cases [5]. Recurrent rearrangements of the *DUSP22-IRF4* locus on 6p25.3 (*DUSP22* rearrangement) or

the *TP63* locus on 3q28, although not specific for ALCL, occur in about 30% and 8% of cases, respectively [4, 5]. The translocation t(6;7)(p25.3;q32.3) was demonstrated in 45% of cases [5, 6]. In addition, gene-expression profiling studies have shown distinct molecular signatures between ALCL, ALK− and PTCL, NOS involving three genes (*TNFRSF8*, *BATF3*, and *TMOD1*) [4, 5].

The prognosis of ALCL, ALK− is poorer than that of ALCL, ALK+, but is superior than of PTCL, NOS [4, 5]. Cases with complex chromosome abnormalities are associated with a significantly shorter overall survival [5]. ALCL, ALK− with *DUSP22* rearrangements has a similar 5-year

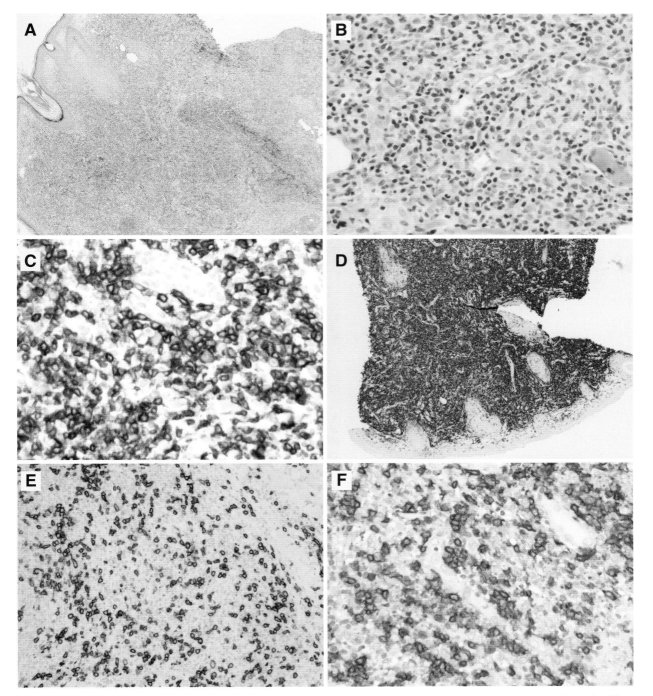

Figure 9.5 Primary cutaneous CD4+ small/medium T-cell lymphoproliferative disorder. A 12-year-old male presented with a solitary cheek lesion. A skin biopsy was performed.

a. The skin biopsy shows a dense and diffuse dermal lymphoid infiltrate with sparing of the epidermis. There is a grenz zone between the infiltrate and the epidermis (H&E, 20x).
b. The lymphoid infiltrate is composed of predominantly small, medium, and scattered larger lymphocytes (usually less than 30%) intermixed with histiocytes and rare plasma cells (H&E, 400x).
c. CD3 is expressed in most lymphocytes (CD3 immunostain, 400x).
d. CD4 is expressed in most T-cells (CD4 immunostain, 40x).
e. CD8 expression is seen in a small subset of T-cells (CD8 immunostain, 200x).
f. CD20 expression is seen in a subset of lymphocytes (CD20 immunostain, 200x).

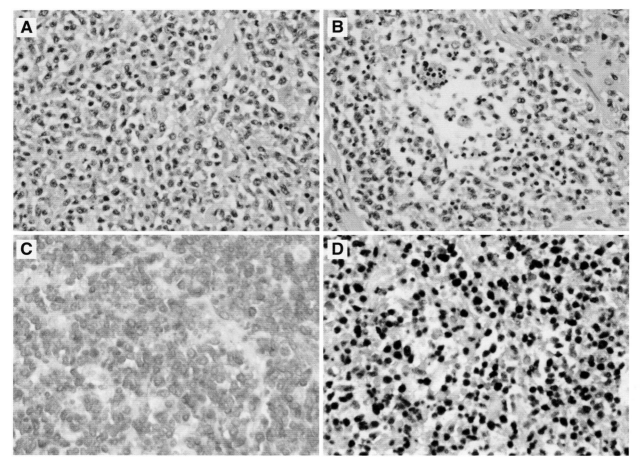

Figure 9.6 Systemic EBV+ T-cell lymphoma of childhood.

a. A lymph node biopsy shows medium-sized atypical lymphocyte proliferation with hyperchromatic and irregular nuclei (H&E, 400x).
b. A biopsy of the lung shows hemophagocytosis (H&E, 400x).
c. The neoplastic cells are CD8 positive (CD8 immunostain, 400x).
d. The neoplastic cells are positive for EBV RNA (EBER in situ hybridization, 400x).

survival rate (90%) to that in ALCL, ALK+ [5]. Cases with *TP63* rearrangement have worse prognoses than those with neither *DUSP22* nor *TP63* rearrangement [4, 5].

Extranodal NK-/T-cell Lymphoma, Nasal Type

Extranodal NK-/T-cell lymphoma (ENKTCL), nasal type is a predominantly extranodal lymphoma of NK-cell or T-cell lineage characterized by vascular damage and destruction, prominent necrosis, cytotoxic phenotype, and association with EBV. It is designated an NK/T-cell lymphoma because although most cases appear to be genuine NK-cell neoplasms, some cases show a cytotoxic T-cell phenotype [1, 7].

ENKTCL is more prevalent in Asians, the indigenous American population of Mexico, Central America and South America, and immunosuppressed patients. It occurs most often in adults and is very rarely seen in children. Males are more frequently affected than females [1, 7].

ENKTCL arises predominantly in extranodal sites, likely in the midline of the body with the upper aerodigestive tract (nasal cavity, nasopharynx, paranasal sinuses palate) being the most common site, but the tumor can also be seen in the skin, soft tissues, gastrointestinal tract, and testis. Unlike

Table 9.2 Comparison of clinicopathologic features among anaplastic large-cell lymphomas, peripheral T-cell lymphoma-NOS, and classical Hodgkin lymphoma

	ALCL, ALK+	ALCL, ALK−	C-ALCL	PTCL, NOS	CHL
Age at diagnosis	First 3 decades	40–65 years	60 years (median age)	Adults	1st peak: 15–34 years; 2nd peak: >60 years
Gender	M:F = 1.5:1	M:F = 1.5:1	M:F = 2–3:1	M:F = 2:1	M ≈ F
Location	LN, skin, bone ST, BM, lung, spleen, liver	LN, bone, ST, GI, skin	Skin	LN, BM, liver, spleen	Mediastinum, cervical LN
Tumor cell growth pattern	Sinuses, interfollicular, or diffuse	Sinuses, interfollicular, diffuse	Diffuse	Diffuse	Nodular, interfollicular, diffuse
Neoplastic cells	A broad morphology, large hallmark cells+	Less broad morphology, large hallmark cells+	Large, pleomorphic, anaplastic	Medium-sized and/or large, pleomorphic	Scattered Reed-Sternberg cells or variants
Immunophenotype	CD30+, ALK+, CD43±, EMA±, EBER−	CD30+, ALK−, CD43+, EMA±, EBER−	CD30+, CD4+, ALK−, EMA−, EBER−	CD3+, CD4+, CD8−, CD30−, ALK−	CD15±, CD30+, PAX5+, EBER±
ALK rearrangement	+	−	−	−	−
Outcome	Favorable	Less favorable	Favorable	Unfavorable	Favorable

ALCL, anaplastic large-cell lymphoma; BM, bone marrow; C, cutaneous; cHL, classical Hodgkin lymphoma; F, female; GI, gastrointestinal; LN, lymph node; M, male; NOS, not otherwise specified; PTCL, peripheral T-cell lymphoma; ST, soft tissue.

adult presentations, pediatric presentations appear to be primarily gastrointestinal or cutaneous [1, 8]. Patients with nasal involvement present with nasal obstruction or epistaxis or with extensive midfacial destructive lesions. Skin lesions are commonly nodular, often with ulceration. Intestinal lesions often manifest as perforation. Although often localized at diagnosis, the tumor may rapidly disseminate to bone marrow, blood, lymph nodes, or other extranodal sites. Some patients may also have hemophagocytosis.

The immunophenotype of the tumor cells is variable. Most lesions show a phenotype of CD2+, CD56+, surface CD3−, and cytoplasmic CD3+, as well as being positive for cytotoxic molecules (granzyme B, TIA-1, and perforin). CD4, CD5, CD8, CD16, and CD57 are usually negative. CD7 and CD30 may display variable positivity. EBER is the most reliable way to demonstrate the presence of EBV. A diagnosis of extranodal NK-/T-cell lymphoma should be accepted with some skepticism if EBV is negative [1, 7, 8].

T-cell receptor (*TCR*) and immunoglobulin (*IG*) genes are in germline configuration in most cases. Rare cases may reveal clonal *TCR* rearrangement. Molecular analysis of EBV shows a clonal, episomal form [1, 8].

If ENKTCL occurs in the gastrointestinal tract and skin, it should be distinguished from enteropathy-associated

T-cell lymphoma and subcutaneous panniculitis-like T-cell lymphoma, respectively. Enteropathy-associated T-cell lymphoma is seen with greater frequency in those areas with a high prevalence of celiac disease, especially in Europe. Most show adult-onset disease with a history of childhood-onset celiac disease. The morphologic features of tumor cells can overlap with those seen in ENKTCL. The neoplastic cells are usually CD3+, CD5−, CD7+, CD8−, and CD103+. They express cytotoxic molecules. EBER is negative. *TCR* is usually clonally rearranged.

Subcutaneous panniculitis-like T-cell lymphoma is slightly more common in female than males with a broad age range. Up to 20% of patients may have associated autoimmune disease, most commonly systemic lupus erythematous. Patients present with multiple subcutaneous nodules. Hemophagocytic syndrome is seen in 15–20% of patients. The tumor cells involve the fat lobules with sparing of septa. The overlying dermis and epidermis are uninvolved. A helpful diagnostic feature is the rimming of the tumor cells surrounding individual fat cells. The tumor cells are usually CD8+ with expression of cytotoxic molecules, but are CD56− and EBER−.

In general, children may have a more favorable outcome. Patients with tumors occurring outside of the nasal cavity appear to have a more aggressive course. Bone marrow transplant may be curative for children and younger patients [1].

Peripheral T-cell Lymphoma, NOS

Peripheral T-cell lymphoma, not otherwise specified (PTCL, NOS) is a heterogeneous category of nodal and extranodal mature T-cell lymphoma that does not correspond to any of the specifically defined entities of mature T-cell lymphoma [9]. PTCL, NOS is infrequently seen in the pediatric population. Most pediatric PTCL, NOS described in the literature arises as mediastinal masses or nodal lesions rather than extranodal lesions [1, 8]. Patients often present with lymphadenopathy and frequently have advanced disease [8, 10].

In nodal cases, tumor cells are primarily CD4+CD8−. Double CD4+/CD8+ or CD4−/CD8− are occasionally seen. CD5 and CD7 are usually downregulated. Cytotoxicity molecules (TIA-1, Granzyme B, or Perforin) are usually expressed. CD30 may be positive in some cases, but it is usually weak. EBV is usually absent in adult cases but appears more prominently in pediatric cases. Genetically, the karyotype is usually complex [1, 9]. PTCL, NOS is a highly aggressive lymphoma. Because of the low numbers of patients in pediatric age groups, the treatment strategy and outcome data are not well defined [1, 9, 10].

Primary Cutaneous CD4+ Small/Medium T-cell Lymphoproliferative Disorder

Primary cutaneous CD4+ small/medium T-cell lymphoproliferative disorder (PCS/M-TCLPD) is an indolent T-cell disorder characterized by a predominance of small to medium-sized CD4+ pleomorphic T-cells and by presentation with a solitary skin lesion in almost all cases, without evidence of the patches and plaques typical of mycosis fungoides [11].

PCS/M-TCLPD can occur at any age but most commonly affects adults. Cases in the pediatric age group have been reported [12]. There is no gender predilection. These lesions frequently present as a solitary plaque or nodule, most often on the face and neck followed by the upper trunk and upper extremities. Lesions are typically asymptomatic [11, 12].

The proliferative lymphoid cells are positive for CD3 and CD4 and negative for CD8, CD30, cytotoxic molecules, and EBER. Loss of pan-T cell antigens (except for CD7) is uncommon. Atypical CD4+ T-cells express PD1, BCL-6 (variable), and CXCL13, suggesting T-follicular helper cell origin. The Ki67 proliferation index typically ranges from 5% to 20% [11].

Monoclonal *TCR* gene rearrangements have been detected in most cases. Specific genetic abnormalities are not detected. The clinical outcome is excellent. Treatment includes intralesional steroids, surgical excision, and radiotherapy. Local recurrences are rare [11, 12].

Systemic EBV+ T-cell Lymphoma of Childhood

Systemic EBV-positive T-cell lymphoma of childhood (previously systemic EBV-positive lymphoproliferative disease of childhood) is a life-threatening disease of children and young adults [1, 13]. The disease is most prevalent in Asia, primarily in Japan, Taiwan, and China. It has been reported in Mexico and in Central and South America [1, 13]. It is characterized by a clonal proliferation of cytotoxic T-cells infected with EBV. Most occur shortly after primary acute EBV infection [1]. This may show overlap with aggressive NK-cell leukemia [14, 15]. A few cases have been in the setting of chronic active EBV infection (CAEBV) [1]. Presenting symptoms include fever, pancytopenia, skin rashes, hepatosplenomegaly, and lymphadenopathy. The disease shows rapid progression, with multiple organ failure, sepsis, and death. The liver and the spleen are the most commonly involved sites, followed by lymph nodes, bone marrow, skin, and lungs [1, 13–15].

The infiltrating T-cells are usually small without substantial cytological atypia. However, pleomorphic medium-sized to large lymphoid cells with irregular nuclei and frequent mitoses have been reported [1, 13]. The liver has prominent portal and sinusoidal infiltration, cholestasis, steatosis, and necrosis. The splenic white pulp is depleted with prominent sinusoidal and nodular T-lymphoid cell infiltrate. The lymph nodes usually show preserved architecture with open sinuses and expansion of paracortical areas that reveal atypical lymphoid cell infiltrate. There is often associated hemophagocytic syndrome. In the blood, there may be an increased number of activated-appearing lymphocytes. The neoplastic cells typically are CD2+, CD3+, TIA-1+, and EBER+, but CD56−. Most cases secondary to acute primary EBV infection are CD8-positive [1, 13–15]. Those cases arising from CAEBV are CD4-positive [1, 13]. Molecular analysis demonstrates clonal *TCR* gene rearrangement. No recurrent cytogenetic abnormalities have been described [1, 13]. Most cases have a fulminant clinical course resulting in death, usually within days to weeks of diagnosis [1, 13–15].

References

1. Perkins SL. Pediatric mature T-cell and NK-cell non-Hodgkin lymphomas. In Proytcheva MA, ed. Diagnostic pediatric hematopathology. Cambridge: Cambridge University Press; 2011:429–64.

2. Falini B, Lamant-Rochaix L, Campo E, Jeffe ES, Gascoyne RD, Stein H, et al. Anaplastic large cell lymphoma, ALK-positive. In Swerdlow SH, Campo E, Harris NL, et al., eds. WHO classification of tumours of haematopoietic and lymphoid tissue. Revised 4th ed. Lyon: IARC Press; 2017:413–18.

3. Liang X, Branchford B, Greffe B, McGavran L, Carstens B, Meltesen L, et al. Dual ALK and MYC rearrangements leading to an aggressive variant of anaplastic large cell lymphoma. J Pediatr Hematol/Oncol. 2013 Jul 1; 35(5): e209–e213.

4. Feldman AL, Harris NL, Stein H, Campo E, Kinney MC, Jeffe ES, et al. Anaplastic large cell lymphoma, ALK-negative. In Swerdlow SH, Campo E, Harris NL, et al., eds. WHO classification of tumours of haematopoietic and lymphoid tissue. Revised 4th ed. Lyon: IARC Press; 2017:418–21.

5. Lamant-Rochaix L, Feldman AL, Delsol G, Brousset P. Anaplastic large cell lymphoma, ALK positive and ALK negative. In Jaffe E, Arber DA, Campo E, et al., eds. Hematopathology. 2nd ed. Philadelphia, PA: Elsevier; 2017:673–91.

6. Ferreri AJ, Govi S, Pileri SA, Savage KJ. Anaplastic large cell lymphoma, ALK-negative. Crit Rev Oncol/Hematol. 2013 Feb 1; 85(2): 206–15.

7. Chan JKC, Quintanilla-Martinez L, Ferry JA. Extranodal NK/T-cell lymphoma, nasal type. In Swerdlow SH, Campo E, Harris NL, et al., eds. WHO classification of tumours of haematopoietic and lymphoid tissue. Revised 4th ed. Lyon: IARC Press; 2017:368–71.

8. Wilberger AC, Liang X. Primary nonanaplastic peripheral natural killer/T-cell lymphoma in pediatric patients: An unusual distribution pattern of subtypes. Pediatr Dev Pathol. 2019 Mar; 22(2): 128–36.

9. Pileri SA, Weisenburger DD, Sng I, Nakamura S, Muller-Hermelink HK, Chan WC, Jaffe ES. Peripheral T-cell lymphoma, NOS. In Swerdlow SH, Campo E, Harris NL, et al., eds. WHO classification of tumours of haematopoietic and lymphoid tissue. Revised 4th ed. Lyon: IARC Press; 2017:403–7.

10. Mellgren K, Attarbaschi A, Abla O, Alexander S, Bomken S, Bubanska E, et al. Non-anaplastic peripheral T cell lymphoma in children and adolescents: An international review of 143 cases. Ann Hematol. 2016 Aug; 95(8): 1295–305.

11. Gaulard P, Berti E, Willemze R, Petrella T, Jaffe ES. Primary cutaneous CD4+ small/medium T-cell lymphoproliferative disorder. In Swerdlow SH, Campo E, Harris NL, et al., eds. WHO classification of tumours of haematopoietic and lymphoid tissue. Revised 4th ed. Lyon: IARC Press; 2017:401–2.

12. Beltraminelli H, Leinweber B, Kerl H, Cerroni L. Primary cutaneous CD4+ small-/medium-sized pleomorphic T-cell lymphoma: A cutaneous nodular proliferation of pleomorphic T lymphocytes of undetermined significance? A study of 136 cases. Am J Dermatopathol. 2009 Jun 1; 31(4): 317–22.

13. Quintanilla-Martinez L, Ko Y-H, Kimura H, Jaffe ES. EBV-positive T-cell and NK-cell lymphoproliferative diseases of childhood. In Swerdlow SH, Campo E, Harris NL, et al., eds. WHO classification of tumours of haematopoietic and lymphoid tissue. Revised 4th ed. Lyon: IARC Press; 2017:355–63.

14. Portsmore S, Chakravorty S, Oppong E, Ahmad R, Bain BJ. Systemic EBV-positive lymphoproliferative disease of childhood. Am J Hematol. 2015 Apr; 90(4): 355.

15. Chen G, Chen L, Qin X, Huang Z, Xie X, Li G, Xu B. Systemic EBV-positive lymphoproliferative disease of childhood with hemophagocytic syndrome. Int J Clin Exp Pathol. 2014 Sep 15; 7(10): 7110–33. eCollection 2014.

Hodgkin Lymphoma

Xiayuan Liang

Hodgkin lymphomas (HLs) encompass two morphologically, immunophenotypically, and clinically distinct subtypes of B-lineage lymphoma – classical Hodgkin lymphoma (cHL) and nodular lymphocyte predominant Hodgkin lymphoma (NLPHL) [1–5]. HLs usually affect lymph nodes. These lymphomas are composed of a small number of large dysplastic mononuclear and multinucleated neoplastic cells (Hodgkin, Reed-Sternberg [RS], and lymphocytic and histiocytic [L&H] cells) set in the background of benign inflammatory elements with or without abundant band-like and/or more diffuse collagen fibrosis [1].

HLs have a bimodal age distribution (two peaks at 15–34 years and after the sixth decade, respectively) [1, 2]. The majority of pediatric cases present in adolescents [2]. HLs occur with increased frequency in the settings of both immunodeficiency and autoimmune lymphoproliferative syndrome [2, 4]. An association with the Epstein-Barr virus (EBV) has been well documented in cHL [1, 2, 5].

Classical Hodgkin Lymphoma

Classical HL includes four histologic subtypes that share some morphologic and immunophenotypic features (CD15+, CD20−, CD30+, CD45−, PAX-5 weakly+, PU-1−, BOB.1, and OCT-2 usually negative) in their neoplastic cells, but differ in the growth pattern and composition of the inflammatory cell background [1, 2, 6].

Nodular Sclerosis Subtype

Nodular sclerosis (NS) cHL is the most common subtype of cHL in Western countries, accounting for about 70% of all cHL [2, 6]. Mediastinum is frequently involved. It is characterized by a nodular growth pattern associated with a patchy distribution of the neoplastic cells and the presence of associated fibrosis and/or sclerosis forming dense collagen bands (Figure 10.1) [2, 6]. There is also often marked capsular fibrosis. The lymphoma contains a variable number of RS cells and variants (lacunar cells and mummified cells) and other inflammatory cells (small lymphocytes, eosinophils, plasma cells, histiocytes, and neutrophils). EBV can be positive in some NS cases [2, 5, 6].

Mixed Cellularity Subtype

The mixed cellularity (MC) subtype accounts for about 20–25% of cHL and is frequently EBV-positive [2, 5, 6]. This subtype is characterized by a diffuse growth pattern, although an interfollicular growth pattern may be seen (Figure 10.2). Neoplastic cells are evenly distributed. The RS cells are typical in appearance with fewer lacunar cells. The background consists of a mixture of inflammatory cells similar to those seen in the NS subtype [2, 6].

Lymphocyte-Rich Subtype

The lymphocyte-rich (LR) subtype accounts for approximately 5% of all cHL and shows considerable clinical and morphologic overlap with NLPHL (Figure 10.3) [2, 6, 7]. There are two growth patterns: (1) the common nodular pattern with many of the nodules containing residual small benign germinal centers, while the neoplastic cells are found within or at the margin of the mantle zone of these follicles, and (2) the rare diffuse pattern. The predominant neoplastic cells are RS cells. The inflammatory background is composed of predominantly small B-lymphocytes with absent or rare eosinophils and granulocytes [2, 6, 8].

Lymphocyte-Depleted Subtype

The lymphocyte-depleted (LD) subtype is rare accounting for <2% of all cHL [2, 6, 7]. It is more common in developing countries, associated with immunocompromised states such as HIV infection, and typically EBV positive [4, 5]. This subtype has a

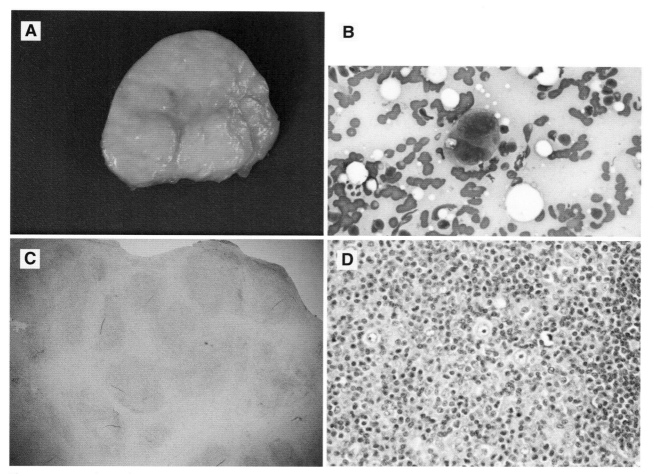

Figure 10.1 NS subtype of cHL.

a. Gross photo of cervical lymph node shows large size and prominent nodularity.

b. Touch imprint of a lymph node shows an RS cell, which is large with abundant cytoplasm, binucleated "owl-eyed" nuclei, and distinct nucleoli (Wright-Giemsa, 400x).

c. Lymph node biopsy shows dense collagen bands dividing the lymph node into nodules (H&E, 20x).

d. High magnification reveals scattered large mononucleated Hodgkin cells with prominent eosinophilic nucleolus are present in a mixed inflammatory background composed of small lymphocytes, eosinophils, and histiocytes (H&E, 400x).

e. Hodgkin cells are positive for CD15 with membrane staining pattern (CD15 immunostain, 400x).

f. Hodgkin cells are positive for CD30 with Golgi and membrane staining pattern (CD30 immunostain, 400x).

g. Hodgkin cells are negative for CD45 (CD45 immunostain, 400x).

h. Hodgkin cells are weakly positive for PAX-5 (PAX-5 immunostain, 400x).

diffuse growth pattern rich in RS cells and/or depleted of non-neoplastic lymphocytes (Figure 10.4). A sarcomatoid appearance can be seen due to large numbers of pleomorphic RS cells. Sometimes the disease shows a diffuse fibrosis with scattered RS cells and rare lymphocytes [2, 6].

No recurrent chromosomal abnormalities are identified in cHL [1, 2, 6]. Cytogenetics usually shows complex karyotype with aneuploidy and hypertetraploidy. Chromosomal copy number alterations seem to be the common finding in cHL, accounting for more than 20% of cases. Gains in 2p, 9p, 16p, 17q, 19q, and 20q as well as losses of 6q, 11q, and 13q were observed [1, 2, 6].

CHL now is essentially curable with modern polychemotherapy protocols and improvements in radiotherapy.

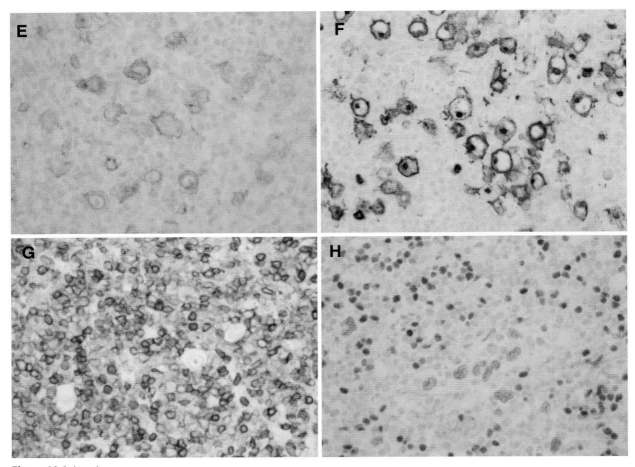

Figure 10.1 (cont.)

Prognosis depends on the tumor stage. In recent years, the CD30-directed antibody-drug conjugate brentuximab vedotin has been used for relapsed/refractory CHL [1, 2, 6, 8].

Nodular Lymphocyte Predominant Hodgkin Lymphoma

Nodular lymphocyte predominant Hodgkin lymphoma (NLPHL) represents approximately 10% of all HL [3, 7] and is characterized by a nodular or a nodular and diffuse proliferation of small lymphocytes with single scattered large neoplastic cells with popcorn appearance known as L&H cells (Figure 10.5) [3]. The neoplastic L&H cells are very large and characterized by marked nuclear lobation, a vesicular chromatin, and multiple and often peripherally located small, amphophilic nucleoli. Expanded meshworks of follicular dendritic cells (FDCs) are commonly seen in the background. The neoplastic L&H cells express CD20, CD79a, PAX-5, BOB.1, OCT-2, PU.1, and CD45, sometimes EMA, but are negative for CD15. CD30 usually is not expressed in L&H cells, but it can be positive in rare cases. Also L&H cells are ringed by PD-1+ and CD57+ T-cells [2, 3, 8, 9].

Six distinct growth patterns have been described. Pattern A is the classical, B-cell-rich nodular pattern. Pattern B is the serpiginous nodular pattern. Pattern C is nodular with prominent extranodular LP cells. Pattern D is T-cell-rich nodular. Pattern E is like T-cell/histiocyte-rich large B-cell lymphoma (THRLBCL). Pattern F is diffuse B-cell rich [3, 9].

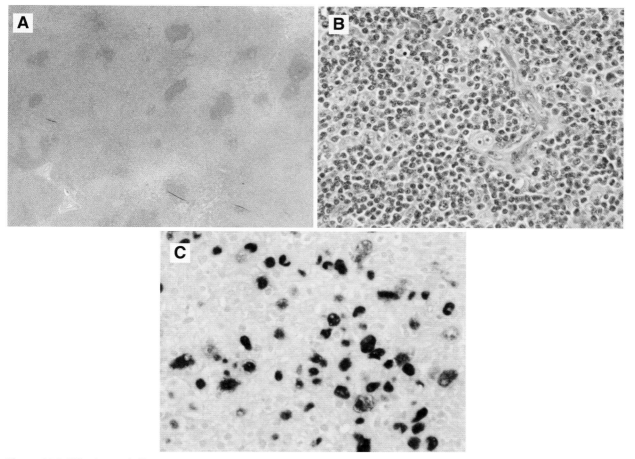

Figure 10.2 MC subtype of cHL.

a. A lymph node biopsy shows an interfollicular expansion (H&E, 20x).
b. Scattered large RS cells with binucleation and prominent eosinophilic nucleolus are present in a mixed inflammatory background composed of small lymphocytes, eosinophils, histiocytes, and plasma cells (H&E, 400x).
c. EBV signals are detected in RS cells and variants (in situ hybridization EBER, 400x).

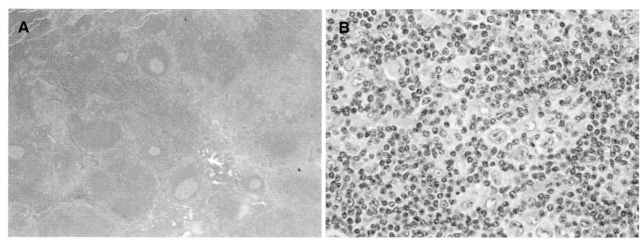

Figure 10.3 LR subtype of cHL.

a. A lymph node biopsy shows well-preserved lymph node architecture (H&E, 20x).
b. High magnification shows rare RS cells surrounded by small lymphocytes (H&E, 400x).

The main differential diagnosis is THRLBCL, as the therapeutic approach and outcome for these two lymphomas is different [2, 3, 10]. Patients with THRLBCL usually present with high-stage disease, while NLPHL tends to be localized. Morphologic features that suggest the possibility of NLPHL in an otherwise diffuse process include the presence of any nodularity, the presence of a large number of small B-cells in the background, the presence of underlying expanded and disorganized dendritic cell meshwork, and immunoglobulin D expression by neoplastic cells, which appears to be distinctive to NLPHL [2, 3, 10].

Historically, patients with NLPHL have been treated based on therapeutic approaches used for cHL. Recently, approaches have diverged on the basis of clinical observations and differences in underlying biology [2, 3].

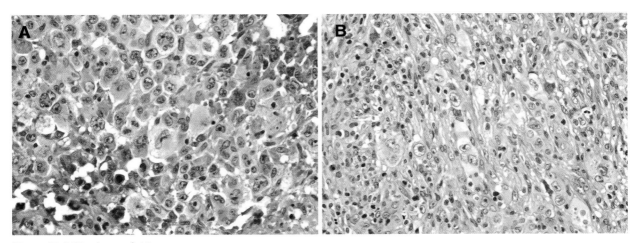

Figure 10.4 LD subtype of cHL.
a. A lymph node biopsy shows sheets of Hodgkin cells with relatively few admixed small lymphocytes visible (H&E, 400x).
b. Hodgkin cells and mummified cells are seen in a prominent fibrillary matrix with fibroblastic proliferation (H&E, 400x).

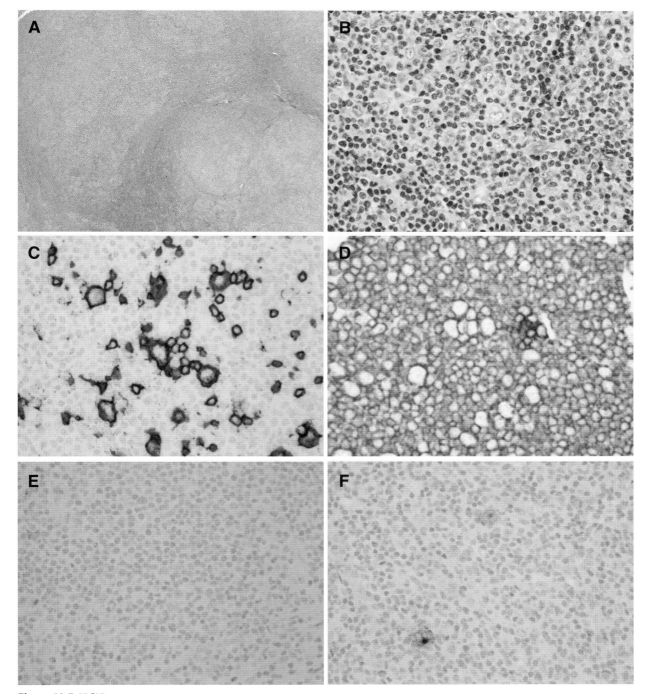

Figure 10.5 NLPHL.

a. A lymph node biopsy shows a delicate nodule growth pattern (H&E, 20x).
b. Rare popcorn cells with lobulated nuclei and small nucleolus are visible in a background of small lymphocytes (H&E, 400x).
c. Popcorn cells are positive for CD20 (CD20 immunostain, 400x).
d. Popcorn cells are positive for CD45 (CD45 immunostain, 400x).
e. Popcorn cells are negative for CD30 (CD30 immunostain, 400x).
f. Popcorn cells are positive for EMA (EMA immunostain, 400x).
g. Popcorn cells are positive for BOB.1 (BOB.1 immunostain, 400x).
h. Popcorn cells are positive for OCT-2 (OCT-2 immunostain, 400x).
i. Popcorn cells are weakly positive for PU.1 (PU.1 immunostain, 400x).
j. CD57-positive cells surround popcorn cells, forming a rosette (CD57 immunostain, 400x).
k. PD-1-positive cells surround popcorn cells, forming a rosette (PD-1 immunostain, 400x).

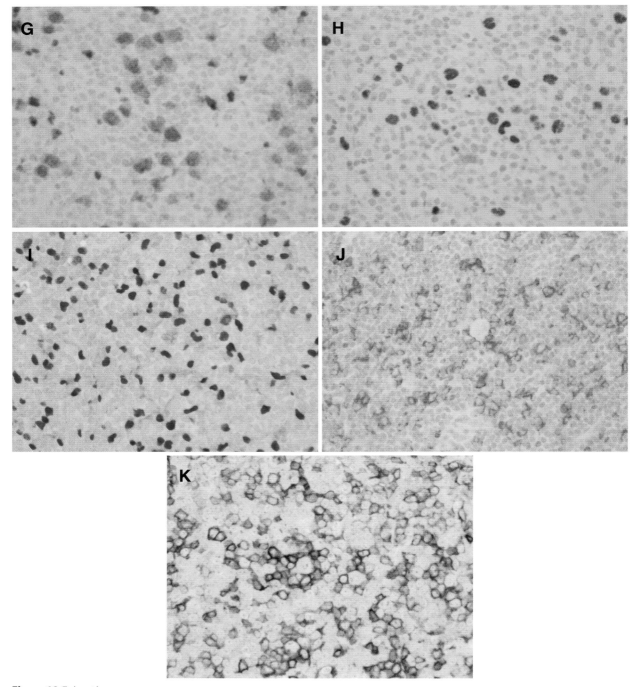

Figure 10.5 (cont.)

References

1. Stein H, Pileri SA, Weiss LM, Poppema S, Gascoyne RD, Jaffe ES. Hodgkin lymphomas. In Swerdlow SH, Campo E, Harris NL, et al., eds. WHO classification of tumours of haematopoietic and lymphoid tissue. Revised 4th ed. Lyon: IARC Press; 2017:424–30.

2. Mihaela O. Hodgkin lymphomas. In Proytcheva MA, ed. Diagnostic pediatric hematopathology. Cambridge: Cambridge University Press; 2011:465–83.

3. Stein H, Swerdlow SH, Gascoyne RD, Popperma S, Jaffe ES, Pileri SA. Nodular lymphocyte predominant Hodgkin lymphoma. In Swerdlow SH, Campo E, Harris NL, et al., eds. WHO classification of tumours of haematopoietic and lymphoid tissue. Revised 4th ed. Lyon: IARC Press; 2017:431–4.

4. Shiels MS, Koritzinsky EH, Clarke CA, Suneja G, Morton LM, Engels EA. Prevalence of HIV infection among US Hodgkin lymphoma cases. Cancer Epidemiol Prev Biomark. 2014 Feb 1; 23(2): 274–81.

5. Zhou XG, Sandvej K, Li PJ, Ji XL, Yan QH, Zhang XP, et al. Epstein-Barr virus (EBV) in Chinese pediatric Hodgkin disease: Hodgkin disease in young children is an EBV-related lymphoma. Cancer. 2001 Sep 15; 92(6): 1621–31.

6. Stein H, Piler SA, MacLennan KA, Poppema S, Guenova M, Gascoyne RD, Jaffe E. Classical Hodgkin lymphoma. In Swerdlow SH, Campo E, Harris NL, et al., eds. WHO classification of tumours of haematopoietic and lymphoid tissue. Revised 4th ed. Lyon: IARC Press; 2017:435–42.

7. Morton LM, Wang SS, Devesa SS, Hartge P, Weisenburger DD, Linet MS. Lymphoma incidence patterns by WHO subtype in the United States, 1992–2001. Blood. 2006 Jan 1; 107(1): 265–76.

8. Shimabukuro-Vornhagen A, Haverkamp H, Engert A, Balleisen L, Majunke P, Heil G, et al. Lymphocyte-rich classical Hodgkin's lymphoma: Clinical presentation and treatment outcome in 100 patients treated within German Hodgkin's study group trials. J Clin Oncol. 2005 Aug 20; 23(24): 5739–45.

9. Fan Z, Natkunam Y, Bair E, Tibshirani R, Warnke RA. Characterization of variant patterns of nodular lymphocyte predominant Hodgkin lymphoma with immunohistologic and clinical correlation. Am J Surg Pathol. 2003 Oct 1; 27(10): 1346–56.

10. Franke S, Wlodarska I, Maes B, Vandenberghe P, Achten R, Hagemeijer A, De Wolf-Peeters C. Comparative genomic hybridization pattern distinguishes T-cell/histiocyte-rich B-cell lymphoma from nodular lymphocyte predominance Hodgkin's lymphoma. Am J Pathol. 2002 Nov 1; 161(5): 1861–7.

Posttransplant Lymphoproliferative Disorder

Xiayuan Liang

Posttransplant lymphoproliferative disorders (PTLDs) comprise a heterogeneous category of lymphoid and plasmacytic proliferations occurring as a result of immunosuppression following solid organ or hematopoietic stem cell transplant [1–5]. PTLDs constitute a spectrum ranging from Epstein-Barr virus (EBV)-driven polyclonal proliferations to monoclonal EBV-positive or EBV-negative proliferations indistinguishable from a subset of B-cell lymphomas, T/natural killer (NK)-cell (less often) lymphomas, or classical Hodgkin lymphoma (cHL) (less often) that occur in immunocompetent individuals [1].

PTLDs occur more frequently in children than adults because children are more often EBV-seronegative at the time of transplantation [1, 2]. Most PTLDs are associated with EBV infection. EBV-negative PTLDs are rare, tend to occur later after transplantation, and are more likely than EBV-positive cases to be monomorphic [1].

PTLDs can occur at almost any site in the body. The histopathology of PTLD is heterogeneous and complex. The 2016 WHO classification defined four categories of PTLDs as described next [1].

Non-destructive Posttransplant Lymphoproliferative Disorders

Non-destructive PTLDs are defined as lymphoid and plasmacytic proliferations in an allograft recipient characterized by preserved architecture of the involved tissue and an absence of features that would be diagnostic of a malignant lymphoma. There are three subtypes – (1) florid follicular hyperplasia, (2) plasmacytic hyperplasia (PH), and (3) infectious mononucleosis (IM) PTLDs [1, 6].

Non-destructive PTLDs are more commonly seen in children, often without a prior EBV infection. They frequently involve Waldeyer ring or lymph nodes. They can regress spontaneously with reduction of immunosuppression or may be successfully treated by surgical excision. However, IM PTLD can be fatal [1].

Morphologically, PH and florid follicular hyperplasia PTLDs (Figure 11.1) are nonspecific. The diagnosis requires the formation of a mass lesion and/or significant EBV positivity. PH is characterized by essentially preserved lymphoid architecture with numerous plasma cells, small lymphocytes, and occasional band-appearing immunoblasts in interfollicular areas. IM PTLD is indistinguishable from typical IM with interfollicular expansion and numerous immunoblasts in a background of T-cells and plasma cells (Figure 11.2). Necrosis can be present. Florid follicular hyperplasia PTLD is a mass lesion with marked follicular hyperplasia that shows different sizes and shapes without evidence suggesting IM. Genetically, non-destructive PTLDs are usually polyclonal [1, 6].

Polymorphic Posttransplant Lymphoproliferative Disorder

Polymorphic posttransplant lymphoproliferative disorder (P-PTLD) is the most common type of PTLD in children [1, 2]. The disease frequently follows primary EBV infection. P-PTLD shows effacement of the architecture of lymph nodes or forms a destructive extranodal mass lesion (Figure 11.3). P-PTLD is histologically heterogeneous lesions composed of small and intermediate-sized lymphocytes, plasma cells, and immunoblasts that do not meet the criteria for any type of lymphomas described in immunocompetent individuals. There may be areas of necrosis or the presence of mitosis.

Immunophenotypically, there is a mixture of B-cells and T-cells, which are usually numerous. CD30 expression is common. EBV infection signals are pronounced [2, 4]. Demonstration of B-cell light chain class restriction is expected in P-PTLDs, although it can be absent in some cases. Reduction in immunosuppression leads to lesion regression in some cases; others may progress and require lymphoma-type therapy [1].

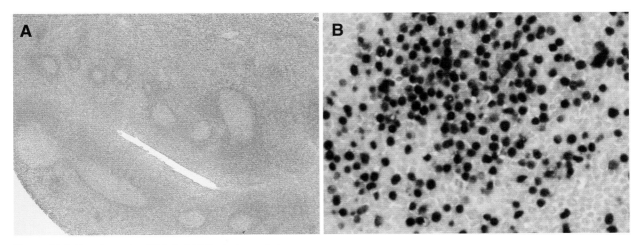

Figure 11.1 Non-destructive PTLD, florid follicular hyperplasia.
a. A tonsil biopsy from an 18-year-old cardiac allograft recipient showed hyperplastic lymphoid follicles with varied sizes and shapes (H&E, 40x).
b. Chromogenic in situ hybridization study showed EBV-encoded small RNA (EBER) expression (in situ hybridization EBER, 400x).

Monomorphic Posttransplant Lymphoproliferative Disorder

Monomorphic posttransplant lymphoproliferative disorder (M-PTLD) fulfills the criteria for one of the B-cell or T/NK-cell neoplasms that are recognized in immunocompetent individuals except for small B-cell lymphoid neoplasms such as follicular lymphoma [1]. The monomorphic B-cell PTLD in children is primarily manifested as a diffuse large B-cell lymphoma (Figure 11.4) or a Burkitt lymphoma (Figure 11.5) (DLBCL > BL) after transplantation [1]. PTLD-related plasma cell neoplasms are extremely rare in pediatric patients [7]. It is important to recognize that B-cell M-PTLDs may not be entirely monotonous proliferations of one cell type because there may be some degree of pleomorphism including the transformed cells, plasmacytic differentiation, and Reed-Sternberg-like cells. Necrosis may be present [1]. EBV infection is detected in the majority of cases. EBV-negative B-cell M-PTLDs are rare and tend to occur later after transplantation [1, 3]. The neoplastic cells express B-cell-associated antigens (CD19, CD20, CD79a, and PAX-5). Both CD10 and BCL-6 are often positive in pediatric cases. Immunoglobulin light chain restriction and clonal *IG* gene rearrangement are observed in almost all cases. BL types of M-PTLDs have *MYC-IG* gene rearrangement. Genetic aberrations

in DLBCL type of M-PTLDs are variable, usually showing complex karyotypes [1].

Monomorphic T/NK-cell PTLDs are uncommon. Most cases present at extranodal sites, sometimes with associated lymphadenopathy. T/NK-PTLDs share features with T/NK-cell lymphomas in immunocompetent individuals. The neoplastic cells express pan-T-cell and sometimes NK-associated antigens. Depending on the tumor type, CD4 or CD8, CD30, ALK-1, and either αβ or γδ T-cell receptors (TCR) may be expressed. EBV positivity is seen in one third of cases. Cases derived from T-cells show clonal *TCR* gene rearrangement [1].

Classical Hodgkin Lymphoma Posttransplant Lymphoproliferative Disorder

Classical **Hodgkin lymphoma** posttransplant **lymphoproliferative** disorder (cHL **PTLD**) is the least common form of PTLD and is almost always EBV-associated (Figure 11.6) [1, 8]. These lesions are frequently mixed cellularity subtype. Since Reed-Sternberg-like cells may be seen in other types of PTLDs, the diagnostic criteria for cHL must be fulfilled based on morphological and immunophenotypical features, including expressions of both CD15 and CD30. CHL PTLD is more likely to express B-cell associated antigens than cHL is in immunocompetent individuals [1, 8].

99

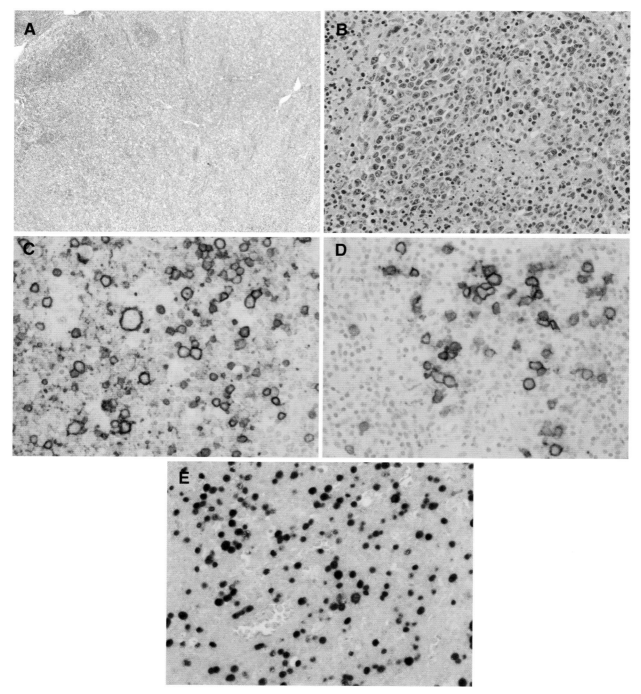

Figure 11.2 Non-destructive PTLD, infectious mononucleosis.

a. A tonsil biopsy from a 14-year-old liver allograft recipient showed marked interfollicular expansion (H&E, 40x).
b. High magnification showed increased large transformed cells and focal necrosis (H&E, 40x).
c. Large transformed cells showed CD20 reactivity (CD20 immunostain, 400x).
d. A number of plasma cells were present in the lesion and showed CD138 positivity (CD138 immunostain, 400x).
e. Chromogenic in situ hybridization for EBV (EBER) showed numerous positive cells (EBER in situ hybridization, 400x).

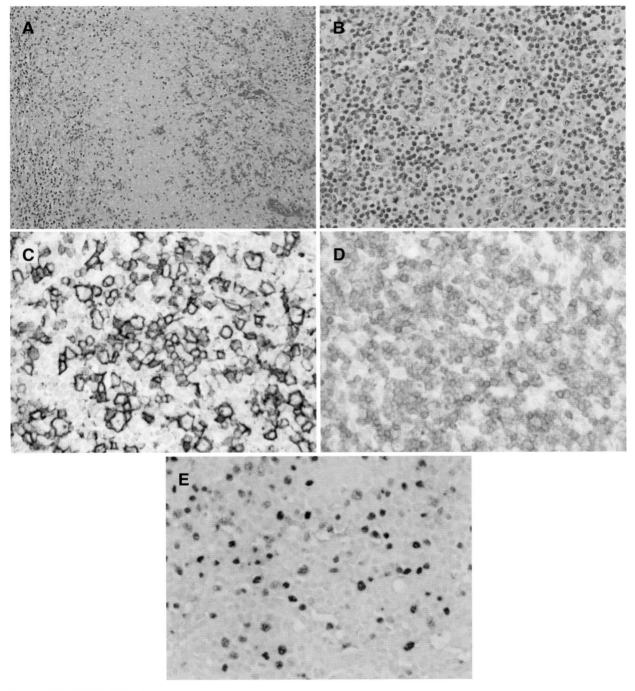

Figure 11.3 P-PTLD, EBV positive.

a. A lymph node biopsy from a 17-year-old renal allograft recipient showed focal necrosis (H&E, 200x).

b. The lesion showed variably sized and shaped lymphoid cells with increased large transformed cells and rare mitotic figures (H&E, 400x).

c. CD20 highlighted the variably sized and shaped B-cells (CD20 immunostain, 400x).

d. CD3 highlighted the T-cells. Most are small in size (CD3 immunostain, 400x).

e. In situ hybridization for EBV (EBER) showed numerous positive cells (EBER in situ hybridization, 400x).

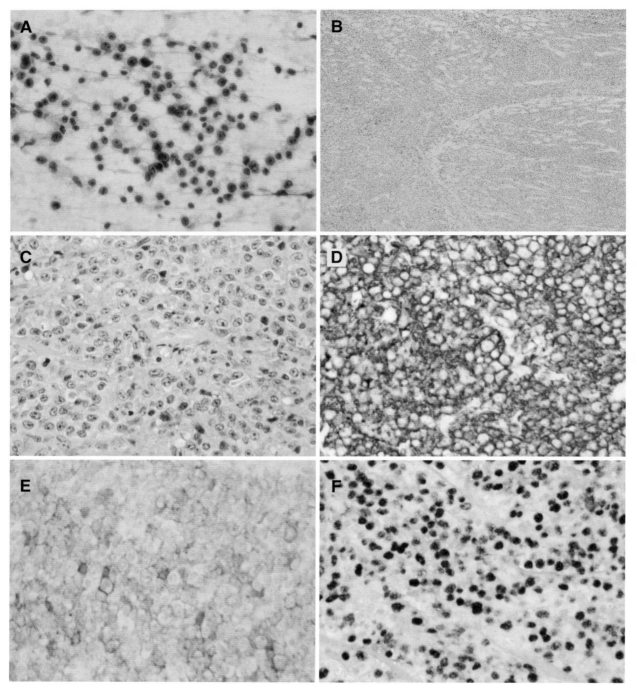

Figure 11.4 M-PTLD, DLBCL, EBV-positive.

a. A 6-year-old female had received a heart transplantation at the age of 3 years. She developed a soft tissue mass in her chest. The touch imprint from the lesion showed a population of discohesive large atypical lymphoid cells with round to oval nuclei, open chromatin, distinct nucleoli, and a moderate amount of cytoplasm (H&E, 400x).

b. Low magnification showed diffuse lymphoid infiltrate (H&E, 40x).

c. High-power view showed monomorphic large neoplastic lymphoid cells with oval to irregular nuclei, vesicular chromatin, distinct nucleoli, and moderate to abundant gray cytoplasm (H&E, 400x).

d. The majority of these cells were positive for CD20 (CD20 immunostain, 400x).

e. A number of large neoplastic cells showed weak and heterogeneous CD30 reactivity (CD30 immunostain, 400x).

f. The large neoplastic lymphoid cells were EBER-positive (EBER in situ hybridization, 400x).

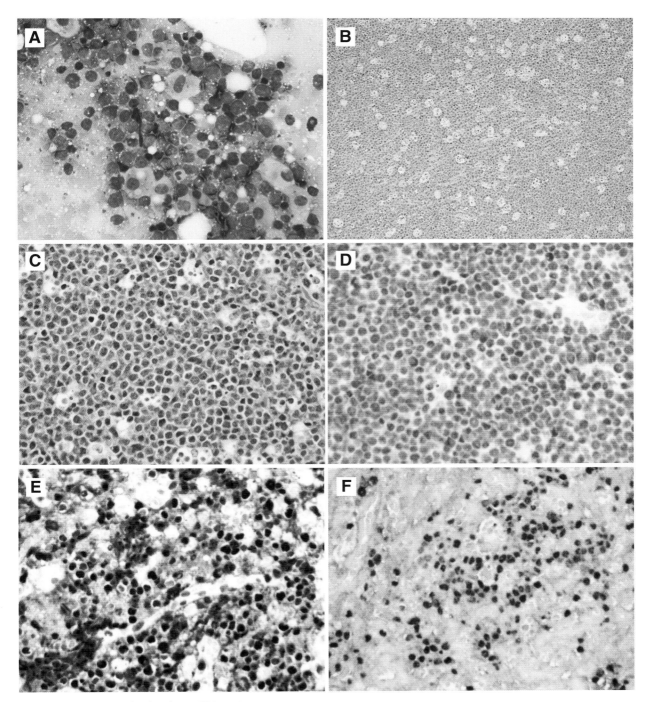

Figure 11.5 M-PTLD, Burkitt lymphoma, EBV-positive.

a. A 10-year-old male received a liver transplantation at age of 3 years. Now he has developed intra-abdominal lymphadenopathy. The touch imprint from a lymph node biopsy showed a population of discohesive monomorphic medium-sized atypical lymphoid cells with deep blue cytoplasm and cytoplasmic vacuoles (Wright-Giemsa, 400x).

b. The lesion showed a diffuse infiltration by intermediate-sized lymphoid cells with a prominent "starry sky" pattern (H&E, 40x).

c. High-power depiction demonstrated relative uniformity of the medium-sized neoplastic lymphoid cells with a modest amount of cytoplasm and inconspicuous nucleoli. Admixed were a number of macrophages ingesting the necrotic cell debris, rendering the "starry sky" pattern (H&E, 400x).

d. The neoplastic cells were positive for PAX-5 (PAX-5 immunostain, 400x).

e. MIB-1 illustrated 100% mitotic activity (MIB-1 immunostain, 400x).

f. The neoplastic lymphoid cells were EBV-positive (EBER in situ hybridization, 400x).

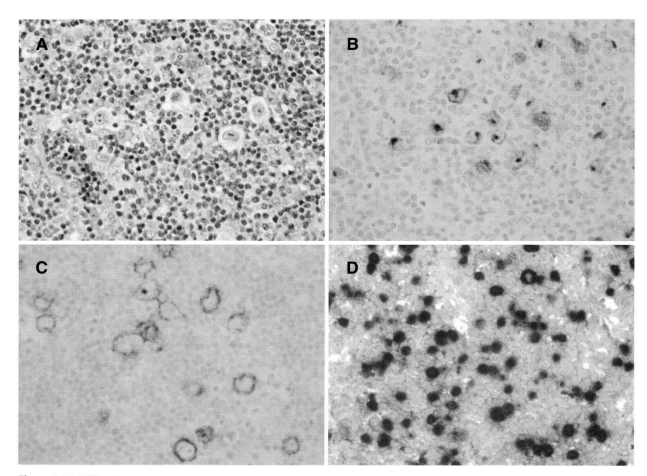

Figure 11.6 PTLD, cHL.

a. A 16-year-old male presented with a mediastinal mass 7 years post liver transplant. A biopsy showed Reed-Sternberg and Hodgkin cells present in a background of mixed inflammatory cells (H&E, 400x).
b. The neoplastic cells were CD15-positive (CD15 immunostain, 400x).
c. The neoplastic cells were CD30-positive (CD30 immunostain, 400x).
d. Both neoplastic cells and reactive lymphocytes were EBER-positive (EBER in situ hybridization, 400x).

References

1. Swerdlow SH, Webber SA, Chadburn A, Ferry LA. Post-transplant lymphoproliferative disorders. In Swerdlow SH, Campo E, Harris NL, et al., eds. WHO classification of tumours of haematopoietic and lymphoid tissue. Revised 4th ed. Lyon: IARC Press; 2017:453–62.

2. Abed N, Casper JT, Camitta BM, Margolis D, Trost B, Orentas R, Chang CC. Evaluation of histogenesis of B-lymphocytes in pediatric EBV-related post-transplant lymphoproliferative disorders. Bone Marrow Transplant. 2004 Feb; **33**(3): 321–7.

3. Nelson BP, Nalesnik MA, Bahler DW, Locker J, Fung JJ, Swerdlow SH. Epstein-Barr virus-negative post-transplant lymphoproliferative disorders: A distinct entity? Am J Surg Pathol. 2000 Mar 1; **24**(3): 375–85.

4. Liu L, Zhang X, Feng S. Epstein-Barr virus-related post-transplantation lymphoproliferative disorders after allogeneic hematopoietic stem cell transplantation. Biol Blood Marrow Transplant. 2018 Jul; **24**(7): 1341–9.

5. Romero S, Montoro J, Guinot M, Almenar L, Andreu R, Balaguer A, et al. Post-transplant lymphoproliferative

disorders after solid organ and hematopoietic stem cell transplantation. Leukemia Lymphoma. 2019 Jan 2; **60**(1): 142–50.

6. Vakiani E, Nandula SV, Subramaniyam S, Keller CE, Alobeid B, Murty VV, Bhagat G. Cytogenetic analysis of B-cell posttransplant lymphoproliferations validates the World Health Organization classification and suggests inclusion of florid follicular hyperplasia as a precursor lesion. Hum Pathol. 2007 Feb 1; **38**(2): 315–25.

7. Epperly R, Ozolek J, Soltys K, Cohen D, Goyal R, Friehling E. Treatment of pediatric plasma cell myeloma type post-transplant lymphoproliferative disorder with modern risk-directed therapy. Pediatr Blood Cancer. 2018 Oct; **65**(10): e27283.

8. Adams H, Campidelli C, Dirnhofer S, Pileri SA, Tzankov A. Clinical, phenotypic and genetic similarities and disparities between post-transplant and classical Hodgkin lymphomas with respect to therapeutic targets. Expert Opin Ther Targets. 2009 Oct 1; **13**(10): 1137–45.

12 Immunodeficiency-Associated Lymphoproliferative Disorders

Michele E. Paessler, Brian Lockhart, Soma Jyonouchi

Immunodeficiency-associated lymphoproliferative disorders (IA-LPDs) encompass a heterogeneous group of disorders that stem from diverse clinical settings and underlying disorders. These disorders may be benign lymphoproliferations to aggressive lymphomas. The World Health Organization (WHO) broadly classifies IA-LPDs into four groups: posttransplant lymphoproliferative disorders (PTLDs), lymphomas associated with HIV, lymphoproliferations associated with primary immune disorders, and other iatrogenic lymphoproliferative disorders. This chapter focuses on IA-LPDs of primary immune deficiencies seen commonly in the pediatric population, HIV-associated lymphoma, and iatrogenic lymphoproliferations.

Lymphoproliferations Associated with Primary Immunodeficiency Disorders

Primary immunodeficiencies are inherited disorders of immune system function that predispose one to an increased rate of infection, immune dysregulation with autoimmune disease and aberrant inflammatory responses, and malignancy [1]. In 1952, Dr. Ogden Bruton described the first case of primary immunodeficiency in a young boy who had recurrent invasive infections and complete absence of gamma globulin in the body (Bruton's agammaglobulinemia). Today, primary immunodeficiency disorders (PIDDs) are a diverse and expanding group of inborn errors of the immune system currently encompassing more than 450 diseases. These disorders are distinct from secondary immunodeficiency states such as HIV infection, or medication-related immune suppression such as chemotherapy or immune suppressants.

The immune system is designed to identify and destroy invading pathogens in order to ensure survival of the host. As a result, patients with PIDDs commonly present with recurrent severe infections often requiring hospitalization and IV antimicrobial therapy. Patients can have infections with unusual pathogens that do not

typically cause infections in immunocompetent hosts, such as *Pneumocystis jiroveci*, *Burkholderia cepacia*, *Serratia marcenscens*, and so forth.

In addition to fighting infections, the immune system must also demonstrate tolerance to the host and prevent excessive immune activation that can cause host damage. Indeed, many PIDDs are associated with early-onset autoimmune disease or inflammatory disease manifestations such as granuloma formation or hemophagocytic lymphohistiocytosis. In this chapter, we review several clinical manifestations and the pathology of PIDDs.

Syndromes of Immune Deficiency

Ataxia Telangiectasia

Ataxia telangiectasia (AT) is an autosomal recessive genomic instability syndrome characterized by neurodegeneration, combined immunodeficiency, dermatologic manifestations such as oculocutaneous telangiectasia and skin granulomas, and predisposition to lymphoid malignancies. AT is due to mutations in the Ataxia-telangiectasia mutated (*ATM*) gene, localized to 11q22.3–23.1, which encodes a protein kinase involved in cell-cycle homeostasis and the cellular response to DNA double-strand breaks and oxidative stress. AT can present as the classic form or with the hyper-IgM type, which reflects a class switch recombination defect. The hyper-IgM type occurs in approximately 10% of AT patients; laboratory studies show low IgG and IgA with high IgM levels similar to hyper-IgM syndrome. A hallmark of AT with the hyper-IgM phenotype is liver disease that manifests as nonalcoholic hepatic steatosis, fibrosis, and granulomatous disease [2]. A subset of patients with AT can develop severe noninfectious cutaneous granulomas that can progress to ulcerating plaques [3] (Figures 12.1–12.4).

Nijmegen Breakage Syndrome

Nijmegen breakage syndrome (NBS) is a rare disease of chromosome instability. It is an autosomal recessive syndrome caused by mutations in the *NBN* gene, which leads to

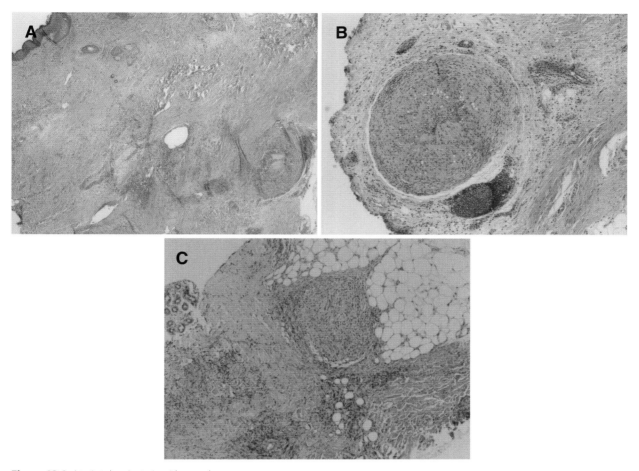

Figure 12.1 Ataxia telangiectasia with granulomas.
A previously healthy 14-month-old boy starts having difficulty with balance and falling. He is diagnosed with cerebral palsy. Starting at 3 years of age, he is treated for "recurrent pink eye" and has skin nodules. He continues to have progressive balance difficulty. He is seen by a neurologist for a second opinion and laboratory testing reveals markedly elevated alpha fetoprotein levels. Genetic testing reveals a diagnosis of ataxia telangiectasia. A skin biopsy is performed on one of the nodules. The epidermis is unremarkable (A, H&E, 2.5x). The dermis and subcutaneous tissue show noncaseating granulomas (B&C, H&E, 5x). Special stains for organisms are negative (not shown).

truncated fragments of the gene product nibrin, which is involved in repairing double-strand DNA breaks. NBS is characterized by microcephaly, dysmorphic facies, short stature, radiation sensitivity, recurrent infections, and a predisposition to lymphoid malignancies (Figures 12.5 and 12.6).

DiGeorge Syndrome, 22q11.2 Deletion Syndrome

DiGeorge syndrome, or 22q11.2 deletion syndrome, is caused by a heterozygous deletion at chromosome 22q11.2. Patients can have a broad range of clinical manifestations including congenital heart disease, palatal abnormalities, immunodeficiency, autoimmune disease, and characteristic facies. Most patients have an immunodeficiency and frequent infections due to impaired T-cell development as a result of thymic hypoplasia/absence (Figure 12.7).

Combined Immunodeficiencies

Hyper-IgM Syndrome

Hyper-IgM syndrome is a rare primary immunodeficiency disorder characterized by low or absent levels of serum IgG, IgA, and IgE and normal or increased levels of serum IgM. Defective interactions of CD40:-CD40 between CD4+ T-cells and antigen presenting cells is the

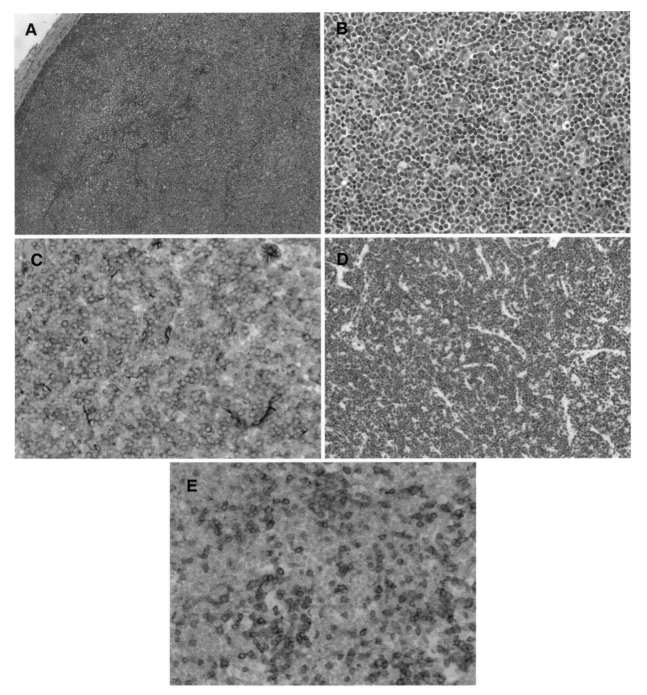

Figure 12.2 Ataxia telangiectasia with T lymphoblastic lymphoma.

An 8-year-old boy with AT has an enlarged cervical lymph node. A biopsy is performed and shows effacement of the normal nodal architecture by a diffuse mononuclear cell infiltrate (A, H&E, 5x). The cells are intermediate in size with scant cytoplasm and round to slightly irregular nuclei and fine chromatin, consistent with blasts (B, H&E, 20X). Immunohistochemistry shows the cells are positive for CD34 (C, CD34, 20x), TdT (D, TdT, 10x), and CD3 (E, CD3, 20x), confirming a diagnosis of T lymphoblastic lymphoma.

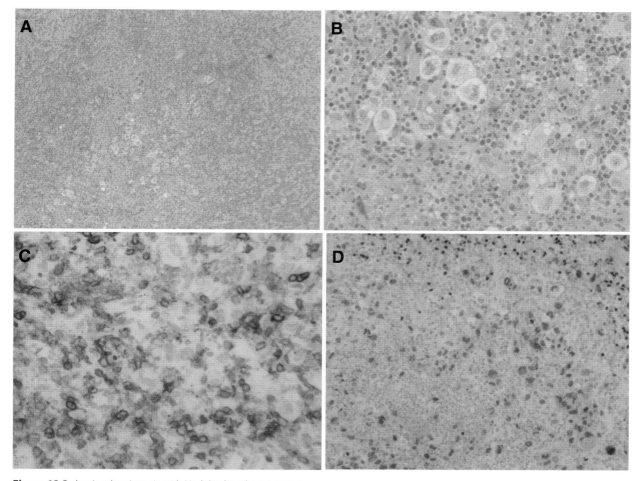

Figure 12.3 Ataxia telangiectasia with Hodgkin lymphoma, EBER+.

A 13-year-old girl with AT has a mediastinal mass and supraclavicular lymphadenopathy. A biopsy of the lymph node shows effacement of the normal nodal architecture by vague nodules (A, H&E, 5x). The nodules are composed of Reed-Sternberg (RS) cells in a mixed inflammatory background of lymphocytes, histiocytes, neutrophils, and eosinophils (B, H&E, 20x). IHC demonstrates the RS cells are negative for CD45 (C, CD45, 20x), while they are dim positive for PAX5 (D, PAX5, 5x), CD30 (E, CD30, 5x), CD15 (F, CD15, 20x), and EBER (G, in situ EBER, 20x).

underlying cause of hyper-IgM syndrome. Various mutations have been reported including both X-linked and autosomal dominant/recessive mutations. Patients present with recurrent infections and a variety of other clinical manifestations including autoimmune and hematologic abnormalities (particularly neutropenia), lymphoproliferation, and malignancies [4] (Figure 12.8).

Severe Combined Immunodeficiency

Severe combined immunodeficiency (SCID) is a life-threatening heterogeneous group of rare, inherited immunodeficiencies with profound defects in the immune system that lead to absence or dysfunction of T- and B-cells; thus, it affects both cellular and humoral immunity. SCID manifests in the first six months of life and, if untreated, is fatal in the first year. Patients usually present with opportunistic infections caused by bacteria and fungi. There are four main categories of SCID based on the presence of T, B, and NK cells and numerous genetic mutations that cause SCID. Hematopoietic stem cell transplant is the only cure for SCID [5] (Figure 12.9).

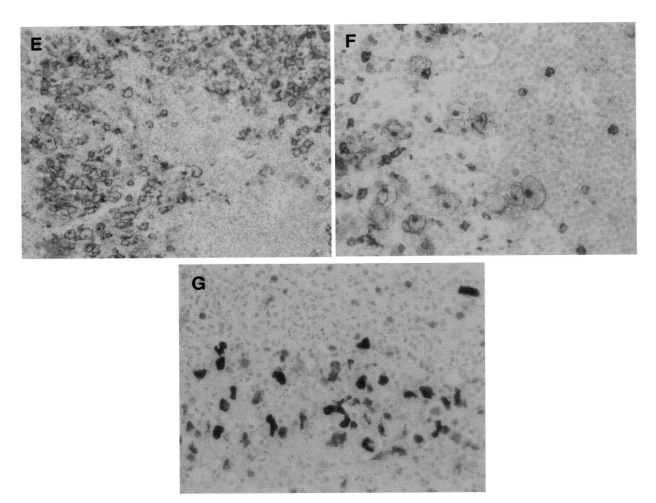

Figure 12.3 (cont.)

Antibody Deficiencies

Common Variable Immunodeficiency

Common variable immunodeficiency (CVID) is a heterogeneous group of primary antibody deficiencies and autoimmune disorders that is associated with recurrent infections and low antibody levels, poor vaccine titers, and low-isotype switched B-cells. Patients present with recurrent sinopulmonary infections, pneumonias, and chronic lung disease [6]. The underlying mechanisms are not fully understood, and a genetic cause is only found in about 20% of cases. Most individuals present with CVID in their 20s, but children and adolescents can be affected. CVID is associated with autoimmune manifestations; up to 20% of patients experience autoimmune cytopenias, enteropathy, lymphadenopathy, and malignancies [7] (Figures 12.10 and 12.11).

Defects of Phagocytes

Chronic Granulomatous Disease

Chronic granulomatous disease (CGD) is caused by defects in any of the five subunits of the NADPH oxidase complex responsible for the respiratory burst in neutrophils. Patients with neutrophil defects can present with severe catalase-positive bacterial and fungal infections of the skin or with lymph node, respiratory tract, and inflammatory

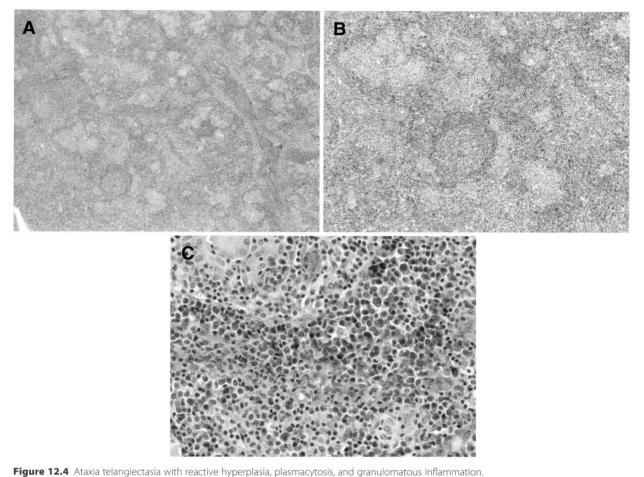

Figure 12.4 Ataxia telangiectasia with reactive hyperplasia, plasmacytosis, and granulomatous inflammation.

A 12-year-old girl with a history of AT has an enlarged mediastinal lymph node. Immune testing reveals low IgG (110), IgA (<5) but elevated IgM (300). A biopsy is performed and shows reactive lymphoid hyperplasia and granulomatous inflammation (A, H&E, 2.5x), germinal centers and non-necrotizing granulomas composed of epithelioid cells (B, H&E, 5x), and interfollicular plasmacytosis (C, H&E, 20x). Granulomatous disease is more likely to develop in AT with the hyper-IgM phenotype [16].

complications such as CGD colitis. Inflammatory complications are a significant contributor to morbidity in CGD and can be refractory to standard therapies. Hematopoietic stem cell transplantation (HSCT) is the only curative treatment [8] (Figures 12.12 and 12.13).

Severe Congenital Neutropenia

Severe congenital neutropenia (SCN) is a rare hematological disease characterized by decreased to absent circulating neutrophils. SCN is genetically heterogeneous with most cases arising sporadically. Autosomal dominant mutations are associated with heterozygous mutations in the gene for neutrophil elastase (ELA2) [9]. Clinically, patients present with mouth ulcers, gingivitis, and infections of the skin, the respiratory tract, and the gastrointestinal tract. The bone marrow shows a maturation arrest in the myeloid series at the promyelocyte stage of development. Patients are treated with G-CSF and may acquire somatic granulocyte colony stimulating factor receptor (G-CSF-R) mutations as severe congenital neutropenia progresses to myelodysplasia and acute myeloid leukemia [10] (Figure 12.14).

Disorders of Immune Dysregulation

The disorders of immune dysregulation include hemophagocytic syndromes, syndromes with autoimmunity and hypersensitivity, and lymphoproliferation.

111

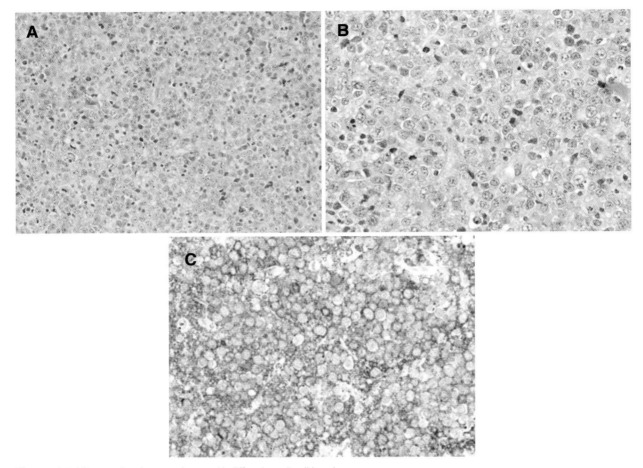

Figure 12.5 Nijmegen breakage syndrome with diffuse large B-cell lymphoma.

A 9-year-old girl with a known history of NBS, with developmental delay, short stature, dysmorphic facies, immunodeficiency, radiation sensitivity, failure to thrive, and chronic pulmonary disease, presents with left neck swelling. An MRI identifies multiple soft tissue masses involving the left posterior neck, retropharyngeal, and nasopharyngeal tissues. A left neck incisional biopsy is performed and shows soft tissue diffusely infiltrated by a hematopoietic neoplasm comprised of intermediate- to large-sized cells with round, slightly irregular nuclear contours, vesicular chromatin, and one or more prominent nucleoli. The cells have a moderate amount of bubbly, eosinophilic cytoplasm. Mitotic figures and apoptotic cells are easily identified. Scattered background small lymphocytes are appreciated (A, H&E, 20x) (B, H&E, 40x). IHC shows that the neoplastic cells are CD20-positive B-cells (C, CD20, 40x) (case courtesy of Dr. Karen Chisholm).

Hemophagocytic Lymphohistiocytosis

Hemophagocytic lymphohistiocytosis (HLH) is a severe systemic inflammatory syndrome that can be fatal. It often has an acute fulminant presentation triggered by infections [1]. HLH is caused by an overactive, uncontrolled hyperinflammatory response of the immune system. HLH can be secondary to infection or autoimmune/inflammatory disorders and is referred to as secondary HLH; it can affect individuals of any age. Familial forms of HLH are due to genetic defects in natural killer cells and cytotoxic T-cells [11]. Patients typically present in the first few months to years of life. There are five subtypes of inherited HLH. Each subtype is caused by a different gene, including PRF1, UNC13Dm STX11, and STXBP2. Patients with primary HLH require chemotherapy and hematopoietic stem cell transplant (Figure 12.15).

X-linked Lymphoproliferative Syndrome

X-linked lymphoproliferative syndrome (XLP) is a rare primary immunodeficiency characterized by a defective immune system that is hyperresponsive to infections with the Epstein-Barr virus (EBV). It can be divided into two

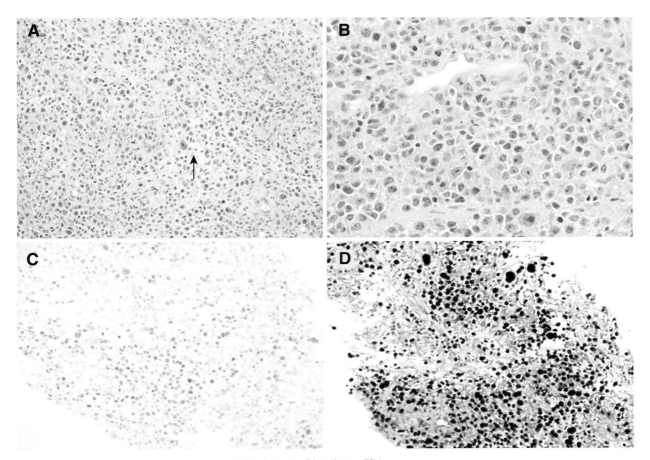

Figure 12.6 Nijmegen breakage syndrome with diffuse large B cell lymphoma, EBV+.

An 18-year-old young man with a history of microcephaly, horseshoe kidney, chronic sinusitis, mild mental retardation, and T-cell acute lymphoblastic leukemia (at age 13) is tested and found to have Nijmegen breakage syndrome after he was diagnosed with hypogammaglobulinemia. He has a paraspinal mass, which is biopsied. Histologic sections reveal fibrous tissue involved by an abnormal hematopoietic proliferation. Much of the proliferation is necrotic but, where viable, there is a mixture of noncohesive cells of varying size. Most of the cells are medium- to large-sized with prominent nucleoli. Some of the cells are multinucleated and simulate Hodgkin cells (arrow) (A, H&E, 20x). Others appear more immunoblastic in size and features with prominent nucleoli (B, H&E, 40x). Additionally, these cells are PAX5-positive B-cells (C, PAX5, 20x) and EBER positive (D, in situ EBER, 20x) (case courtesy of Dr. Karen Chisholm).

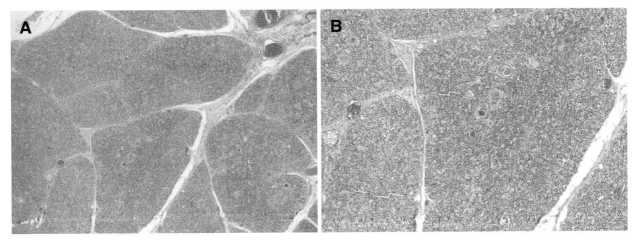

Figure 12.7 DiGeorge syndrome.

A 27-day-old baby with multiple cardiac anomalies undergoes a cardiac procedure and a hypoplastic thymus is removed. Low power shows severe hypoplasia of the thymus and a marked reduction in size and weight (0.9 g). Low-power views show normal thymic architecture and lobulation (A, H&E, 2.5x). High power shows the presence of Hassle's corpuscles (B, H&E, 20x).

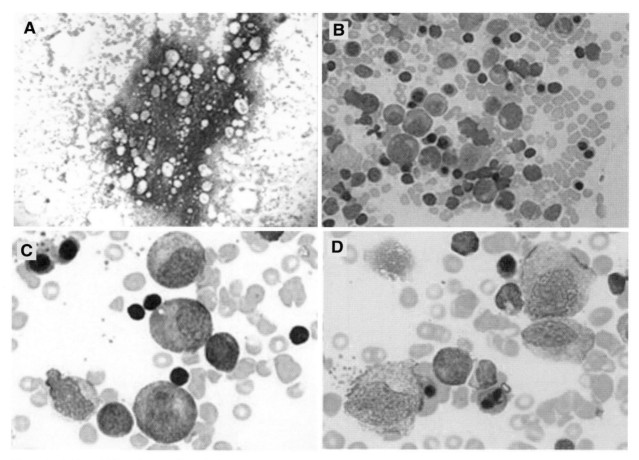

Figure 12.8 Hyper-IgM syndrome with myeloid maturation arrest.

A 9-month-old boy presents to the ER with a fever and neutropenia. He has a history of pneumocystis pneumonia, recurrent bacterial pneumonia, sinus infections, and intermittent neutropenia (lowest ANC 90). A bone marrow aspiration is performed to rule out leukemia. The marrow shows a left shift in myeloid elements with maturation arrest at the promyelocyte stage of development (A, Wright-Giemsa, 5x) and increased eosinophils (B, Wright-Giemsa, 20x) (C&D, Wright-Giemsa, 100x). Immune testing reveals low IgG (120) IgA (<5) but elevated IgM (296). Tetanus, diphtheria, and pneumococcal vaccine titers are all absent. CD40 L protein expression on stimulated T-cells (by flow cytometry) is absent. Genetic testing reveals a mutation in the CD40 L gene consistent with X-linked hyper-IgM syndrome.

types: SAP deficiency (XLP1) and XIAP deficiency (XLP2), caused by mutations in the SH2D1a or the XIAP gene, respectively, and is inherited in an X-linked manner. Mutations in SAP result in reduced NK cell function and lead to an increased vulnerability to EBV infection and tumors. Males with XLP can become seriously ill when infected with EBV and develop a fatal mononucleosis infection with HLH, lymphadenopathy, hepatosplenomegaly, hepatitis, and lymphoma (Figure 12.16).

Autoimmune Lymphoproliferative Syndrome

Autoimmune lymphoproliferative syndrome (ALPS) is a rare disorder characterized by massive enlargement of the lymphoid organs, autoimmune cytopenias, and a predisposition to developing lymphoid malignancies. The basic defect is a disturbance of lymphocyte apoptosis, and the hallmark of ALPS is an increase in circulating double negative T-cells (TCR a/b+, CD3+, CD4−, CD8−). The genetic defect found in most patients is a mutation in the FAS gene that induces programmed cell death. Patients usually present in childhood with autoimmune cytopenias, diffuse lymphadenopathy, and hepatosplenomegaly and have an increased incidence of lymphoma [12]. Inherited conditions can predispose to Rosai-Dorfman disease (RDD) and have clinical overlap. Autoimmune lymphoproliferative

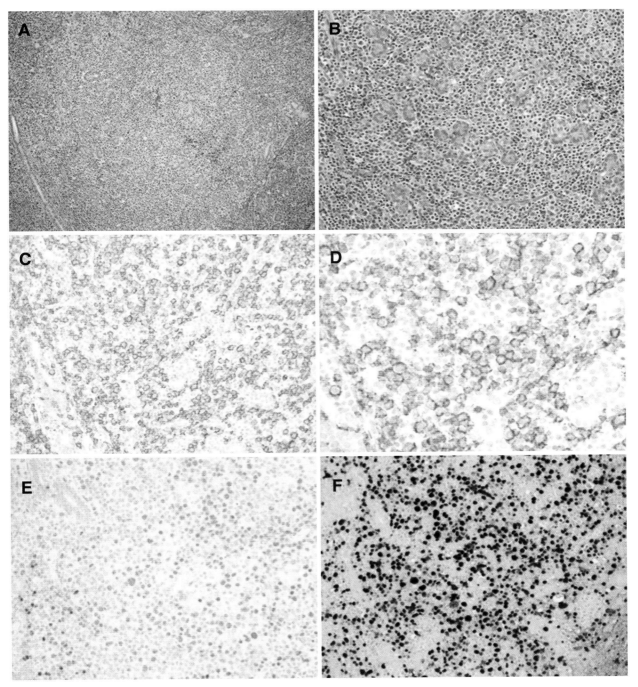

Figure 12.9 Severe combined immunodeficiency, EBV-driven atypical lymphoproliferation.

A 4-year-old boy with a history of combined immunodeficiency, recurrent infections, and T-cell dysfunction is found to have compound heterozygous mutations in RASGRP1 by whole-exome sequencing. He presents with abdominal pain and is found to have pelvic masses, multiple lung masses, cervical, submandibular, and pericaval lymphadenopathy, and enlarged bilateral parotid glands. Histologic sections demonstrate a salivary gland involved by an infiltrate, including mature lymphocytes, plasma cells, histiocytes, immunoblasts, and large, atypical lymphocytes (A, H&E, 10x). Lymphoepithelial lesions are present (B, H&E, 20x). IHC shows increased B-cells that are CD20 positive (C, CD20, 20x), (D, CD20, 40x), PAX5 dim positive (E, PAX5, 20x), and EBER positive (F, in situ EBER, 20x). (case courtesy of Dr. Karen Chisholm).

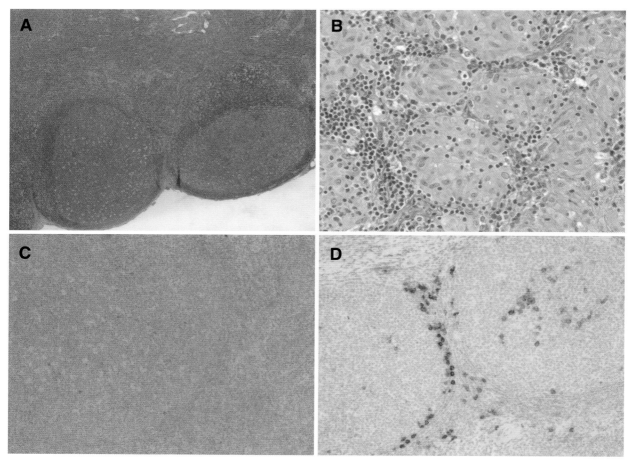

Figure 12.10 CVID with follicular hyperplasia and granulomas.

A 15-year-old female with a history of monthly sinus infections starting at age 11 presents with lymphadenopathy. She has had multiple ear infections and pneumonia as well. Two years ago, she was treated for autoimmune hemolytic anemia. Immune testing revealed low IgG, IgA, and IgM and poor responses to vaccinations consistent with a diagnosis of common variable immune deficiency (CVID). A lymph node biopsy shows preservation of the nodal architecture, follicular hyperplasia (A, H&E, 2.5x), and noncaseating granulomas (B, H&E, 40x). The CD138 stain shows absent plasma cells in the germinal centers (C, CD138, 5x) as compared to CD138 on the normal control, which shows plasma cells in germinal centers and interfollicular areas (D, CD138, 10x).

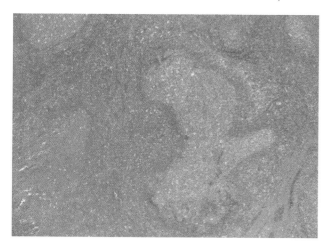

Figure 12.11 CVID with follicular hyperplasia.

A 16-year-old male with CVID and autoimmune cytopenias presents with lymphadenopathy. An excisional biopsy shows irregularly shaped, enlarged germinal centers (A, H&E, 2.5x). Hyperplastic, irregularly shaped germinal centers specifically correlate with patients with CVID and autoimmune cytopenias [17].

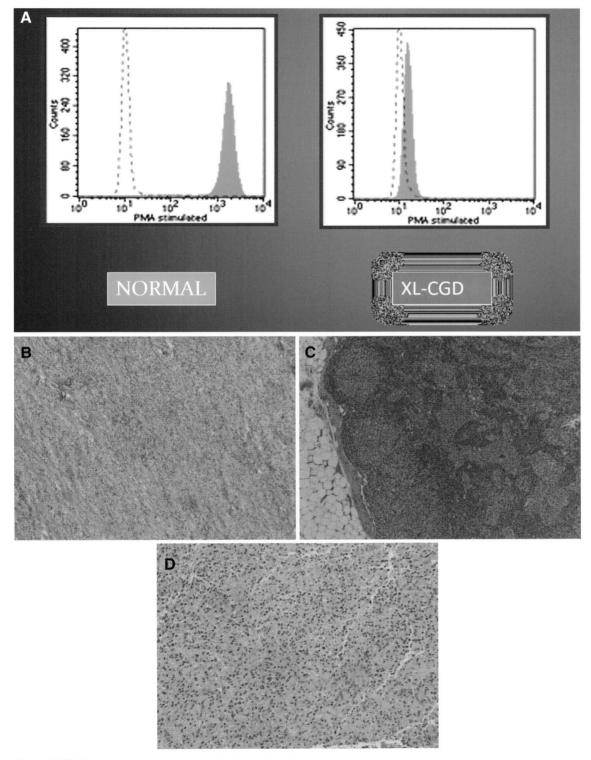

Figure 12.12 Chronic granulomatous disease in the lymph node.

An 18-month-old boy with a history of pneumonia requiring IV antibiotics and staph skin infections presents with painful swelling of the left neck. Incision and drainage of the lymph node reveals Serratia. Absolute neutrophil count is normal but the flow cytometry assay (dihydrorhodamine assay, DHR) for neutrophil oxidative burst is completely absent (A, DHR plot). The DHR assay shows a dotted red peak, which represents the resting neutrophils, and a green peak, which represents the stimulated neutrophils. When stimulated, normal neutrophils will generate an oxidative burst, causing the nonfluorescent DHR-123 dye to oxidize to Rhodamine-123 and fluoresce, which can be detected by flow cytometry. The peak will show an increased syndrome (ALPS)-related RDD is caused by germline mutations in the FAS gene *TNFRSF6*. These patients have a more aggressive clinical course, are predominantly male, and present at a very young age. Many of these patients have nodal RDD but the RDD-like changes are usually self-limited [13] (Figures 12.17 and 12.18).

Lymphoproliferations Associated with HIV Infection

Lymph nodes of patients with HIV are associated with a spectrum of morphologic changes running the gamut from follicular hyperplasia, the most common finding,

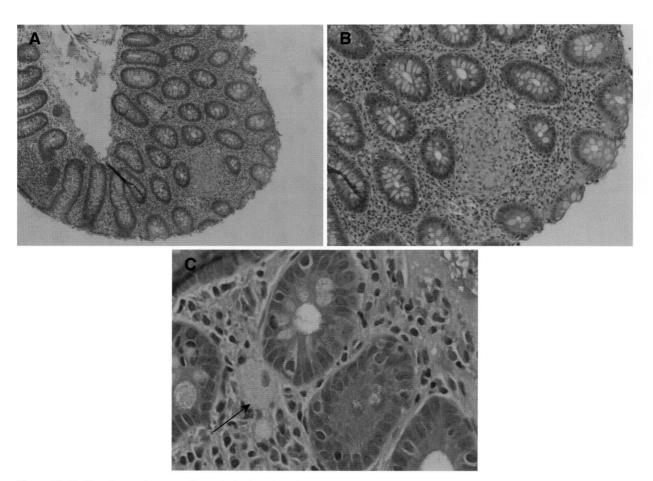

Figure 12.13 Chronic granulomatous disease in the large bowel.

A 5-year-old boy with a history of inflammatory bowel disease was diagnosed at 2 years of age. He has a history of fungal osteomyelitis and recurrent pneumonia. A colonoscopy is performed for inflammatory bowel disease and shows colonic mucosa with noncaseating granulomas (A, H&E, 5X), (B, H&E, 10x), foamy histiocytes (see arrow) in the lamina propria, and noncaseating granulomas (C, H&E, 40x).

Caption for Figure 12.12 (cont.)

mean channel fluorescence (right plot). In X-linked CGD, the neutrophils have a mutation in the cytochrome oxidase complex and cannot generate the oxidative burst; thus the green shaded peak does not fluoresce since DHR-123 will not get oxidized to Rhodamine-123, and the green peak is seen adjacent to the resting peak (left plot). Genetic testing confirms a mutation in the CYBB gene (part of the NADPH oxidase complex) consistent with a diagnosis of X-linked CGD. Excisional biopsy of the neck mass shows fibro-connective tissue and skeletal muscle infiltrated by a brisk mixed inflammatory infiltrate of histiocytes, lymphocytes, neutrophils, plasma cells, and focal necrosis (B, H&E, 5x). Loose granulomas (C, H&E, 5x) and granulomatous inflammation are present (D, H&E, 20x).

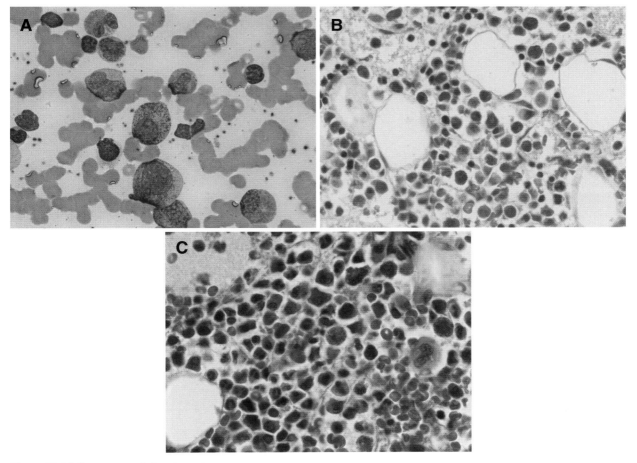

Figure 12.14 Severe congenital neutropenia.

An 18-month-old girl with a history of a skin abscess and mouth ulcerations presents with a skin ulceration and fever. A CBC shows ANC of 0. A bone marrow biopsy and aspirate show trilineage hematopoiesis and a maturation arrest at the promyelocyte stage in the myeloid series. Aspirate and biopsy show myeloid arrest at the promyelocyte stage (A, Wright-Giemsa, 50x), increased eosinophils (B, H&E, 40x), and a left shift in myeloid maturation with a paucity of mature neutrophils and increased eosinophils (C, H&E, 40x).

paracortical hyperplasia, and follicular lysis to follicular involution and profound lymphocyte depletion. Histologic features of HIV are classified into three patterns: type I pattern shows follicular and paracortical hyperplasia, type II shows loss of germinal centers and increased interfollicular areas, and type III shows lymphocytic depletion, involution of the germinal centers, and hyalinized follicles, plasma cells, and small vessels. HIV patients are at risk to develop lymphomas, particularly B-cell lymphomas, which may be the initial manifestation of the disease and are considered AIDS-defining conditions [14]. The lymphomas seen in HIV patients may be seen in immunocompetent patients, while there are several others that are more unique to HIV patients. The most common lymphomas that develop in HIV patients are aggressive B-cell lymphomas; however, other common lymphomas include Burkitt lymphoma, diffuse large B-cell lymphoma, CNS lymphoma, primary effusion lymphoma, and plasmablastic lymphoma (Figures 12.19 and 12.20).

Iatrogenic Immunodeficiency-Associated Lymphoproliferative Disorders

Iatrogenic immunodeficiency-associated lymphoproliferative disorders are lymphoproliferations or lymphomas that arise in patients treated with immunosuppressive drugs, most commonly for autoimmune diseases, and are not

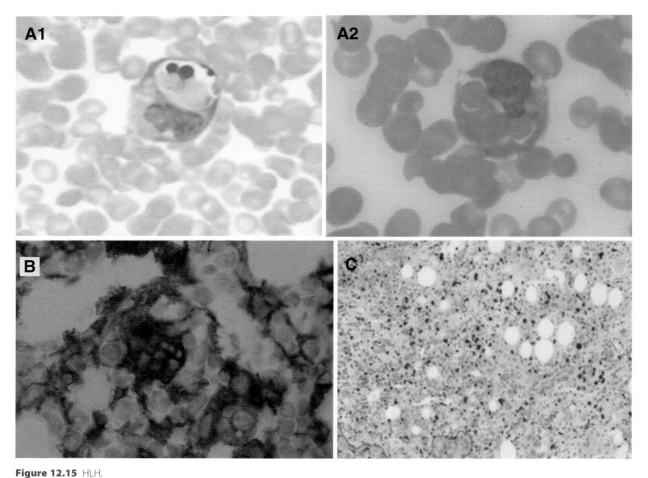

Figure 12.15 HLH.

A 16-month-old male presents with fever, hepatosplenomegaly, cytopenias, and markedly increased ferritin. The bone aspirate shows increased hemophagocytic macrophages (A, Wright-Giemsa, 100x). The tandem biopsy shows increased hemophagocytosis highlighted by CD163 (B, CD163, 50x) and positive cells by in situ hybridization for EBER (C, in situ EBER, 20x).

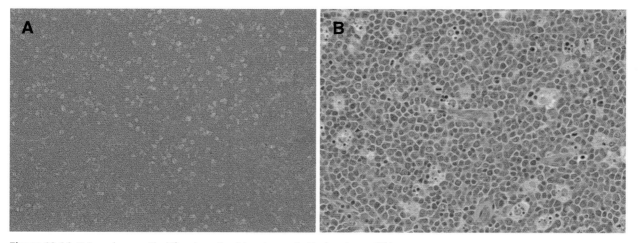

Figure 12.16 XLP syndrome with diffuse large B-cell lymphoma, Burkitt lymphoma, EBV+.

A 6-year-old boy presents with an enlarging neck mass. A lymph node biopsy is performed and shows a diffuse infiltrate of medium- to large-sized cells with a starry sky pattern (A, H&E, 5x). The cells have multiple small inconspicuous nucleoli, frequent mitoses, and tingible body macrophages (B, H&E, 20x). Flow cytometry shows the neoplastic cells expressed CD20, CD10, and kappa light chain restriction. Flow cytometry for SAP is absent and NK function is reduced (flow cytometry not shown). XLP and Burkitt lymphoma, EBV+ are diagnosed and he is treated with chemotherapy. He receives a bone marrow transplant due to high susceptibility of lymphoma and HLH with XLP.

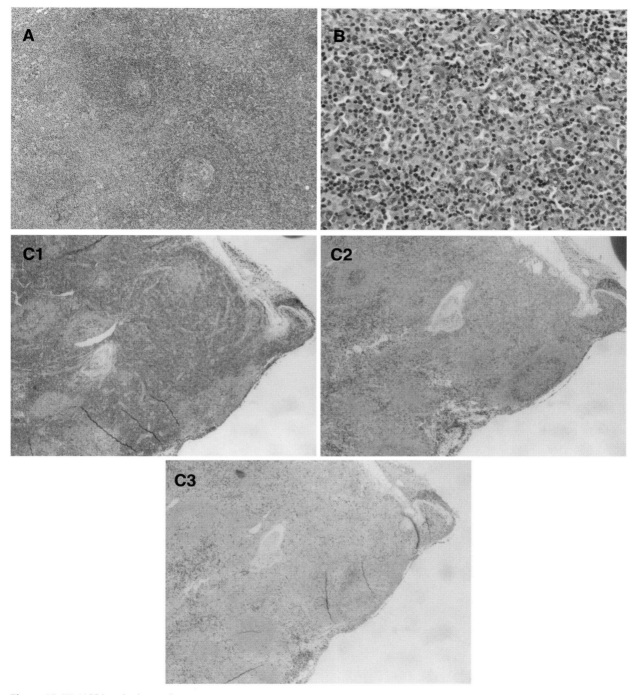

Figure 12.17 ALPS lymphadenopathy.

A 6-year-old with a history of Evans syndrome presents with diffuse lymphadenopathy. A lymph node biopsy is performed and shows preservation of the normal nodal architecture with follicular and interfollicular hyperplasia (A, H&E, 5X). The interfollicular area is expanded with lymphocytes, occasional immunoblasts, and histiocytes (B, H&E, 5x). Immunohistochemistry shows the interfollicular area is composed predominantly of CD3-positive T-cells (C, CD3, 5x) and a subset of CD4-, CD8-double negative T cells (DNTs), as the CD4- and CD8-positive T-cells appear less than the number of CD3-positive cells (D, CD4, 5x) (E, CD8, 5x). (Flow cytometry on the peripheral blood shows an increased population of DNTs [15%]). Molecular studies confirm a mutation in the FAS gene.

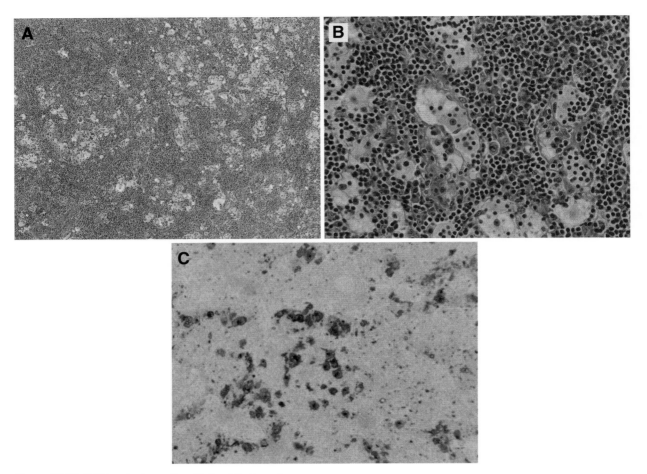

Figure 12.18 ALPS lymphadenopathy with Rosai-Dorfman disease.

An 18-month-old male with splenomegaly, anemia, neutropenia, and diffuse lymphadenopathy has an excisional biopsy of a cervical lymph node. The biopsy shows histiocytes with emperipolesis (A, H&E, 5x). The histiocytes have a central nucleus and contain lymphocytes (B, H&E, 40x) and are positive for S100 (C, S100, 5x). A TNFSF6 mutation is identified and a diagnosis of RDD-associated ALPS is rendered.

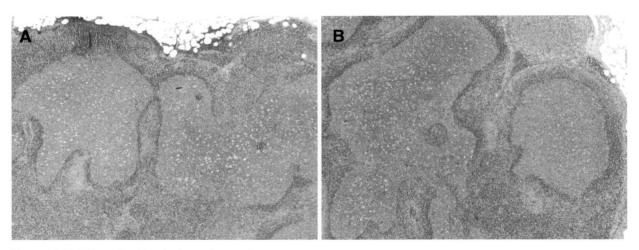

Figure 12.19 HIV-associated lymphadenopathy, type I pattern.

A 16-year-old HIV+ male presents with diffuse lymphadenopathy and fevers. A lymph node biopsy shows follicular hyperplasia with large irregular follicles, tingible body macrophages, and preserved mantle zones consistent with early HIV lymphadenopathy, type I pattern (A, B, H&E, 2.5x) (photo courtesy of Dr. Dale Frank).

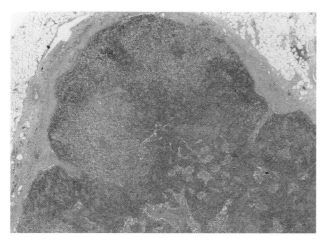

Figure 12.20 HIV-associated lymphadenopathy, type III pattern.
An 18-year-old HIV+ male presents with an enlarged axillary lymph node. A biopsy was performed and shows loss of secondary follicles, small atretic and hyalinized follicles, and increased vasculature consistent with type III pattern (A, 2.5x, H&E) (photo courtesy of Dr. Dale Frank).

given in posttransplant settings [14]. These lymphoproliferations are like PTLDs in that they arise in a background of immunodeficiency and show a spectrum of morphology that includes polymorphic lymphoproliferations to overt lymphoma. These lymphoproliferations include diffuse large B-cell lymphoma, which may be associated with EBV or HHV8, peripheral T/NK cell lymphoma, and Hodgkin lymphoma.

Hepatosplenic T-cell lymphoma (HSTCL) is a rare, extranodal lymphoma that has a rapidly progressive course and a high mortality. It is derived from cytotoxic T-cells that are gamma-delta positive. It shows sinusoidal infiltration of the liver and red pulp of the spleen and bone marrow. HSTCL has been associated with immunosuppression especially in young male patients on immunomodulators for inflammatory bowel disease and in immunocompromised patients [15] (Figure 12.22).

References

1. Bonilla FA, Khan DA, Ballas ZK, Chinen J, Frank MM, Hsu JT, et al. Practice parameter for the diagnosis and management of primary immunodeficiency. J Allergy Clin Immunol. 2015; **136**(5): 1186–205.

2. Szczawińska-Poplonyk A, Ossowska L, Jończyk-Potoczna K. Granulomatous liver disease in ataxia-telangiectasia with the hyper-IgM phenotype: A case report. Front Pediatr. 2020; **8**: 570330.

3. Rothblum-Oviatt C, Wright J, Lefton-Greif MA, McGrath-Morrow SA, Crawford TO, Lederman HM. Ataxia telangiectasia: A review. Orphanet J Rare Dis. 2016; **11**(1): 159. https://doi.org/10.1186/s13023-016-0543-7.

4. Yazdani R, Fekrvand S, Shahkarami S, Azizi G, Moazzami B, Abolhassani H, et al. The hyper IgM syndromes: Epidemiology, pathogenesis, clinical manifestations, diagnosis and management. Clin Immunol. 2019; **198**: 19–30.

5. Aluri J, Desai M, Gupta M, Dalvi A, Terance A, Rosenzweig SD, et al. Clinical, immunological, and molecular findings in 57 patients with severe combined immunodeficiency (SCID) from India. Front Immunol. 2019; **10**: 23.

6. Ghafoor A, Joseph SM. Making a diagnosis of common variable immunodeficiency: A review. Cureus. 2020; **12**(1): e6711.

7. Romberg N, Lawrence MG. Birds of a feather: Common variable immune deficiencies. Ann Allergy Asthma Immunol. 2019; **123**(5): 461–7.

8. Arnold DE, Heimall JR. A review of chronic granulomatous disease. Adv Ther. 2017; **34**(12): 2543–57.

9. Horwitz M, Benson KF, Person RE, Aprikyan AG, Dale DC. Mutations in ELA2, encoding neutrophil elastase, define a 21-day biological clock in cyclic haematopoiesis. Nat Genet. 1999; **23**(4): 433–6.

10. Tidow N, Pilz C, Teichmann B, Müller-Brechlin A, Germeshausen M, Kasper B, et al. Clinical relevance of point mutations in the cytoplasmic domain of the granulocyte colony-stimulating factor receptor gene in patients with severe congenital neutropenia. Blood. 1997; **89**(7): 2369–75.

11. George MR. Hemophagocytic lymphohistiocytosis: Review of etiologies and management. J Blood Med. 2014; **5**: 69–86.

12. Fisher GH, Rosenberg FJ, Straus SE, Dale JK, Middleton LA, Lin AY, et al. Dominant interfering FAS gene mutations impair apoptosis in a human autoimmune lymphoproliferative syndrome. Cell. 1995; **81**(6): 935–46.

13. Maric I, Pittaluga S, Dale JK, Niemela JE, Delsol G, Diment J et al. Histologic features of sinus histiocytosis with massive lymphadenopathy in patients with autoimmune lymphoproliferative syndrome. Am J Surg Pathol. 2005; **29**(7): 903–11.

14. Swerdlow SH, Campo E, Harris NL, Jaffe ES, Pileri SA, Stein H, et al. Immunodeficiency-associated lymphoproliferative disorders. In Swerdlow SH, Campo E, Harris NL, Jaffe ES, Pileri SA Stein H, et al., eds. WHO classification of tumours and haematopoietic and lymphoid tissues. Revised 4th ed. Lyon: IARC Press; 2017: 449, 462.

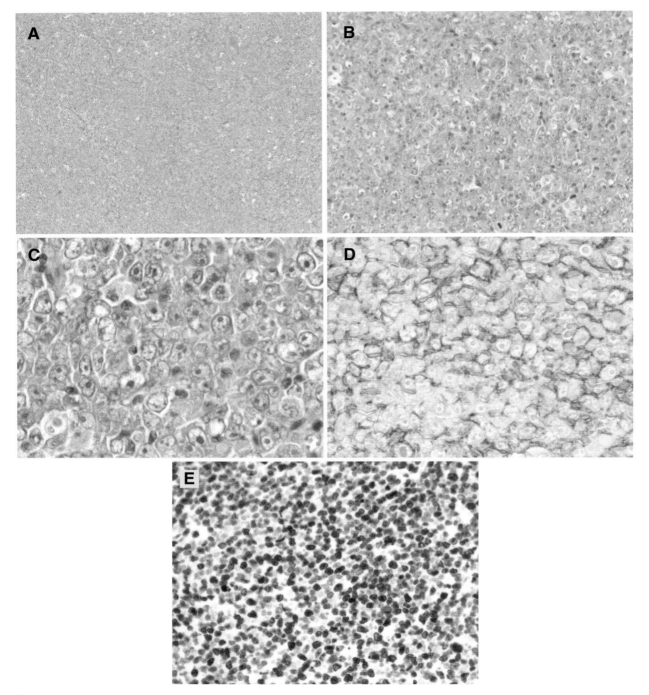

Figure 12.21 HIV-associated high-grade B-cell lymphoma.

A 12-year-old girl with a history of HIV diagnosed at birth develops a rapidly enlarging lymph node. A biopsy is performed and shows a high-grade B-cell lymphoma. The lymph node is replaced with sheets of large, monomorphic cells with vesicular chromatin, large nucleoli, and frequent mitoses (A, H&E, 5x), (B, H&E, 20x) (C, H&E, 40x). Immunohistochemistry shows the cells are positive for CD20 (D, CD20, 20x) and a high proliferative index on a Ki67 stain (E, Ki67, 20x).

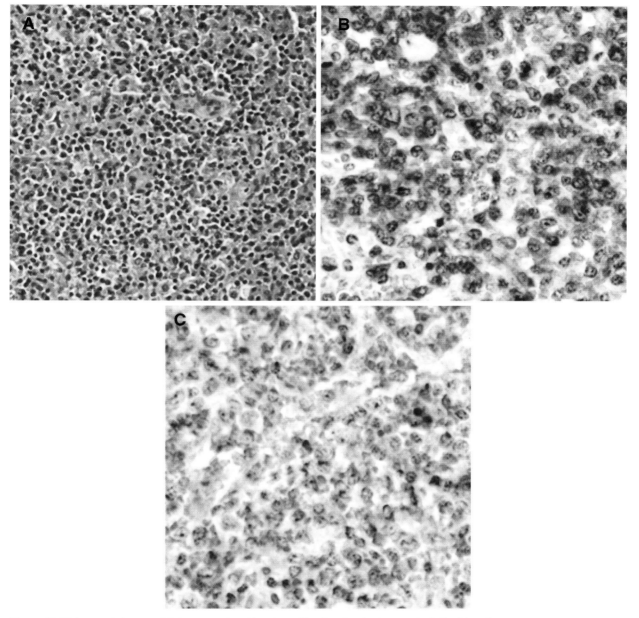

Figure 12.22 Iatrogenic immunodeficiency-associated lymphoproliferative disorder, hepatosplenic T-cell lymphoma.

A 19-year-old male with a long history of Crohn's disease on infliximab therapy presents with malaise, cytopenias, and hepatomegaly. A liver biopsy shows a sinusoidal infiltrate composed of medium-sized lymphocytes (A, H&E, 40x). IHC shows the lymphoid cells are CD3-positive T-cells (B, CD3, 20x) that lack CD5 (C, CD5, 20x). The spleen shows diffuse involvement of the red pulp (D, H&E, 10x) by medium-sized lymphoid cells with scant cytoplasm and inconspicuous nucleoli (E, H&E, 40x). IHC shows the cells are CD3 positive (F, CD3, 40x). (images courtesy of Dr. Megan Lim).

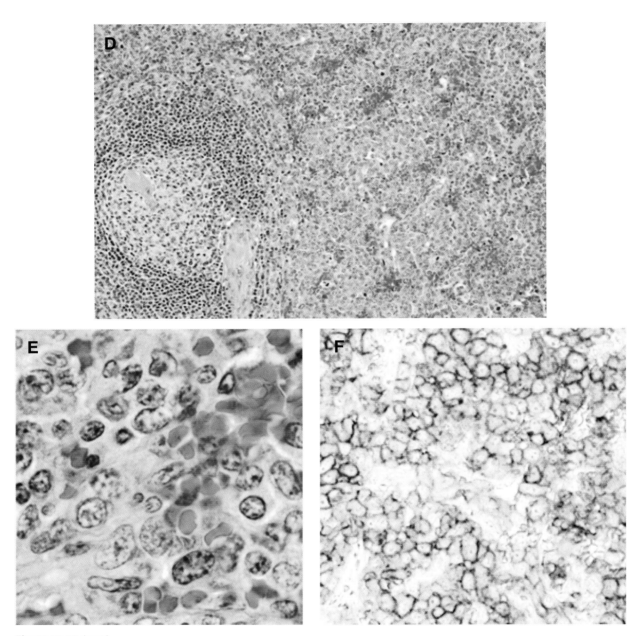

Figure 12.22 (cont.)

15. Thai A, Prindiville T. Hepatosplenic T cell lymphoma and inflammatory bowel disease. J Crohns Colitis. 2010; **4**(5): 11–22.

16. Amirifar P, Yazdani R, Shad TM, Ghanadan A, Abolhassani H, Lavin M, et al. Cutaneous granulomatosis and class switching defect as a presenting sign in ataxia-telangiectasia: First case from the national Iranian registry and review of the literature. Immunol Invest. 2020; **49**(6): 597–610.

17. Romberg N, Le Coz C, Glauzy S, Schickel JN, Trofa M, Nolan BE, et al. Patients with common variable immunodeficiency with autoimmune cytopenias exhibit hyperplastic yet inefficient germinal center responses. J Allergy Clin Immunol. 2019; **143**(1): 258–65.

Precursor Lymphoblastic Leukemia/Lymphoma

Virginia Knez, Billie Carstens, Xiayuan Liang

Precursor lymphoid neoplasms comprise lymphoblastic leukemias (ALLs) and lymphoblastic lymphomas (LBLs), of either B- or T-cell origin. As a general rule, ALLs and LBLs are considered biologically equivalent. The distinction between ALLs and LBLs is arbitrary. Bone marrow or peripheral blood blasts ≥25% are defined as ALL. Neoplasms with predominant extramedullary involvement, bone marrow, or peripheral blood blasts <25% are classified as LBL.

B-lymphoblastic Leukemia/Lymphoma

B-lymphoblastic leukemia/lymphoma (B-ALL/B-LBL) is a neoplasm of lymphoblasts committed to the B-cell lineage [1]. B-ALL is primarily a disease of children; 75% of cases occur in patients <6 years of age [1]. Most patients present with evidence of bone marrow failure: thrombocytopenia, anemia, and/or neutropenia. The

leukocyte count may be decreased, normal, or markedly elevated. Bone pain and arthralgia may be prominent symptoms [1], sometimes prompting patients to seek orthopedic care. Occasionally extramedullary disease may be present in sites such as the central nervous system, lymph nodes, spleen, liver, and gonads [1–6].

B-LBL is an uncommon type of lymphoma and constitutes approximately 10% of LBL cases [1]. The most frequent sites are the skin, followed by the bone, soft tissue, and lymph nodes [1]. Mediastinal masses are uncommon [1].

Morphologic Features

In a majority of cases, lymphoblasts vary from small to medium in size with scanty cytoplasm, described as L1 morphology (Figure 13.1) in French-American-British (FAB) classification [7]. In a minority of cases, blasts are

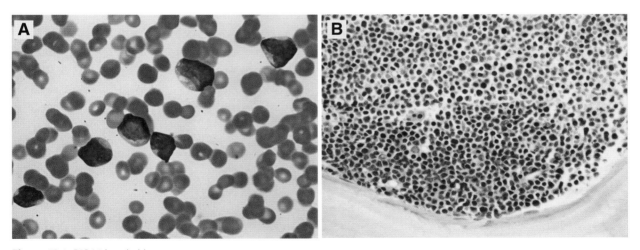

Figure 13.1 FAB L1 lymphoblasts.

a. Bone marrow aspirate smear shows blasts with small in size, high nuclear: cytoplasmic ratio, minimal cytoplasm, slightly fine chromatin, and inconspicuous nucleolus (Wright-Giemsa, 1,000x).

b. Bone marrow biopsy shows 100% cellularity with the morphology similar to that seen in the aspirate smear (H&E, 400x).

larger and show a moderate amount of cytoplasm, described as L2 morphology (Figure 13.2) in FAB classification [7]. There are other morphologic variants (Figures 13.3–13.7). B-ALLs may associate with fibrosis, resulting in hypocellular aspirate smears (Figure 13.8), which may raise the differential diagnosis of acute megakaryoblastic leukemia. Occasionally, B-ALL may present with extensive marrow necrosis (Figure 13.9). Re-biopsy in another area of bone marrow or immunophenotypic analysis of peripheral blood blasts allows for diagnosis. Rare cases of B-ALL may be preceded by transient bone marrow aplasia/aplastic anemia, with progression to B-ALL within 6 to 15 months [4]. LBL is generally characterized by a diffuse pattern of lymph node or other tissue involvement (Figure 13.10) [1]. A single-file pattern of infiltration in soft tissue is common [1]. In most cases, mitotic figures are numerous and, in some cases, there may be a focal "starry sky" pattern [1, 8].

Hypereosinophilia may occasionally be seen and is thought to represent a reactive process in response to cytokines generated by the lymphoblasts [7]. Molecular

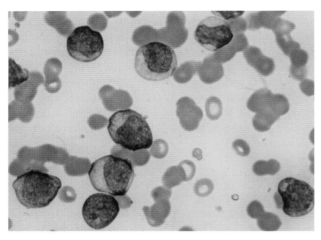

Figure 13.2 FAB L2 lymphoblasts in bone marrow are larger than L1 blasts with moderate amounts of cytoplasm, fine chromatin, and conspicuous nucleolus (Wright-Giemsa, 1,000x).

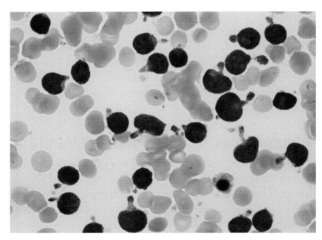

Figure 13.3 Hand mirror cells in ALL show cytoplasmic pseudopods (Wright-Giemsa, 1,000x).

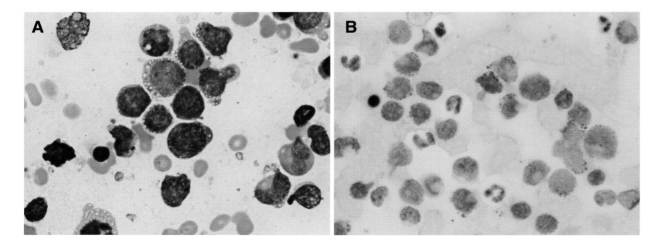

Figure 13.4 Morphological variant of ALL with cytoplasmic vacuoles in blasts.

a. Lymphoblasts show a small amount of cytoplasm and a number of different-sized cytoplasmic vacuoles (Wright-Giemsa, 1,000x).
b. Vacuoles in lymphoblasts are periodic acid-Schiff (PAS) staining positive (PAS, 1,000x).

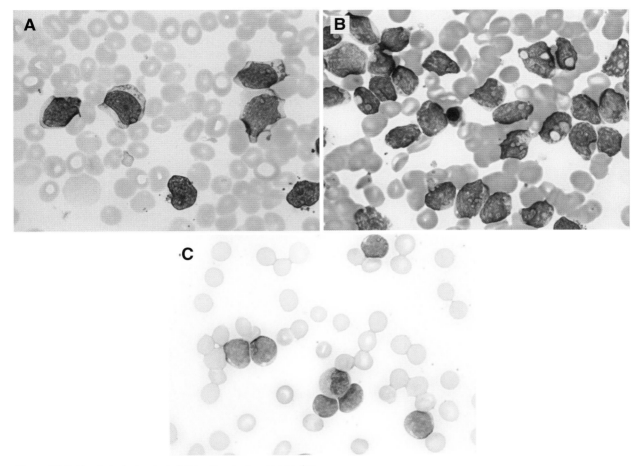

Figure 13.5 Morphological variant of ALL with cytoplasmic granules.

a. Lymphoblasts display pink granules within the cytoplasm (Wright-Giemsa, 1,000x).
b. Blasts display large, pink, coarse, Chédiak-Higashi-like granules, which can cause morphologic confusion with myeloblasts. The granules show activity suggestive of lysosomes, but they are negative for myeloperoxidase. This variant may be associated with t(9;22)(q34;q11.2) (Wright-Giemsa, 1,000x).
c. Cytoplasmic Chédiak-Higashi-like granules in lymphoblasts are PAS positive (PAS, 1,000x).

testing should be done to exclude rearrangements of t(5;14)(q31.1;q32.1)/*IGH-IL3* (Figure 13.11), *PDGRA*, *PDGFRB*, *FGFR1*, and *PCM1-JAK2*. If any of these rearrangements are found, the disease should be reclassified as myeloid/lymphoid neoplasms with the specific gene rearrangement listed in the diagnosis [1].

Immunophenotype

The blasts have an immature B-cell phenotype expressing TdT, HLA-DR, CD19, cytoplasmic CD22, and cytoplasmic CD79a [1]. Most cases are positive for CD10, CD24, and PAX5. CD10 is absent in some cases, especially in infant B-ALL, and correlates with *KMT2A* rearrangements [1, 7]. There is variable expression of CD20 and CD34 [1, 7]. CD45 may be absent, and if present, is nearly always dimmer than the mature B-cells [1]. Aberrant expressions of myeloid antigens CD13 and/or CD33 are found in some cases of B-ALL and should not be used as evidence for a diagnosis of mixed-phenotype acute leukemia, B/myeloid [1, 7].

Furthermore, occasionally, myeloperoxidase can be weakly expressed; however, if it is the only myeloid marker in a typical B-ALL, this should not be classified as B/myeloid leukemia [1]. In B-LBL, the major differential diagnosis is Burkitt lymphoma in children [1]. Burkitt lymphoma generally doesn't express CD34 and TdT, but expresses a monoclonal surface light chain. Identification of the diagnostic t(8;14) in Burkitt lymphoma is an important distinction.

Genetic Features

Nearly all cases of B-ALL/B-LBL have clonal rearrangements of *IGH*; however, T-cell receptor gene rearrangements may be seen in up to 70% of cases [1]. Immunoglobulin light-chain rearrangement is thought to be a more specific marker for B-cell differentiation [8].

Precursor B-cell lymphoid neoplasms without recurrent genetic abnormalities are classified as B-ALL/B-LBL,

Figure 13.6 Anaplastic variant of ALL. Lymphoblasts are large, displaying variable amounts of blue-gray cytoplasm, markedly enlarged and irregular nuclei, heterogeneous chromatin, and multiple prominent nucleoli. This variant is frequently associated with hypodiploidy, a poor prognostic factor (Wright-Giemsa, 1,000x).

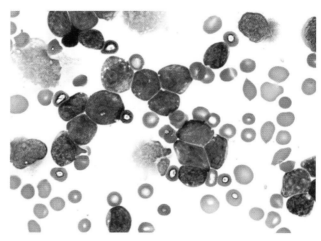

Figure 13.7 Blasts in ALL form clusters mimicking metastatic solid tissue tumor in bone marrow (Wright-Giemsa, 1,000x).

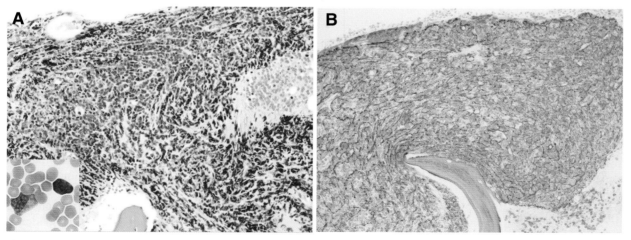

Figure 13.8 a. A bone marrow biopsy shows packed marrow with interstitial fibrosis (H&E, 400x). Inset shows hypocellular aspirate with a blast. b. Marked reticulin fibrosis (reticulin stain, 400x).

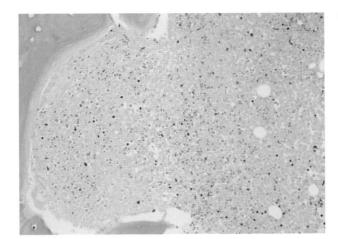

Figure 13.9 A bone marrow biopsy in a patient with ALL shows bone marrow necrosis. The necrotic blasts are pink with loss of nuclei and do not show clear cell borders (H&E, 200x).

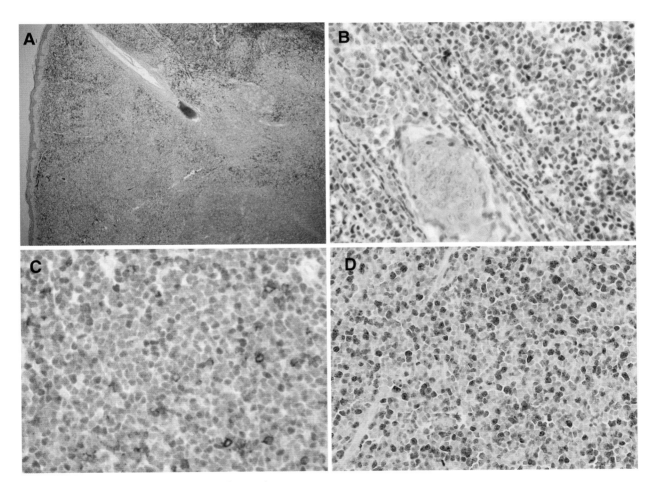

Figure 13.10 B-lymphoblastic lymphoma involving scalp.
a. A scalp biopsy reveals subepithelial grenz zone and diffuse and dense dermal infiltration by lymphoblasts (H&E, 20x).
b. Medium power shows sheets of lymphoblasts with homogeneity, scant cytoplasm, high nuclear: cytoplasmic ratio, and fine chromatin with occasionally visible nucleoli in an interstitial distribution (H&E, 200x).
c. Lymphoblasts are TdT positive with nuclear staining pattern (immunostain, 400x).
d. Lymphoblasts are PAX5 positive with nuclear staining pattern, consistent with B-cell lineage (immunostain, 400x).

Table 13.1 Prognostic parameters in pediatric B-lymphoblastic neoplasms

	Favorable	Unfavorable
Clinical factors	1–9 years	<1 year or ≥10 years
	Female	Male
	Caucasian, Asian	African American, Hispanic
	WBC < 50,000/mm^3	WBC ≥ 50,000/mm^3
	CNS not involved	CNS involvement
	Testes not involved	Testes involvement
	Non-Down syndrome	Down syndrome
Cytogenetics	High hyperdiploidy (51–65 chromosomes)	Hypodiploidy (< 44 chromosomes)
	t(12;21)(p13.2;q22.1); *ETV6-RUNX1*	t(9;22)(q34.1;q11.2); *BCR-ABL1*
		t(v;11q23.3); *KMT2A*-rearranged
		BCR-ABL1-like
		iAMP21[*]
		t(1;19)(q23;p13.3); *TCF3-PBX1*[*]
MRD	<0.01%	≥0.01%

[*] Can be overcome by risk-stratified or modern chemotherapy.

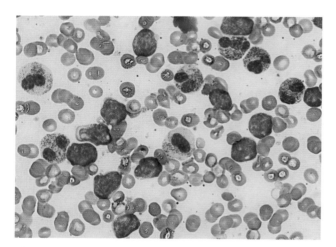

Figure 13.11 B-ALL/LBL with t(5;14) (q31.1; q32.1); *IGH-IL3*. Numerous eosinophils are present along with lymphoblasts in a bone marrow aspirate. Eosinophils range from immature to mature or hypersegmented forms (Wright-Giemsa stain, 1,000x).

not otherwise specified [1, 8]. Table 13.1 summarizes the different genetic subtypes and prognosis. Due to the challenges of adequate leukemic blast metaphases by conventional cytogenetic analysis, fluorescence in situ hybridization is usually needed at diagnosis to identify various genetic subtypes.

Prognosis

B-ALL/LBL has a more favorable outcome in children than in adults. The prognosis is determined by patients' age, white blood cell (WBC) count, central nervous system (CNS) involvement, cytogenetic abnormalities, and minimal residual disease (MRD) (Table 13.1) [1, 2, 8–10].

Infant and Congenital B-lymphoblastic Leukemia

Infant lymphoblastic leukemia occurs within the first year of life. It is a rare and biologically different disease from general pediatric ALL (≥1 year) [11, 12]. Congenital ALL, occurring within the first month of life, is exceedingly rare, arising in fewer than 5 births per 1 million [11–13]. Infant ALL cases are usually B-cell in origin (Figure 13.13). They are characterized by a high frequency of t(v;11q23.3) involving rearrangements of the *KMT2A* gene. *KMT2A* rearrangement, occurring in the highest frequency in the congenital group, has been identified in neonatal blood spots, suggesting it can occur in utero. The most common partner gene is *AFF1* on chromosome 4q21 [1, 12, 14]. Other common partners include *MLLT1* on chromosome 19p13 and *MLLT3* on chromosome 9p21 [1, 3, 12].

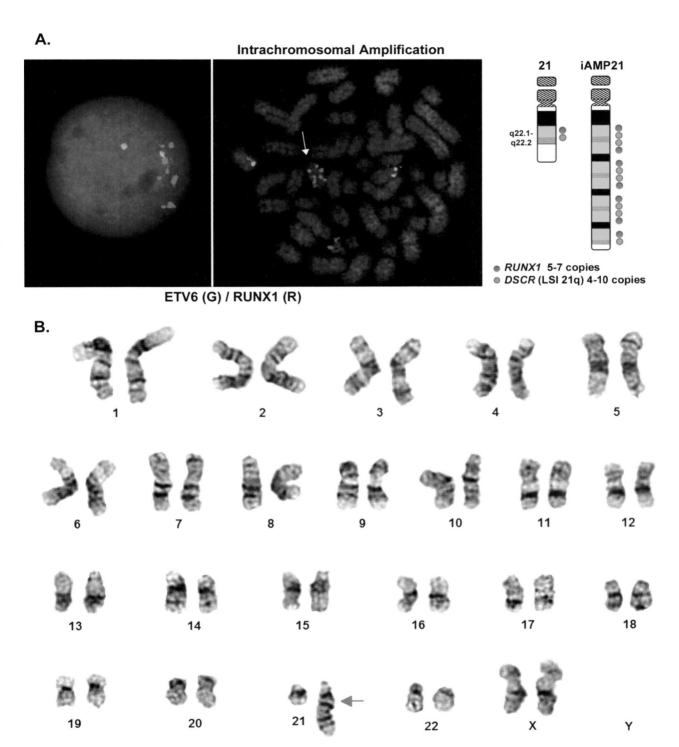

Figure 13.12 Cytogenetics of B-ALL/LBL with iAMP21. The upper panel is FISH analysis. *RUNX1* probe is labeled red and *ETV6* probe is labeled green. The upper left is interphase FISH revealing ≥5 copies of *RUNX1* gene signals. The upper middle is metaphase FISH demonstrating ≥5 copies of *RUNX1* gene signals. The upper right is the schematic representation. The lower image shows the iAMP21 karyotype, which is characterized by intrachromosomal amplification of a portion of long arm of chromosome 21 involving *RUNX1*.

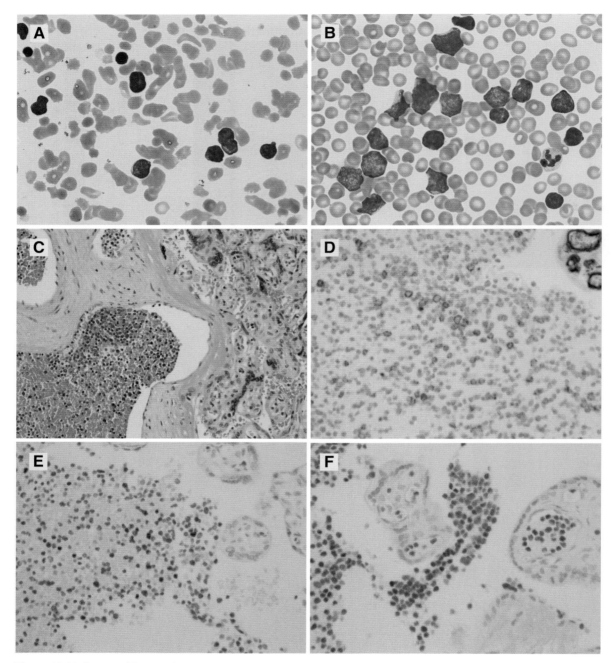

Figure 13.13 Congenital B-ALL with t(v;11q23.3); *KMT2A* rearranged.

a. A smear from cord blood shows lymphoblasts that display high nuclear: cytoplasmic ratio, slightly dense chromatin, and indistinct nucleoli (Wright-Giemsa, 1,000x).

b. Bone marrow from a 10-day-old newborn shows numerous lymphoblasts (Wright Giemsa, 1,000x).

c. A section of placenta demonstrates numerous lymphoblasts within blood vessels (H&E, 400x).

d. Blasts in the placenta are CD34 positive (immunostain, 400x).

e. Blasts in the placenta are TdT positive (immunostain, 400x).

f. Blasts in the placenta are PAX-5 positive, indicating B-cell lineage (PAX-5 immunostain, 400x).

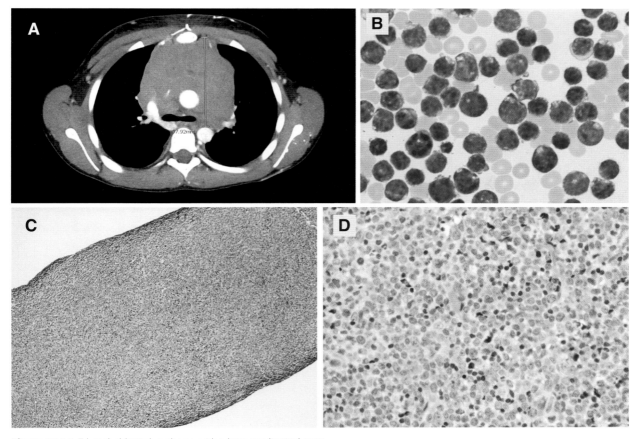

Figure 13.14 T-lymphoblastic lymphoma with a large mediastinal mass.

a. Chest-computed tomography shows a vastly enlarged mediastinal mass.

b. Pleural effusion reveals a monomorphic population of cells composed of blasts with high nuclear: cytoplasmic ratio, scanty blue cytoplasm, and inconspicuous nuclei (Wright-Giemsa, 1,000x).

c. A core biopsy of a mediastinal mass reveals a confluent sheet of immature cells consistent with blasts (H&E, 100x).

d. Higher-power view of blasts shows intermediate to large size and occasionally visible nucleoli (H&E, 400x).

e. Blasts are CD3 positive (immunostain, 400x).

f. Blasts are TdT positive with nuclear staining fashion (immunostain, 400x).

g. Blasts are CD1a positive, indicating common (cortical) stage II maturation (immunostain, 400x).

Patients typically present with a very high WBC count, frequently >100 × 10^9/L. There is a high frequency of CNS involvement at the time of diagnosis [12, 14, 15]. The lineage switch from B-ALL to AML occurs in congenital B-ALL more often than non-congenital infant B-ALL [14, 16–18].

With increasing age in infants, non-*KMT2A* cytogenetic abnormalities start significantly emerging around 9 months, essentially driving the clinicopathologic features of B-ALL/B-LBL to merge with that in pediatric patients ≥1 year old [14].

Infant B-ALL with *KMT2A* rearrangement portends a poor prognosis. Poor prognostic factors include age <6 months, hyperleukocytosis, and CNS involvement [12, 14, 15]. Mortality is highest in the congenital group, probably because of its high rate of lineage switch to AML [11, 14].

T-lymphoblastic Leukemia/Lymphoma

T-lymphoblastic leukemia/lymphoma (T-ALL/LBL) is a neoplasm of lymphoblasts committed to the T-cell lineage [19]. The disease involves the bone marrow or blood (T-ALL), or presents with primary involvement of the thymus (Figure 13.14), nodal, or extranodal sites (T-LBL) [19].

T-ALL accounts for about 15% of childhood ALL cases [19–21]. T-LBL accounts for about 85–90% of LBLs [19].

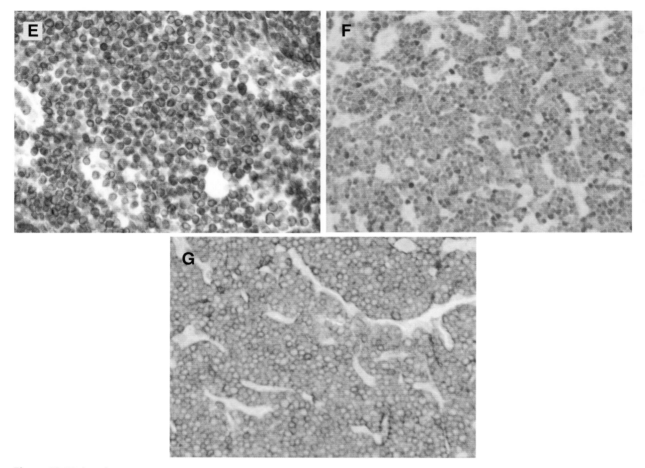

Figure 13.14 (cont.)

Both are most common in male adolescents [19, 21]. T-ALL typically presents with a high leukocyte count, anemia, thrombocytopenia, organomegaly, bone pain, and frequent CNS involvement [19]. T-LBL often presents with a large mediastinal mass or other tissue mass [19].

Immunophenotype

The blasts are usually positive for T-cell markers, CD1a, CD2, CD3, CD4, CD5, CD7 (bright), CD8, and variable positive for TdT [19]. Surface expression of CD3 can be absent, but all cases express cytoplasmic CD3 [7, 8, 19]. CD4 and CD8 are frequently coexpressed, mimicking the cortical stage of thymocytes [19]. CD10 may also be positive [19]. CD34 expression is less frequent [19]. Myeloid-associated antigens CD13 and/or CD33 may also be expressed in approximately 20–30% of cases, and should not be used as

evidence for a diagnosis of mixed-phenotype acute leukemia, T/myeloid [19]. CD117 is positive in occasional cases and is associated with *FLT3* mutations [19].

Genetic Features

Genetic profile almost always shows clonal rearrangements of the T-cell receptor genes (*TCR*) on chromosomes 7 and 14, as well as immunoglobulin-heavy locus gene rearrangements in approximately 20% of cases [19]. The most common *TCR* abnormalities involve the alpha and delta loci at 14q11.2, beta locus at 7q35, and gamma locus at 7p14-15, with a variety of partners [3, 19]. The most commonly involved genes include transcription factors *TLX1* (also called *HOX11*) at 10q24 in 7% of childhood cases, and *TLX3* (also called *HOX11L2*) at 5q35 in 20% of childhood cases [19].

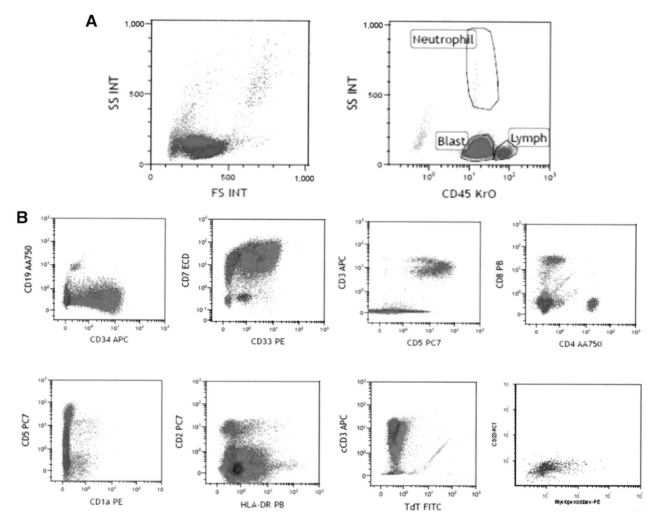

Figure 13.15 Flow cytometry plots of early T-cell precursor lymphoblastic leukemia (ETP-ALL).

a. The left panel shows a two-parameter dot plot illustrating forward scatter (FS) versus side scatter (SS) characteristics of a bone marrow (BM) specimen in a patient with ETP-ALL. The red region represents blast population, the green region represents mature lymphocytes, and the pink/purple region represents granulocytes. The right panel shows a dot plot illustrating CD45 versus side scatter (SS) gating. The red region represents blast population, the green region represents mature lymphocytes, and the gray region represents granulocytes including neutrophils.

b. The panel of dot plots demonstrates antigen expression using CD45 versus SS gating indicated in the right panel of a. The red region represents blast population which are CD34+, CD33+, CD5 dimly+, CD7+, cytoplasmic CD3 (cCD3)+, HLA-DR dimly+, CD19−, CD22−, CD1a−, CD2−, CD3−, CD4−, CD8−, TdT−, and MPO−.

Deletions also occur in T-ALL/T-LBL, the most important of which is del(9p), resulting in loss of tumor suppressor gene *CDKN2A*, which is detected in about 30% of cases by cytogenetic analysis and in greater frequency by molecular testing [19, 21]. About 50% of cases have activating mutations involving *NOTCH1*, which encodes a protein critical for early T-cell development [19, 21].

Prognosis

T-ALL in childhood is generally considered a higher-risk disease than B-ALL, partially due to older age and high WBC [19]. Compared to B-ALL, T-ALL is associated with a higher risk of induction failure, early relapse, large mediastinal mass, and isolated CNS relapse [19]. MRD following therapy is generally a strong adverse prognostic factor.

Early T-cell Precursor Lymphoblastic Leukemia

Early T-cell precursor lymphoblastic leukemia (ETP-ALL) is a unique subtype of T-ALL derived from a subset of thymocytes that represent recent immigrants from the bone marrow to the thymus and retain multilineage differentiation potential. ETP-ALL has a characteristic expression profile and immunophenotype [22]. By definition, blasts in ETP-ALL lack CD1a and CD8 expression but express CD7 and one or more of the myeloid/stem cell markers CD34, CD117, HLA-DR, CD13, CD33, CD11b, and CD65 (Figure 13.15) [8, 19]. They also express other T-cell markers such as cytoplasmic or rarely surface CD3, and sometimes CD2 and/or CD4 [19]. CD5 is often dim or negative. Dim CD5 expression is defined by at least one log dimmer than the residual normal T-cells or less than 75% of the blasts are positive for CD5. Recent studies using intensive therapy have demonstrated that, despite the higher rate of MRD in ETP-ALL compared to T-ALL patients, there is no significant difference in overall outcome [8,19].

References

1. Borowitz MJ, Chan JKC, Downing JR, Le Beau MM, Arber DA. B-lymphoblastic leukaemia/lymphoma with recurrent genetic abnormalities. In Swerdlow SH, Campo E, Harris NL, Jaffe ES, Pileri SA, Stein H, et al., eds. WHO classification of tumours of haematopoietic and lymphoid tissues. Revised 4th ed. Lyon: IARC Press; 2017:203–9.

2. Geethakumari PR, Hoffmann MS, Pemmaraju N, Hu S, Jorgensen JL, O'Brien S, Daver N. Extramedullary B lymphoblastic leukemia/lymphoma (B-ALL/LBL): A diagnostic challenge. Clin Lymphoma, Myeloma Leukemia. 2014 Aug; 14(4): e115.

3. Cortelazzo S, Ponzoni M, Ferreri AJ, Hoelzer D. Lymphoblastic lymphoma. Crit Rev Oncol/Hematol. 2011 Sep 1; 79(3): 330–43.

4. Lin P, Jones D, Dorfman DM, Medeiros LJ. Precursor B-cell lymphoblastic lymphoma: A predominantly extranodal tumor with low propensity for leukemic involvement. Am J Surg Pathol. 2000 Nov 1; 24(11): 1480–90.

5. Soslow RA, Baergen RN, Warnke RA. B-lineage lymphoblastic lymphoma is a clinicopathologic entity distinct from other histologically similar aggressive lymphomas with blastic morphology. Cancer. 1999 Jun 15; 85(12): 2648–54.

6. Maitra A, McKenna RW, Weinberg AG, Schneider NR, Kroft SH. Precursor B-cell lymphoblastic lymphoma: A study of nine cases lacking blood and bone marrow involvement and review of the literature. Am J Clin Pathol. 2001 Jun 1; 115(6): 868–75.

7. Perkins SL, McKenna R. Precursor lymphoid neoplasms. In Kjeldsberg CR, Perkins SL, eds. Practical diagnosis of hematologic disorders, 5th ed., Volume 2, Malignant disorders. Singapore: American Society for Clinical Pathology; 2010:691–719.

8. Duffied AS, Racke FK, Borowitz MJ. Precursor B- and T-cell neoplasms. In Jaffe E, Arber D, Campo E, Harris NL, Quintanilla-Martinez L, eds. Hematopathology. 2nd ed. Philadelphia, PA: Elsevier; 2017:761–73.

9. Inaba H, Mulligan CG. Pediatric acute lymphoblastic leukemia. Haematologica. 2020 Nov 1; 105(11): 2524–39.

10. Hunger SP, Mulligan CG. Acute lymphoblastic leukemia in children. N Engl J Med. 2015 Oct 15; 373(16): 1541–52.

11. Van der Linden MH, Valsecchi MG, De Lorenzo P, Möricke A, Janka G, Leblanc TM, et al. Outcome of congenital acute lymphoblastic leukemia treated on the Interfant-99 protocol. Blood. 2009 Oct 29; 114(18): 3764–8.

12. Pieters R, Schrappe M, De Lorenzo P, Hann I, De Rossi G, Felice M, et al. A treatment protocol for infants younger than 1 year with acute lymphoblastic leukaemia (Interfant-99): An observational study and a multicentre randomised trial. Lancet. 2007 Jul 21; 370(9583): 240–50.

13. Van der Linden MH, Creemers S, Pieters R. Diagnosis and management of neonatal leukaemia. Semin Fetal Neonatal Med. 2012 Aug 1; 17(4): 192–5.

14. Knez V, Liu X, Schowinsky J, Pan Z, Wang D, Lorsbach R, et al. Clinicopathologic and genetic spectrum of infantile B-lymphoblastic leukemia: A multi-institutional study. Leukemia Lymphoma. 2019 Mar 21; 60(4): 1006–13.

15. Kang H, Wilson CS, Harvey RC, Chen I, Murphy MH, Atlas SR, et al. Gene expression profiles predictive of outcome and age in infant acute lymphoblastic leukemia: A Children's Oncology Group study. Blood. 2012 Feb 23; 119 (8): 1872–81.

16. Sakaki H, Kanegane H, Nomura K, Goi K, Sugita K, Miura M, et al. Early lineage switch in an infant acute lymphoblastic leukemia. Int J Hematol. 2009 Dec; 90(5): 653–5.

17. Rossi JG, Bernasconi AR, Alonso CN, Rubio PL, Gallego MS, Carrara CA, et al. Lineage switch in childhood acute leukemia: An unusual event with poor outcome. Am J Hematol. 2012 Sep; 87(9): 890–7.

18. Park M, Koh KN, Kim BE, Im HJ, Jang S, Park CJ, et al. Lineage switch at relapse of childhood acute leukemia: A report of four cases. J Korean Med Sci. 2011 Jun; 26(6): 829–31.

19. Borowitz MJ, Chan JKC, Béné M-C, Arber A. T-lymphoblastic leukaemia/lymphoma. In Swerdlow SH, Campo E, Harris NL, Jaffe ES, Pileri SA, Stein H, et al., eds. WHO classification of tumours of haematopoietic and lymphoid tissues. Revised 4th ed. Lyon: IARC Press; 2017:209–12.

20. Raetz EA, Perkins SL, Bhojwani D, Smock K, Philip M, Carroll WL, Min DJ. Gene expression profiling reveals intrinsic differences between T-cell acute lymphoblastic leukemia and T-cell lymphoblastic lymphoma. Pediatr Blood Cancer. 2006 Aug; 47(2): 130–40.

21. Uyttebroeck A, Vanhentenrijk V, Hagemeijer A, Boeckx N, Renard M, Wlodarska I, et al. Is there a difference in childhood T-cell acute lymphoblastic leukaemia and T-cell lymphoblastic lymphoma? Leukemia Lymphoma. 2007; 48(9): 1745–54.

22. Coustan-Smith E, Mullighan CG, Onciu M, Behm FG, Raimondi SC, Pei D, et al. Early T-cell precursor leukaemia: A subtype of very high-risk acute lymphoblastic leukaemia. Lancet Oncol. 2009 Feb 1; 10(2): 147–56.

Blastic Plasmacytoid Dendritic Cell Neoplasm

Stephanie D. Schniederjan, Aurelia Meloni-Ehrig, Caroline An, Kristian T. Schafernak

Introduction

Blastic plasmacytoid dendritic cell neoplasm (BPDCN) is a rare, aggressive malignancy that is notable for frequently presenting with skin lesions and for its unfavorable prognosis. The revised fourth edition of the World Health Organization classification places BPDCN in a separate, stand-alone chapter between acute myeloid leukemia and acute leukemias of ambiguous lineage in recognition of its distinct lineage and aggressive clinical behavior. [1]. Knowledge of the cell of origin and the increasing availability of markers specific for plasmacytoid dendritic cells has recently allowed the recognition of heterogeneity in the clinical presentation and immunophenotype of BPDCN [2].

BPDCN is more common in older adults than in pediatric populations and has a male-to-female ratio of approximately 3:1 [2]. The prognosis has historically been dismal, although new anti-CD123 therapy appears to improve survival, and younger age predicts a better outcome [3, 4]. While BPDCN frequently manifests initially as skin lesions, which are most commonly nodular, cases may present with leukemia, lymphadenopathy, and/or cytopenias; of note, 24% of pediatric cases presented without skin involvement in one recently reported series [2, 4, 5].

Using standard immunophenotypic profiling by flow cytometry or immunohistochemistry, there is considerable overlap with other hematolymphoid neoplasms, including myeloid/monocytic sarcoma or "leukemia cutis," acute myeloid leukemia with monocytic differentiation (AML-MD), aggressive NK-cell leukemia, NK-lymphoblastic leukemia/lymphoma, extranodal NK/T-cell lymphoma, and T-lymphoblastic lymphoma [1, 6]. The distinction between myeloid sarcoma/AML-MD and BPDCN is clinically significant, as AML-like

therapy may be associated with inferior outcomes in BPDCN [7]. Although BPDCN and AML-MD share a proclivity for extramedullary manifestations, gene-expression profiling and array comparative genomic hybridization have provided evidence supporting distinct lineages [8].

Another diagnostic consideration, depending on the presentation, is a mature plasmacytoid dendritic cell proliferation (MPDCP), which expresses a similar immunoprofile and may have a greater propensity for expression of aberrant lymphoid and myeloid/monocytic markers. In MPDCP, CD56 is negative and the Ki-67 proliferation index is lower than in BPDCN (less than 10% versus greater than 30% in BPDCN) [9, 10].

Due to the overlapping immunophenotype with other categories of hematologic malignancies, a comprehensive panel of antibodies is used for the diagnosis of BPDCN. Positivity for at least four of the following markers has been proposed as allowing for reliable diagnosis: CD4, CD56, CD123, CD303, TCL1, and TCF4 [9]. TCF4 and CD123 have shown high sensitivity and specificity [11].

Karyotypes of children with BPDCN are often complex, as seen in adults. Studies that analyzed cytogenetic abnormalities found pediatric cases predominantly showed deletions of 5q, 12p,13q, 6q, and 15q, as well as monosomies, primarily of chromosome 9 [12, 13]. Next-generation sequencing and whole-exome sequencing studies performed on BPDCN found mutations primarily involving TET2 (57%), ZRSR2 (57%), ASXL1 (28%), NPM1 (20%), NEA (20%), IKZF1/2/3 (20%), ZEB2 (16%), and TP53 (14%) [14, 15]. About 50% of the tumors are characterized by mutations involving DNA methylation or chromatin remodeling genes, and these mutations are associated with a worse outcome and lower survival [14, 15].

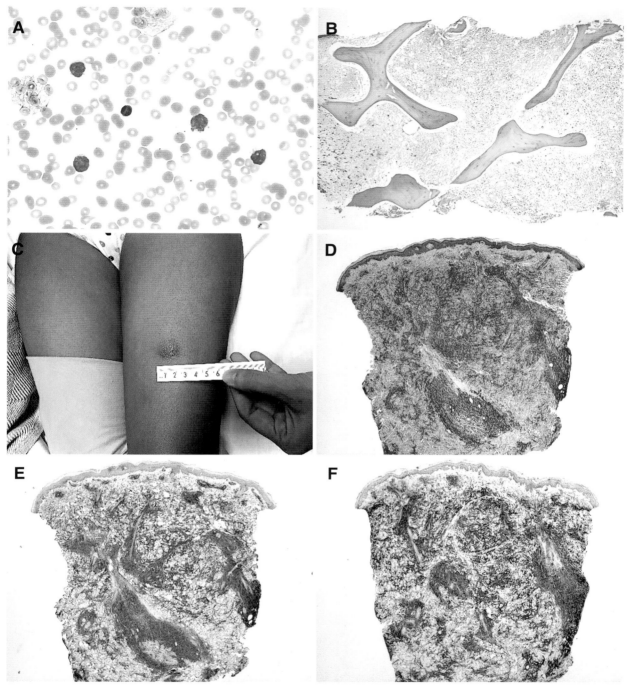

Figure 14.1 An 11-year-old girl presented with profound normocytic anemia and marked thrombocytopenia (a, 400x). The peripheral blood smear was remarkable for leukocytosis with many circulating "blasts." The "blasts" were intermediate-sized with rather scant cytoplasm. Some cells have vacuoles and highly irregular nuclear contours. The bone marrow was largely necrotic (b, 40x). She also had an enlarging thigh skin lesion (c) and increasing generalized lymphadenopathy. The skin punch biopsy (d, 40x) showed a mostly crushed dermal infiltrate of mononuclear cells separated from the epidermis by a Grenz zone dissecting collagen bundles and surrounding but sparing skin appendages. The tumor cells were diffusely positive for CD4 (e, 40x), CD56 (f, 40x), CD123, CD43, MUM1, and BCL2, with weak or partial staining for CD7 (finely granular), CD68 (dot-like), CD117, and BCL6 (not shown).

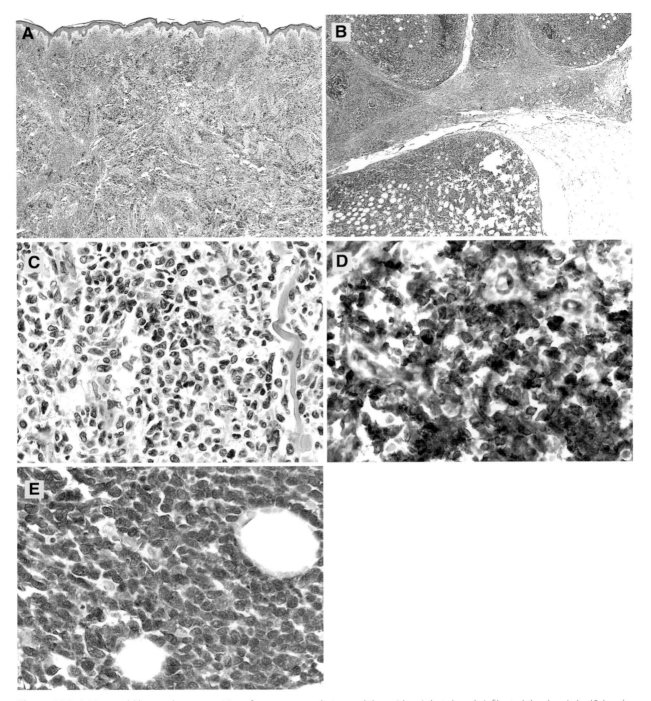

Figure 14.2 A 16-year-old boy underwent excision of an arm tumor that spared the epidermis but densely infiltrated the dermis (a, 40x) and subcutaneous fat (b, 40x). The tumor cells were intermediate in size, with scant cytoplasm and irregular to twisted nuclei containing coarse to vesicular chromatin and inconspicuous nucleoli (c, 400x). The tumor cells were positive for CD123 (d, 400x) and TCL1 (e, 400x).

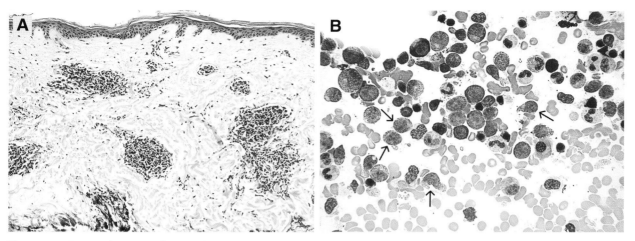

Figure 14.3 Perivascular tumor infiltrate in shave biopsy (a, 40x) and bone marrow involvement: tumor cells in the aspirate smear (b, 400x) have an elongated, hand-mirror appearance with pseudopodia and vacuolated cytoplasm.

References

1. Facchetti FP, Petrella T, Pileri, SA. Blastic plasmacytoid dendritic cell neoplasm. In Swerdlow SH, Campo E, Harris NL, Jaffe ES, Pileri, SA, Stein H, et al. eds. WHO classification of tumours of haematopoietic and lymphoid tissues. 4th ed., revised ed. Lyon: International Agency for Research on Cancer; 2017:174–7.

2. Martín-Martín LLA, Vidriales B, Caballero MD, Rodrigues AS, Ferreira SI, Lima M, et al. Classification and clinical behavior of blastic plasmacytoid dendritic cell neoplasms according to their maturation-associated immunophenotypic profile. Oncotarget. 2015; **6**(22): 19204–16.

3. Gurbaxani S. Blastic plasmacytoid dendritic cell neoplasm. In Larson RA, ed. UpToDate. Waltham, MA: Wolters Kluwer; 2019.

4. Jegalian AG, Buxbaum NP, Facchetti F, Raffeld M, Pittaluga S, Wayne AS, et al. Blastic plasmacytoid dendritic cell neoplasm in children: Diagnostic features and clinical implications. Haematologica. 2010; **95**(11): 1873–9.

5. Tzankov A, Hebeda K, Kremer M, Leguit R, Orazi A, Van der Walt J, et al. Plasmacytoid dendritic cell proliferations and neoplasms involving the bone marrow: Summary of the workshop cases submitted to the 18th Meeting of the European Association for Haematopathology (EAHP) organized by the European Bone Marrow Working Group, Basel 2016. Ann Hematol. 2017; **96**(5): 765–77.

6. Bekkenk MW, Jansen PM, Meijer CJLM, Willemze R. CD56+ hematological neoplasms presenting in the skin: A retrospective analysis of 23 new cases and 130 cases from the literature. Ann Oncol. 2004; **15**(7): 1097–1108.

7. Pagano L, Valentini CG, Pulsoni A, Fisogni S, Carluccio P, Mannelli F, et al. Blastic plasmacytoid dendritic cell neoplasm with leukemic presentation: An Italian multicenter study. Haematologica. 2013; **98**(2): 239–46.

8. Dijkman R, Van Doorn R, Szuhai K, Willemze R, Vermeer MH, Tensen CP. Gene-expression profiling and array-based CGH classify CD4+CD56+ hematodermic neoplasm and cutaneous myelomonocytic leukemia as distinct disease entities. Blood. 2007; **109**(4): 1720–7.

9. Suzuki Y, Kato S, Kohno K, Satou A, Eladl AE, Asano N, et al. Clinicopathological analysis of 46 cases with CD4(+) and/or CD56(+) immature haematolymphoid malignancy: Reappraisal of blastic plasmacytoid dendritic cell and related neoplasms. Histopathology. 2017; **71**(6): 972–84.

10. Facchetti F, Cigognetti M, Fisogni S, Rossi G, Lonardi S, Vermi W. Neoplasms derived from plasmacytoid dendritic cells. Mod Pathol. 2016; **29**(2): 98–111.

11. Sukswai N, Aung PP, Yin CC, Li S, Wang W, Wang SA, et al. Dual expression of TCF4 and CD123 is highly sensitive and specific for blastic plasmacytoid dendritic cell neoplasm. Am J Surg Pathol. 2019; **43**(10): 1429–37.

12. Leroux D, Mugneret F, Callanan M, Radford-Weiss I, Dastugue N, Feuillard J, et al. CD4(+), CD56(+) DC2 acute leukemia is characterized by recurrent clonal chromosomal changes affecting 6 major targets: A study of 21 cases by the Groupe Francais de Cytogenetique Hematologique. Blood. 2002; **99**(11): 4154–9.

13. Lucioni M, Novara F, Fiandrino G, Riboni R, Fanoni D, Arra M, et al. Twenty-one cases of blastic plasmacytoid dendritic cell neoplasm: Focus on biallelic locus 9p21.3 deletion. Blood. 2011; **118**(17): 4591–4.

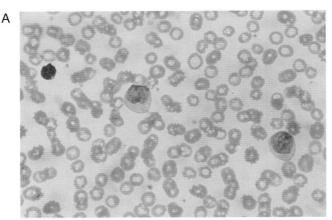

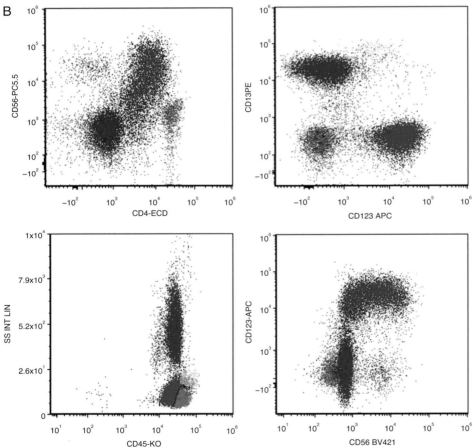

Figure 14.4 A 17-year-old boy presented with circulating blasts and lymphadenopathy (a, 400x) blast in peripheral smear, Wright stain; (b), PDCs are shown in blue, granulocytes in purple, lymphocytes in red. CD4 versus CD56; CD123 versus CD13; CD45 versus side scatter; CD56 versus CD123. Note the redCD4-positive T-cells and the CD56-positive NK-cells. CD4, CD56 and CD123 are coexpressed; the BPDC population lacks CD13.

14. Menezes J, Acquadro F, Wiseman M, Gomez-Lopez G, Salgado RN, Talavera-Casanas JG, et al. Exome sequencing reveals novel and recurrent mutations with clinical impact in blastic plasmacytoid dendritic cell neoplasm. Leukemia. 2014; **28**(4): 823–9.

15. Taylor J, Kim SS, Stevenson KE, Yoda A, Kopp N, Louissaint A, et al. Loss-of-function mutations in the splicing factor ZRSR2 are common in blastic plasmacytoid dendritic cell neoplasm and have male predominance. Blood. 2013; **122**(21): 741.

A

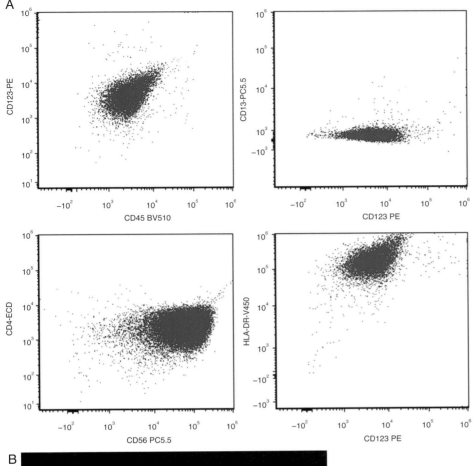

B

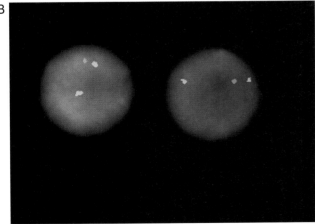

Figure 14.5 A 21-year-old woman with a history of BPDCN treated with hyper-CVAD achieved complete remission. Ten months later, testing showed CSF involvement: (a) flow cytometry CD45 versus CD123 CD123 versus HLA-DR, CD123 versus CD13, and CD56 versus CD4 scatterplots; chromosome analysis showed a complex karyotype. (b) Deletion 5q was confirmed by FISH (missing one red signal).

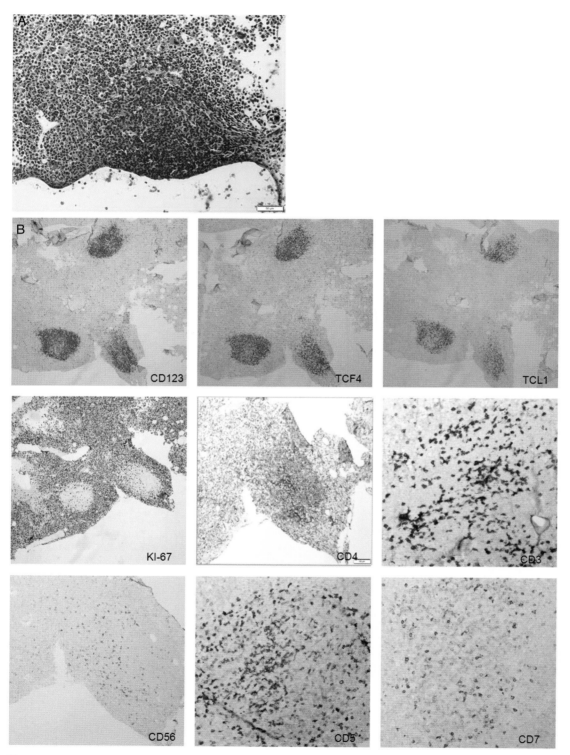

Figure 14.6 MPDCP in an adult with a history of MPN who later developed AML: bone marrow biopsy showed multiple foci of dense "lymphoid" aggregates (a, H&E, 400x); (b), CD123, TCF4, TCL1, Ki-67, CD4, CD56 (mostly negative), CD7, and CD5 are aberrantly expressed (weakly) by the PDCs.

Chapter 15

Acute Myeloid Leukemia and Related Precursor Neoplasms

Virginia Knez, Xiayuan Liang, Billie Carstens, Silvia T Bunting

Acute myeloid leukemia (AML) is a heterogeneous group of diseases representing a clonal expansion of immature, non-lymphoid, bone marrow-derived cells that involve the bone marrow, blood, and extramedullary tissues. In general, blood or bone marrow blast counts ≥20% (Figure 15.1) are required for diagnosing AML, except for AML with t(8;21) (q22; q22.1), AML with inv (16) (p13.1q22) or t(16;16) (p13.1; q22), and acute promyelocytic leukemia (APML) with *PML-RARA* [1–4]. The World Health Organization (WHO) classification incorporates morphologic, immunophenotypic, genetic, and clinical features to define prognostically significant disease [3–5].

Acute Myeloid Leukemia with Recurrent Genetic Abnormalities

Table 15.1 summarizes the clinical and pathologic features of AML with recurrent genetic abnormalities (Figures 15.2–15.9) [2–6].

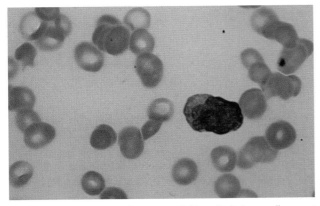

Figure 15.1 Blood smear shows a myeloblast displaying small amount of cytoplasm, a prominent Auer rod, fine chromatin, and distinct nucleoli (Wright-Giemsa, 1,000x).

Acute Myeloid Leukemia with Myelodysplasia-Related Changes

AML with myelodysplasia-related changes (AML-MRC) is defined as ≥20% blood or bone marrow blasts with morphological features of myelodysplasia, or occurring in patients with a prior history of myelodysplastic syndrome (MDS) or myelodysplastic/myeloproliferative neoplasm (MDS/MPN), or with MDS-related cytogenetic abnormalities. Furthermore, the specific genetic abnormalities characteristic of AML with recurrent genetic abnormalities are absent [3]. AML-MRC is uncommon in children. Patients usually present with pancytopenia. In children, the clinical course likely is slowly progressive. Therefore, cases with 20–29% marrow blasts and stable clinical course for ≥2 months can be considered as either MDS or AML [7].

The diagnostic criteria of AML-MRC are that dysplasia must be present in ≥50% of the cells in at least two hematopoietic lineages (Figure 15.10) [3]. For cases without sufficient elements for assessing for multilineage dysplasia or that do not meet the aforementioned morphologic criteria, AML-MRC can be diagnosed on the basis of detection of MDS-related cytogenetic abnormalities such as -7, del(7q), del(5q) or t(5q) etc. and/or a history of MDS or MDS/MPN [3].

The genetic abnormalities are similar to those seen in MDS. Trisomy 8 and del(20q) (common in MDS) are not by themselves sufficient to classify a case as AML-MRC [3]. *NPM1*, *FLT3*, or *CEBPA* mutations may be identified in cases of AML with multilineage dysplasia. When an MDS-related cytogenetic abnormality is absent, such cases should be classified as AML with mutated *NPM1* or AML with biallelic mutation of *CEBPA*, rather than AML-MRC [2, 4]. AML-MRC has a worse prognosis than other AML subtypes.

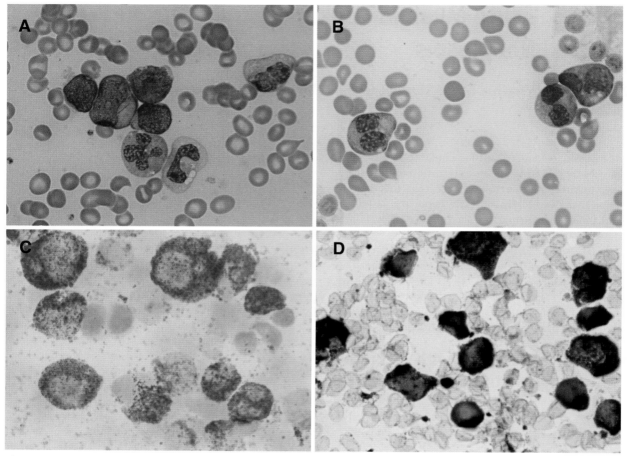

Figure 15.2 AML with t(8;21) (q22; q22.1); *RUNX1-RUNX1T1*.

a. Bone marrow shows blasts with deep blue rim of cytoplasm, prominent nucleolus, and a single long, sharp Auer rod and maturing granulocytes with orange-colored granules (Wright-Giemsa, 1,000x).
b. Dysplasia is present with pseudo-Pelger-Huet neutrophils (Wright-Giemsa, 1,000x).
c. Myeloblasts are myeloperoxidase-positive (MPO cytochemical stain, 1,000x).
d. Myeloblasts are Sudan Black B-positive (SBB histochemical stain, 1,000x).
e. Cytogenetics. The upper panel shows FISH analysis. *RUNX1* probe is labeled green. *RUNX1T1* probe is labeled red. The upper left is a normal pattern (separate red and green signals). The upper-middle images show *RUNX1-RUNX1T1* rearrangement (red-green fusion signals). The upper right is a schematic representation. The lower image shows the karyotype of t(8;21) (q22; q22.1).

Therapy-Related Myeloid Neoplasms

Therapy-related myeloid neoplasms (t-MNs) are a late complication of chemotherapy and radiation therapy. They consist of t-AML, t-MDS, and t-MDS/MPN [4]. The pathogenesis of t-MNs in children is probably secondary to a combination of age at the time of primary cancer diagnosis, genetic susceptibility (neurofibromatosis type 1, Fanconi anemia, Bloom syndrome, Schwachman syndrome, etc.), environmental exposure, and prior therapeutic regimens

[8]. Two subsets of t-MNs are recognized clinically (Table 15.2) [4, 8].

The morphologic diagnostic criteria for t-MDS, t-AML, and t-MDS/MPN should follow the guidelines for primary MDS, MDS/MPN, or de novo AML [8]. Most cases are associated with multilineage dysplasia and myelomonocytic or monoblastic/monocytic differentiation (Figure 15.11). Genetic information must be incorporated into the diagnosis in t-MNs. The prognosis

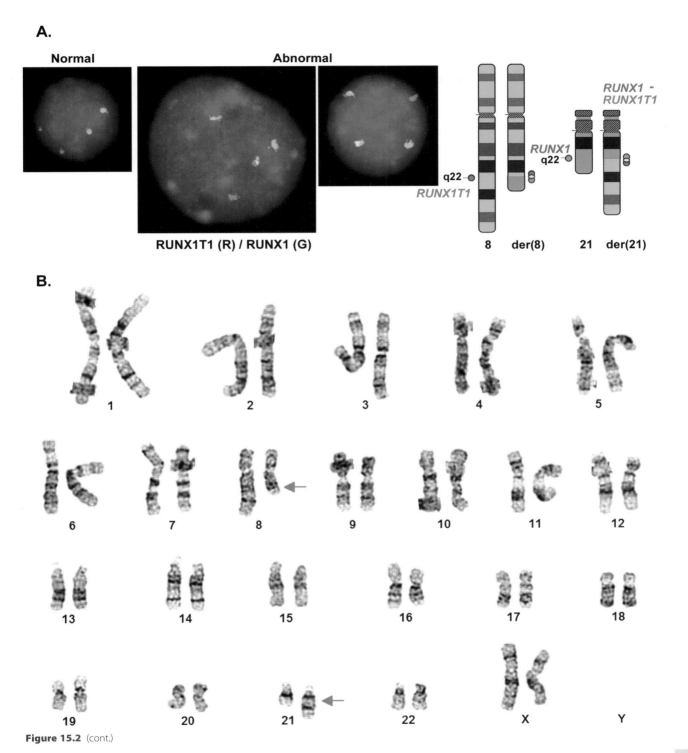

Figure 15.2 (cont.)

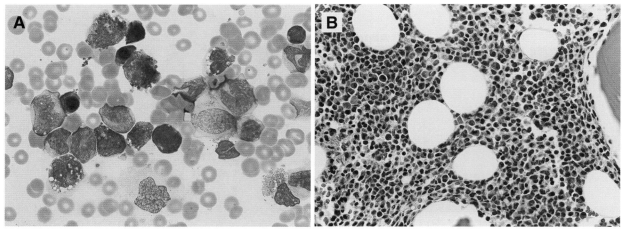

Figure 15.3 AML with inv (16) (p13.1q22) or t(16;16) (p13.1; q22); *CBFB-MYH11*.

a. Bone marrow shows blasts with myeloid and monocytic differentiation. Myeloblasts display scant cytoplasm, fine chromatin, and distinct nucleoli. Monocytic blasts/promonocytes show abundant cytoplasm and irregular nuclei. Eosinophils are increased with large basophilic-colored granules (Wright-Giemsa, 1,000x).

b. The biopsy shows increased blasts and eosinophilia (H&E, 400x).

c. Cytogenetics. The upper panel is a FISH analysis. 3'*CBFB* probe is labeled green. 5'*CBFB/MYH11* probe is labeled red. The upper left is a normal pattern (red-green fusion signals). The upper middle shows *CBFB-MYH11* rearrangement (red and green split signals). The upper right is a schematic representation. The lower image shows the karyotype of inv (16) (p13.1q22).

is poor. Cases with *TP53* mutations and a complex karyotype have a particularly poor outcome [4].

Acute Myeloid Leukemia, Not Otherwise Specified

Table 15.3 summarizes the clinical and pathologic features of AML in this category (Figures 15.12 and 15.13) [2]. Mutation analysis and cytogenetic studies are required before a case can be placed into this category.

Myeloid Sarcoma

Myeloid sarcoma (MS) is an extramedullary tumor mass consisting of myeloid blasts with or without maturation. Infiltration of any site of the body by myeloid blasts in a patient with leukemia is not classified as MS unless it presents with tumor masses in which the tissue architecture is effaced [5].

It is more common in pediatric patients. The frequency may reflect association with the t(8;21), inv(16), and 11q23 translocation subtypes. The frequently affected sites include skin, lymph nodes (Figure 15.14), gastrointestinal tract, bone, soft tissue, and gonads [5]. The myeloblasts of MS usually form sheets. In most cases, blasts display myelomonocytic or pure monoblastic features [5].

Acute Myeloid Leukemia with t(8;16) (p11; p13); *KAT6A-CREBBP*

AML with t(8;16) (p11; p13) comprises <1% of AML [9]. Possibly because of the low incidence, it is not yet recognized as a recurrent genetic abnormality by the WHO system [9]. Almost half of the cases were <2 years at diagnosis and a third were diagnosed in newborns [9]. Cases show a female predominance [9]. Leukemia cutis, erythrophagocytosis, and disseminated intravascular coagulation (DIC) are present frequently [9]. The central nervous system may also be involved [9]. Most cases demonstrate blasts with myelomonocytic or monocytic morphology (Figure 15.15) [9]. Erythrophagocytosis (leukemic blasts ingest red blood cells) is found in 70% of cases.

The t(8;16) (p11; p13) results in the fusion of *KAT6A* located on chromosome 8p11 and CREB- binding protein (*CREBBP*) located on chromosome 16p13 [9], resulting in leukemogenesis.

The disease has an intermediate survival [9]. Early recognition of this disease is important because patients have a high death rate from DIC. Although nonspecific, the presence of hemophagocytosis should raise suspicion for this disease. Spontaneous remissions have occurred in a subset of neonatal cases [9].

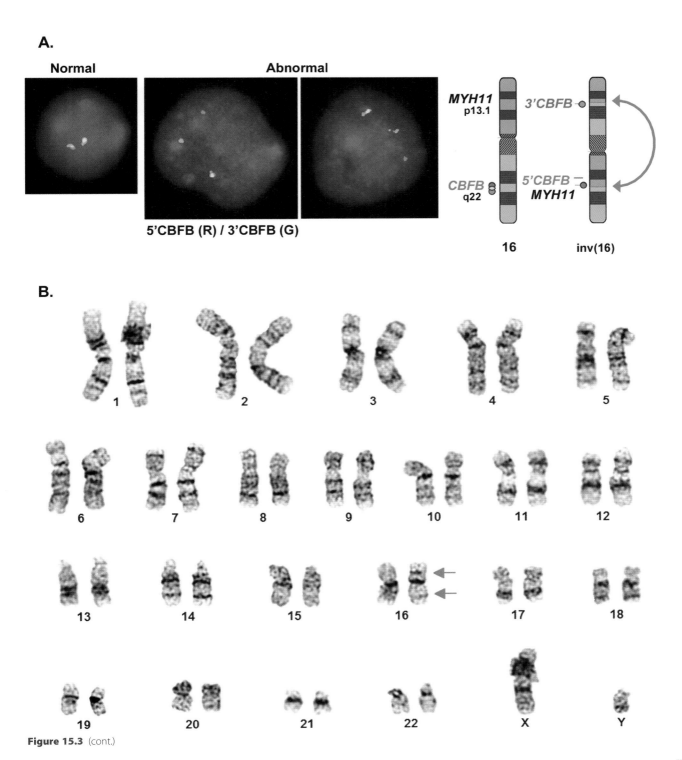

Figure 15.3 (cont.)

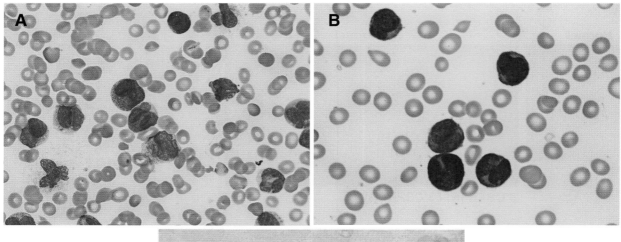

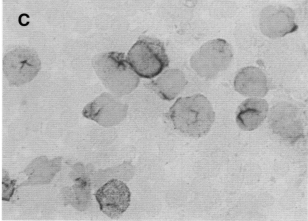

Figure 15.4 APML with *PML-RARA*.

a. Hypergranular variant: neoplastic promyelocytes show numerous cytoplasmic granules and bilobed nuclei. A Faggot cell with a bundle of Auer rods is seen in the middle of the image (Wright-Giemsa, 1,000x).

b. Hypogranular variant: neoplastic promyelocytes reveal absence of cytoplasmic granules and predominantly bilobed nuclei that may cause confusion with neoplastic monocytes (Wright-Giemsa, 1,000x).

c. Neoplastic promyelocytes are positive for myeloperoxidase (MPO cytochemical stain, 1,000x).

d. Cytogenetics. The upper panel shows a FISH analysis. The *PML* probe is labeled red. The *RARA* probe is labeled green. The upper left shows a normal pattern (separate red and green signals). The upper middle shows *PML-RARA* gene rearrangement (red-green fusion signals). The upper right is a schematic representation. The lower image is the karyotype showing t(15;17) (q24.1; q21.2).

Acute Leukemia of Ambiguous Lineage

Acute leukemia of ambiguous lineage (ALAL) is rare and comprises <4% of acute leukemia. It is a high-risk leukemia and has a poor prognosis. The classification is based on criteria outlined in the WHO classification [10]. Table 15.4 shows the different subtypes of ALAL.

Flow cytometric immunophenotyping plays an important role in the classification of ALAL. Table 15.5 delineates the requirements for assigning more than one lineage to a single blast population [10, 11].

MPO is considered the specific hallmark of the myeloid component of mixed phenotype acute leukemia (MPAL). Some MPO antibodies have been shown to react with B- or T-ALL cells nonspecifically by flow cytometry (Figure 15.16). Thus, it is recommended not to classify a typical B-ALL with sole MPO expression as MPAL. A typical B/myeloid leukemia shows a pattern of heterogeneity (Figure 15.17). To assign T-cell lineage, the brightest cCD3-positive blasts should reach the similar intensity of the normal residual T-cells (Figure 15.18). The CD3 antibody should detect a CD3 epsilon

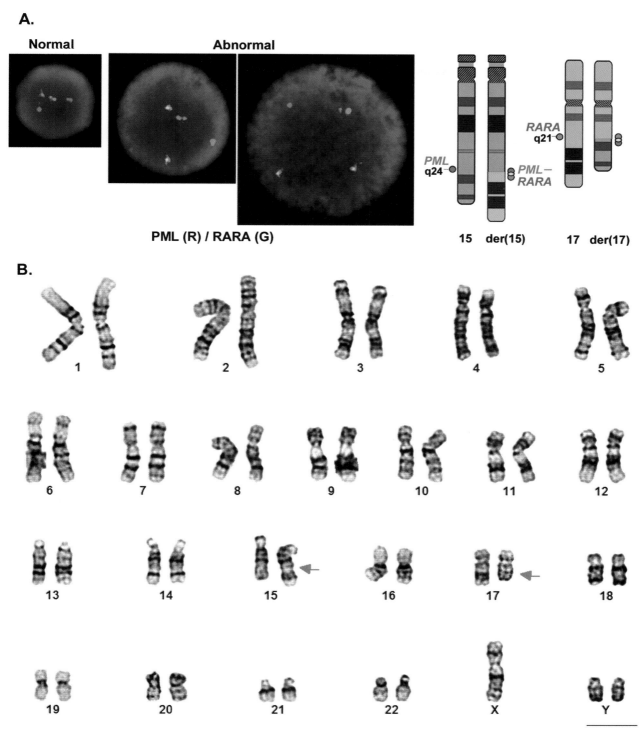

Figure 15.4 (cont.)

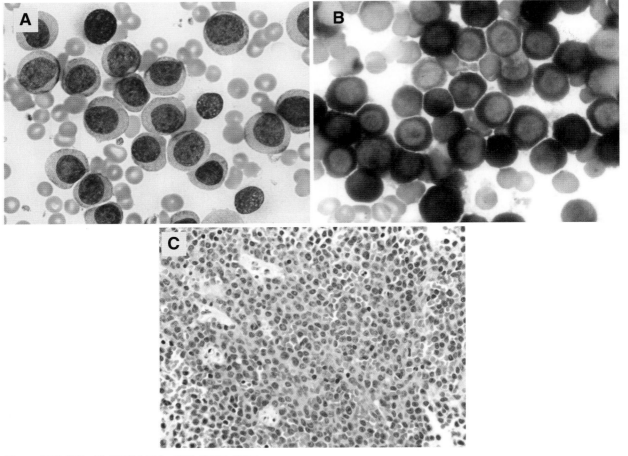

Figure 15.5 AML with t(9;11) (p21.3; q23.3); *KMT2A-MLLT3*.

a. Monoblasts show very abundant cytoplasm, round nuclei and fine chromatin (Wright-Giemsa, 1,000x).
b. Monoblasts are nonspecific esterase-positive (NSE cytochemical stain, 1,000x).
c. Bone marrow biopsy shows increased monoblasts with abundant cytoplasm, oval nuclei, fine chromatin and conspicuous nucleoli (H&E, 400x).
d. Cytogenetics. The upper panel shows a FISH analysis. 3'*KMT2A* probe is labeled red. *MLLT3*/5'*KMT2A* probe is labeled green. The upper left shows a normal pattern (red-green fusion signals). The upper middle shows *KMT2A-MLLT3* gene rearrangement (red and green split signals). The upper right is a schematic representation. The lower image shows the karyotype of t(9;11) (p21.3; q23.3).

chain. If the antibody can also detect a CD3 zeta chain, which is typically used in a immunohistochemical study, it is not specific to T-cells because a CD3 zeta chain can also present in activated natural killer cells. Occasionally, an acute leukemia shows no evidence of lineage differentiation. There is no expression of lineage specific markers such as cytoplasmic CD3, MPO, or cCD79a (Figure 15.19).

The therapeutic strategies and outcomes for different subtypes of AML are based on their risk category, which is determined by genetic and molecular characters. The revised European Leukemia Net (ELN) version of risk stratification based on genetics has been widely adopted (Table 15.6) [11, 12].

References

1. Arber DA, Brunning RD, Le Beau MM, Falini B, Vardiman JW, Porwit A, et al. Acute myeloid leukemia with recurrent genetic abnormalities. In Swerdlow SH, Campo E, Harris NL, et al., eds. WHO classification of tumours of haematopoietic and lymphoid tissues. Revised 4th ed. Lyon: IARC Press; 2017:130–49.

2. Arber DA, Brunning RD, Orazi A, Porwit A, Peterson LC, Thiele J, et al. Acute myeloid leukemia, NOS. In Swerdlow

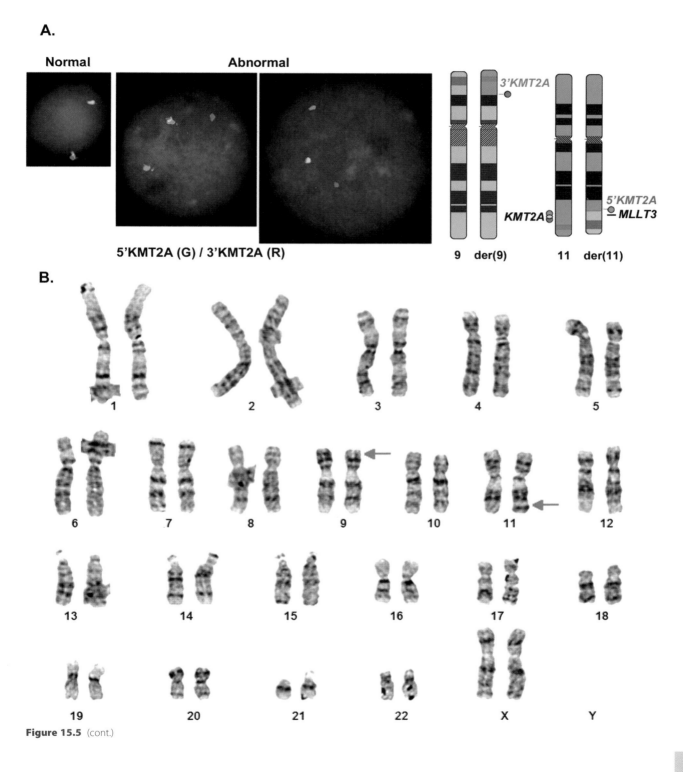

A.

Normal   Abnormal

5'KMT2A (G) / 3'KMT2A (R)

3'KMT2A

KMT2A

5'KMT2A
MLLT3

9   der(9)   11   der(11)

B.

Figure 15.5 (cont.)

SH, Campo E, Harris NL, et al., eds. WHO classification of tumours of haematopoietic and lymphoid tissues. Revised 4th ed. Lyon: IARC Press; 2017:156–66.

3. Arber DA, Brunning RD, Orazi A, Bain BJ, Porwit A, Le Beau MM, Greenberg PL. Acute myeloid leukemia with myelodysplasia-related changes. In Swerdlow SH, Campo E, Harris NL, et al., eds. WHO classification of tumours of haematopoietic and lymphoid tissues. Revised 4th ed. Lyon: IARC Press; 2017:150–2.

4. Vardiman JW, Arber DA, Brunning RD, Larson RA, Matutes E, Baumann I, Kvasnicka HM. Therapy-related myeloid neoplasms. In Swerdlow SH, Campo E, Harris NL, et al., eds. WHO classification of tumours of haematopoietic and lymphoid tissues. Revised 4th ed. Lyon: IARC Press; 2017:153–5.

5. Pileri SA, Orazi A, Falini B. Myeloid sarcoma. In Swerdlow SH, Campo E, Harris NL, et al., eds. WHO classification of tumours of haematopoietic and lymphoid tissues. Revised 4th ed.Lyon: IARC Press; 2017:167–8.

6. Matynia AP, Szankasi P, Shen W, Kelley TW. Molecular genetic biomarkers in myeloid malignancies. Arch Pathol Lab Med. 2015 May; 139(5): 594–601.

7. Greenberg PL, Stone RM, Bejar R, Bennett JM, Bloomfield CD, Borate U, et al. Myelodysplastic syndromes, version

2.2015. J Natl Compr Canc Netw. 2015 Mar 1; 13(3): 261–72.

8. Wang SA. Myelodysplastic syndromes and therapy-related myeloid neoplasms. In Proytcheva MA, ed. Diagnostic pediatric hematopathology. Cambridge: Cambridge University Press; 2011:253–71.

9. Coenen EA, Zwaan CM, Reinhardt D, Harrison CJ, Haas OA, de Haas V, et al. Pediatric acute myeloid leukemia with t (8; 16) (p11; p13), a distinct clinical and biological entity: A collaborative study by the International-Berlin-Frankfurt-Münster AML-study group. Blood. 2013 Oct 10;122(15): 2704–13.

10. Borowitz MJ, Bene MC, Harris NL, Porwit A, Matutes E, Arber DA. Acute leukemias of ambiguous lineage. In Swerdlow SH, Campo E, Harris NL, et al., eds. WHO classification of tumours of haematopoietic and lymphoid tissues. Revised 4th ed. Lyon: IARC Press; 2017:180–7.

11. Döhner H, Estey E, Grimwade D, Amadori S, Appelbaum FR, Büchner T, et al. Diagnosis and management of AML in adults: 2017 ELN recommendations from an international expert panel. Blood. 2017 Jan 26; 129(4): 424–47.

12. Alexander TB, Gu Z, Iacobucci I, Dickerson K, Choi JK, Xu B, et al. The genetic basis and cell of origin of mixed phenotype acute leukaemia. Nature. 2018 Oct; 562(7727): 373–9.

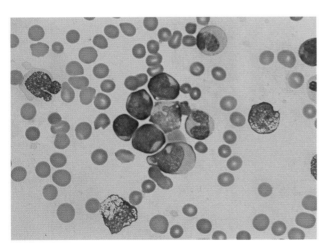

Figure 15.6 AML with t(6;9) (p23; q34.1); *DEK-NUP214*.

a. Blasts reveal a small amount of cytoplasm, round to slightly irregular nuclei, fine chromatin, and distinct nucleoli (Wright-Giemsa, 1,000x).
b. Cytogenetics. The upper panel shows a FISH analysis. The *NUP214* probe is labeled red. The *DEK* probe is labeled green. The upper left shows a normal pattern (red and green split signals). The upper middle shows *DEK-NUP214* gene rearrangement (red-green fusion signals). The upper right is a schematic representation. The lower image shows the karyotype of t(6;9) (p23; q34.1).

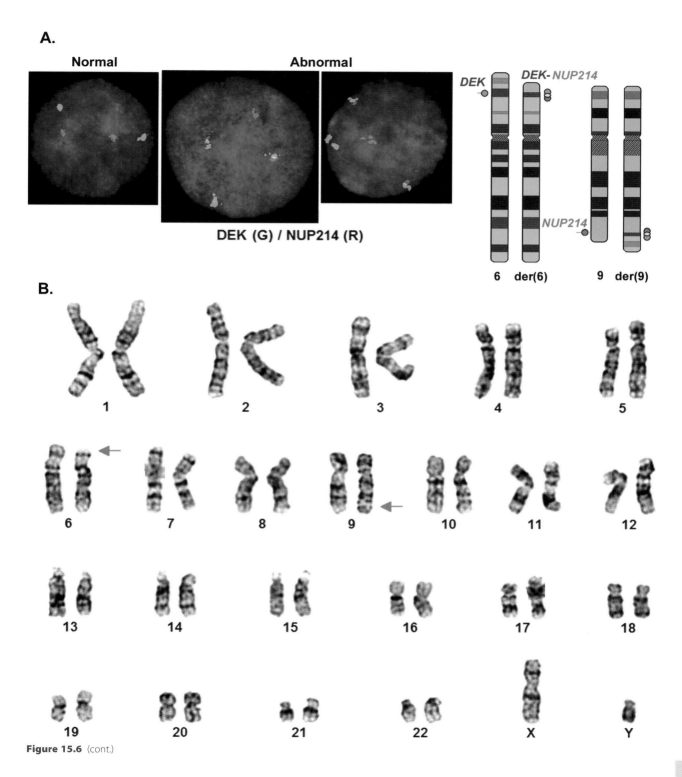

Figure 15.6 (cont.)

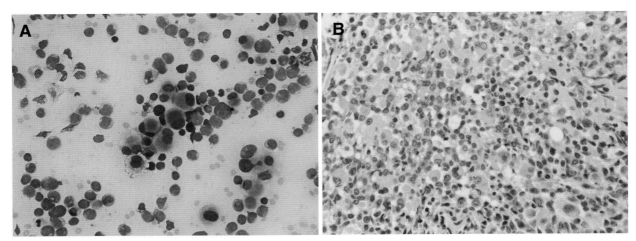

Figure 15.7 AML with inv (3) (q21.3q26.2) or t(3;3) (q21.3; q26.2); *GATA2, MECO.*

a. Bone marrow shows myeloblast proliferation and megakaryocytic hyperplasia with dysplasia (small, non-lobated or bilobed forms and micromegakaryocytes) (Wright-Giemsa, 1,000x).

b. The biopsy illustrates numerous dysplastic megakaryocytes (H&E, 400x).

c. Cytogenetics. The upper panel shows a FISH analysis. The FISH probe is designed with an aqua/blue signal proximal to *EVI1*, a green signal covering *EVI1* (*MECOM*), and red signal distal to *EVI1* (*MYNN*). The upper left shows a normal pattern (red-green-aqua fusion signals). The upper middle shows a *MECOM* rearrangement (one aqua signal separated from the red/green pair). The upper right is a schematic representation. The lower image (karyotype) reveals inv (3) (q21q26) and monosomy 7.

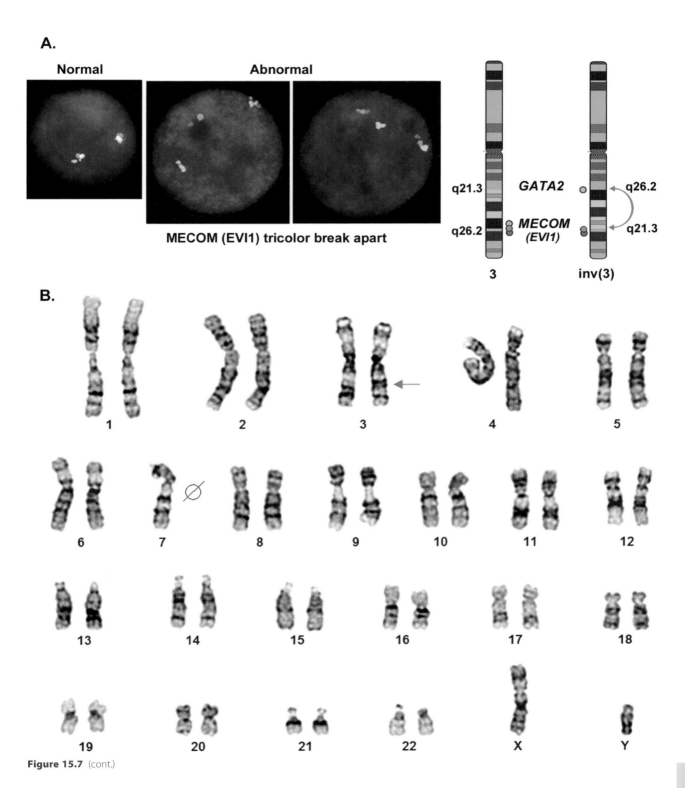

A.

Normal   Abnormal

MECOM (EVI1) tricolor break apart

q21.3   *GATA2*

q26.2   *MECOM*
         (EVI1)

q26.2

q21.3

3   inv(3)

B.

Figure 15.7 (cont.)

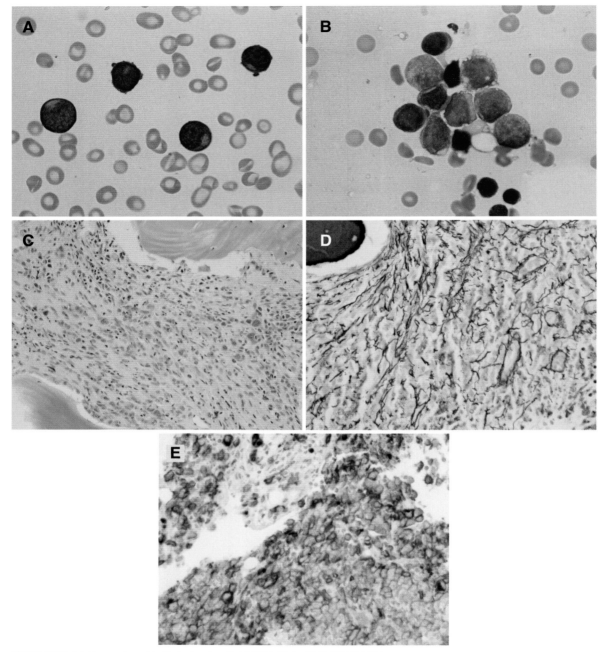

Figure 15.8 Acute megakaryoblastic leukemia with t(1;22) (p13.3; q13.1); *RBM15-MKL1*.

a. Megakaryoblasts show scant cytoplasm mimicking lymphoblasts and distinct cytoplasmic blebs (Wright-Giemsa, 1,000x).
b. Megakaryoblasts display undifferentiated morphology with a small amount of cytoplasm, round nuclei, fine chromatin, and indistinct nucleolus (Wright-Giemsa, 1,000x).
c. Bone marrow biopsy shows megakaryoblast proliferation with dysplasia and fibrosis (H&E, 400x).
d. Bone marrow fibrosis (reticulin stain, 400x).
e. Megakaryoblasts and megakaryocytes are CD42-positive (CD42 immunostain, 400x).
f. Chromosomal analysis reveals t(1;22) (p13.3; q13.1).

A.

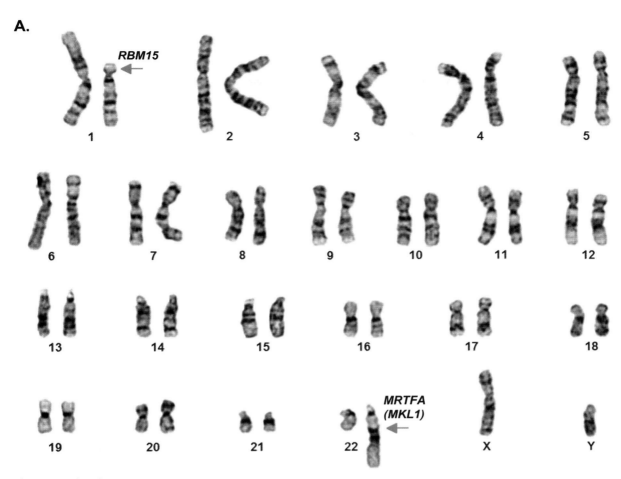

Figure 15.8 (cont.)

Table 15.1 Clinicopathologic features of AML with recurrent genetic abnormalities

	Clinical Features	Pathological Features	Outcome
AML with t(8;21) (q22; q22.1); *RUNX1-RUNX1T1* (Figure 15.2)	- associated with myeloid sarcoma (MS)	- neutrophilic maturation - blasts with big salmon-colored cytoplasmic granules and perinuclear clearing - Auer rods frequently found - CD56+ in some cases	- favorable
AML with inv (16) (p13.1q22) or t(16;16) (p13.1; q22); *CBFB-MYH11* (Figure 15.3)	- infants and toddlers uncommon - MS often	- monocytic and granulocytic differentiation - ↑ abnormal eosinophils	- favorable
Acute promyelocytic leukemia (APML) with *PML-RARA* (Figure 15.4)	- rarely occurring < 10 years - ↑DIC - hypergranular variant: 60–70% - hypogranular/ microgranular variant: ↑WBC	- abnormal reniform/bilobed nuclei - aurophilic granulation in hypergranular variant - Faggot cells may be present in hypergranular variant - HLA-DR−, CD34−	- favorable
AML with t(9;11) (p21.3; q23.3); *KMT2A-MLLT3* (Figure 15.5)	- typically, in children - DIC may present - MS/tissue infiltration often	- monoblastic or monocytic	- limited to de novo cases - intermediate survival
AML with t(6;9) (p23; q34.1); *DEK-NUP214* (Figure 15.6)	- 1% of AML cases	- basophilia may present - most cases CD34+ and CD117+ - 50% cases TdT+	- very poor - *FLT3-ITD* occurring in 69% of pediatric cases
AML with inv (3) (q21.3q26.2) or t(3;3) (q21.3; q26.2); *GATA2, MECO* (Figure 15.7)	- 1–2% of AML cases	- multilineage dysplasia - ↑dysplastic megakaryocytes (small non-lobated or bilobed forms)	- dismal - -7, -5q and complexed karyotype common with worse prognosis
AML (megakaryoblastic) with t(1;22) (p13.3; q13.1); *RBM15-MKL1* (Figure 15.8)	- <1% of AML cases - in young children without DS	- hypocellular aspirate - heterogeneous blast morphology - cytoplasm blebs or pseudopod - dysplastic megakaryocytes - marrow fibrosis - cCD41+ or cCD61+ more specific	- worse than cases without t (1;22)
AML with mutated *NPM1* (Figure 15.9)	- relatively specific for AML - normal karyotype - female > male - ↑WBC and ↑ platelet count - extramedullary involvement often	- blasts with a distinct cup-like nuclear invagination - multilineage dysplasia often - CD34− and HLA-DR− often	- favorable without *FLT3-ITD* mutation

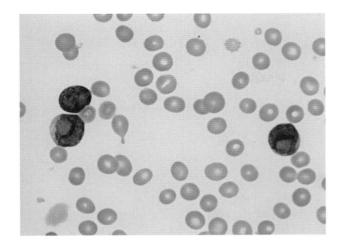

Figure 15.9 AML with mutated *NPM1*.

Blasts exhibit a distinct cuplike (fish mouth) nuclear invagination, fine chromatin, and visible nucleoli (Wright-Giemsa, 1,000x).

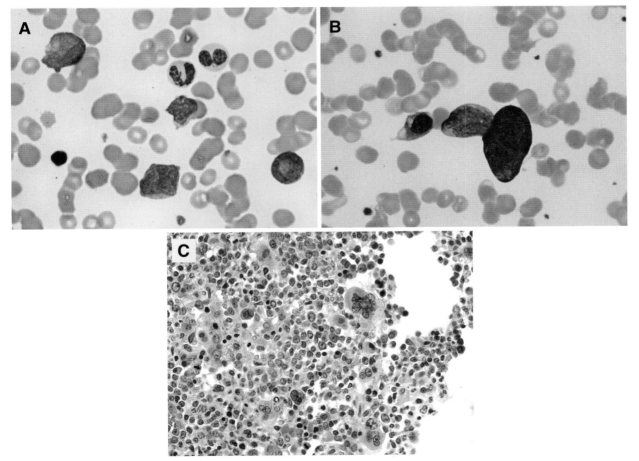

Figure 15.10 AML with myelodysplasia-related changes (AML-MRC).

a. Myeloblasts, pseudo-Pelger-Huet neutrophils, and hypogranulated band (Wright-Giemsa, 1,000x)
b. Myeloblasts and dysplastic erythroid precursors (Wright-Giemsa, 1,000x)
c. Myeloblasts and dysplastic megakaryocytes (small and monolobated forms) (H&E 400x)

Table 15.2 Therapy-related myeloid neoplasms

Etiology	Frequency	Latency Period	Presentations	Cytogenetic Abnormalities
Alkylating agents and/or ionizing radiation	70%	5–10 years	t-MDS, t-MDS/MPN, t-AML	Unbalanced including -5, -7, 7q-, 5q-; complex karyotype; *TP53* mutation
Topoisomerase II inhibitors	20–30%	1–5 years	t-AML	Balanced involving 11q23 (*KMT2A*) rearrangement; t(8;21), t(15;17), inv(16)/t(16;16)

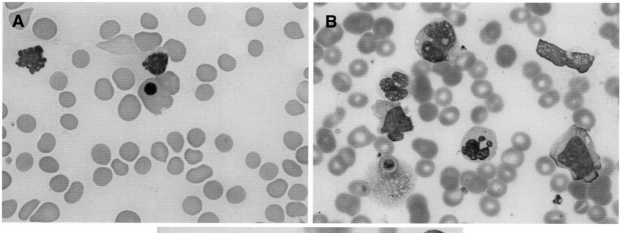

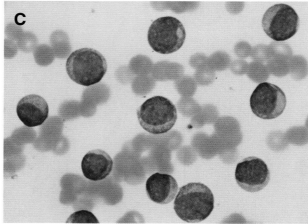

Figure 15.11 Therapy-related myeloid neoplasms.

a. Dyserythropoiesis with megaloblastoid change (Wright-Giemsa, 1,000x)

b. Myeloblasts and dysmyelopoiesis (abnormal segmentation in a neutrophil) (Wright-Giemsa, 1,000x)

c. Monoblastic proliferation (Wright-Giemsa, 1,000x)

d. Cytogenetics. The upper panel shows a FISH analysis (*EGR1*, at 5q31 is labeled red; a probe at 5p15.2 is green). The upper left (two interphase cells) shows loss of one long arm in chromosome 5 (one red and two green signals). The upper middle (metaphase cell) demonstrates one normal chromosome 5 (two red and two green signals) and a deleted 5q at arrow (loss of red signal). The upper right is a schematic representation. The lower image shows a complex karyotype with loss of 5q and 7q.

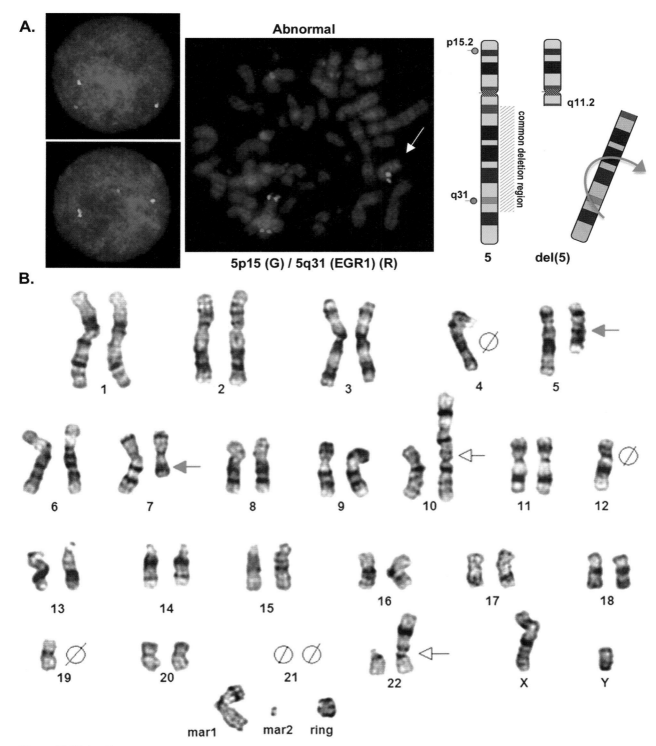

A.

Abnormal

5p15 (G) / 5q31 (EGR1) (R)

p15.2

q11.2

q31

common deletion region

5   del(5)

B.

1   2   3   4   5   6   7   8   9   10   11   12   13   14   15   16   17   18   19   20   21   22   X   Y   mar1   mar2   ring

Figure 15.11 (cont.)

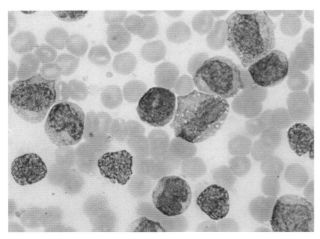

Figure 15.12 Acute monocytic leukemia.
Bone marrow smear shows proliferation of promonocytes that have delicate nuclear folds and abundant cytoplasm with rare cytoplasmic vacuoles (Wright-Giemsa, 1,000x).

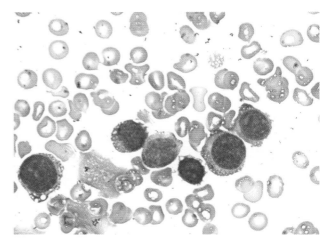

Figure 15.13 Pure erythroid leukemia.
Bone marrow smear shows a number of neoplastic pronormoblasts with round nuclei and blue cytoplasm containing cytoplasmic vacuoles (Wright-Giemsa, 1,000x) (image courtesy Dr. Karen Chisholm).

Table 15.3 Acute myeloid leukemia, NOS (≥20% blasts)

	Pathologic Features	Clinical Features
AML with minimal differentiation	- MPO cytochemical stain + blasts <3% - ≥2 myeloid-associated markers positive	Poor prognosis
AML without maturation	- Myeloblasts ≥90% of nucleated cells in bone marrow (BM) (MPO+ blasts ≥3%) - Maturing granulocytes <10% of BM cells	
AML with maturation	- Myeloblasts <90% of nucleated cells in BM (MPO+ blasts ≥3%) - Maturing granulocytes ≥10% of BM cells	
Acute myelomonocytic leukemia	- Promonocytes are blast equivalent - MPO+ blasts ≥3% - Neutrophils and their precursors ≥20% of BM cells - Monocytes and their precursors ≥20% of BM cells	

Acute monoblastic and monocytic leukemia	- ≥80% of leukemic cells (monoblasts, promonocytes, monocytes) are of monocytic lineage
	  • Acute monoblastic leukemia: ≥80% of leukemic cells are monoblasts
	  • Acute monocytic leukemia: most of leukemic cells are promonocytes or monocytes (Figure 15.12)
	- Expressing ≥2 monocytic markers
		Bleeding, extramedullary masses and CNS+ common

Pure erythroid leukemia	- Erythroid components >80% in BM cells with ≥30% proerythroblasts (Figure 15.13) - No significant myeloblastic component - Positive for alpha-naphthyl acetate esterase, acid phosphatase, and PAS - Expressing glycophorin and hemoglobin A, CD71, E-cadherin	A rapid clinical course, median survival 3 months
Acute megakaryoblastic leukemia	- Megakaryoblasts ≥50% of all blasts - Cases with DS, AML-MRC, t-AML are excluded - Dry tap due to marrow fibrosis	Poor prognosis
Acute basophilic leukemia	- Blasts and immature basophils (may be detected only by electron microscopy) - Skin involvement, organomegaly, lytic lesion and symptoms related to hyperhistaminemia - CD13+, CD33+, CD123+, CD203c+, and CD11b+	Very rare
Acute panmyelosis with myelofibrosis	- Acute panmyeloid proliferation and fibrosis in BM - Marked pancytopenia - BM aspirate usually unsuccessful	Very rare, poor prognosis

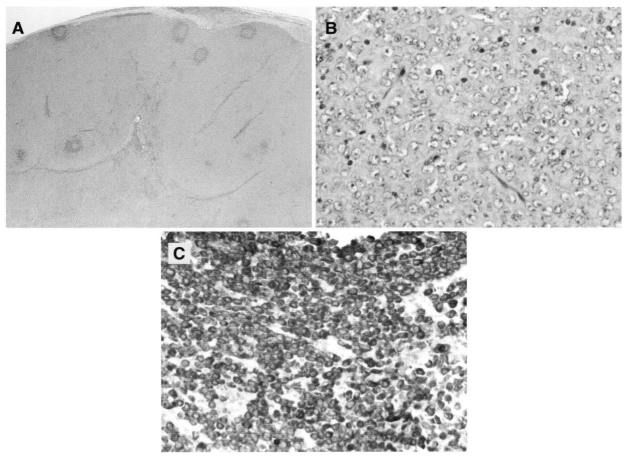

Figure 15.14 Myeloid sarcoma.

a. A lymph node biopsy shows interfollicular expansion by neoplastic cells (H&E, 20x).
b. Neoplastic cells show blast features with scant to small amounts of cytoplasm, fine chromatin, and distinct nucleoli (H&E, 400x).
c. Myeloblasts are positive for myeloperoxidase (MPO immunostain, 400x).

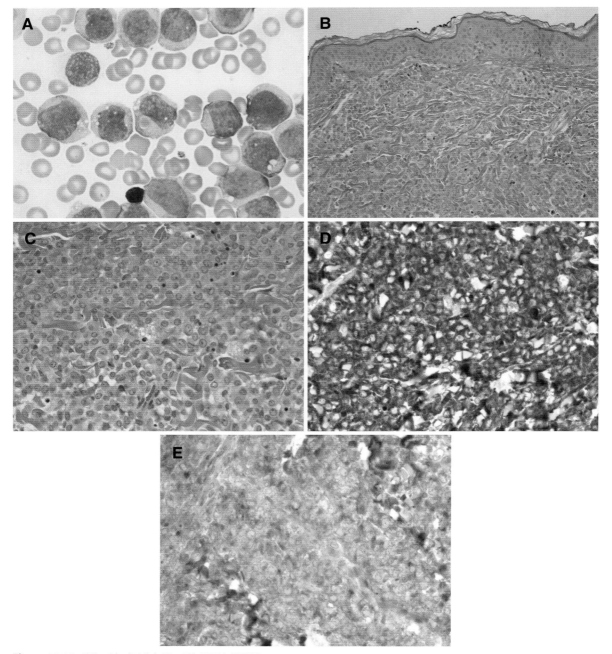

Figure 15.15 AML with t(8;16) (p11; p13); *KAT6A-CREBBP*.

a. A number of large blasts show abundant cytoplasm, scattered cytoplasmic vacuoles, large round nuclei, fine chromatin, and faintly visible nucleoli. Erythrophagocytosis is present (Wright-Giemsa, 1,000x).

b. A skin nodule biopsy shows diffuse infiltration of dermis by blasts (H&E, 200x).

c. Blasts display generous pink cytoplasm, round to oval to slightly folded nuclei, fine chromatin, and visible nucleoli (H&E, 400x).

d. Lysozyme positive in blasts (Lysozyme immunostain, 400x).

e. CD4 positive in blasts (CD4 immunostain, 400x).

f. Chromosome analysis shows t(8;16) (p11; p13).

A.

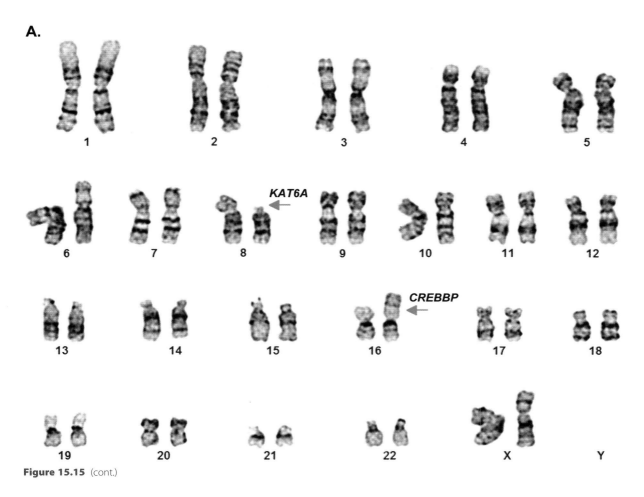

Figure 15.15 (cont.)

Table 15.4 The types of acute leukemia of ambiguous lineage and characteristics

Types	Definition	Comments
Acute undifferentiated leukemia	The blasts show no lineage-specific antigens.	A comprehensive phenotype by flow cytometry or immunohistochemical stains is needed.
MPAL – Bilineage	Two/three distinct blast populations	Each population will be classified as the respective lineage.
MPAL – Biphenotypic	One blast population with multiple antigens of different lineages	See Table 15.5.
MPAL with t(9;22) (q34.1; q11.2); *BCR-ABL*	Should fulfill the criteria of MPAL	Should not be made in patients who are known to have had CML
MPAL – t(v;11q23.3); *KMT2A*-rearranged	Should fulfill the criteria of MPAL	B-ALL with myeloid phenotype or AML with lymphoid phenotype and that have translocation with *KMT2A* should not be considered.
ZNF384-rearranged leukemia [12]	Seen in B/myeloid MPAL and also B-ALL. The partner genes include *TCF3*, *EP300*, and *TAF15*.	A distinct subtype of acute leukemia with immunophenotype ranging from B-ALL to B/myeloid MPAL.

Table 15.5 Requirements for assigning more than one lineage to a single blast population*

Myeloid lineage
Myeloperoxidase (by flow cytometry, immunohistochemistry, or cytochemistry);
Or
Monocytic differentiation (>/= 2 of the following: nonspecific esterase, CD11c, CD14, CD64, lysozyme)

T-cell lineage
cCD3 (by flow cytometry with antibodies to CD3 epsilon chain). Immunohistochemistry using polyclonal anti-CD3 antibody may detect CD3 zeta chain, which is not T-cell specific.
Or
CD3 (rare in mixed phenotypic acute leukemias)

B-cell lineage
Strong CD19
With >/= 1 of the following strongly expressed: CD79a, cCD22, CD10
Or
Weak CD19
With >/= 2 of the following strongly expressed: CD79a, cCD22, CD10

* Copyright permission.

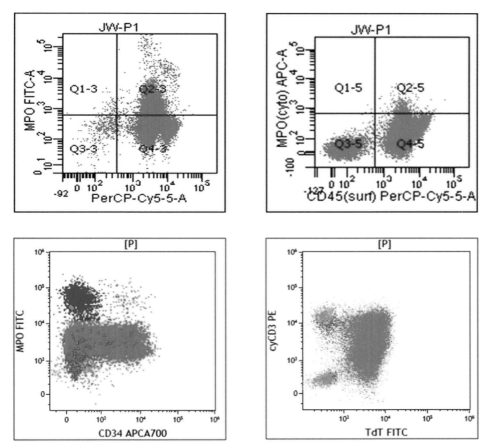

Figure 15.16 Flow cytometry demonstrating nonspecific MPO staining in B-ALL and T-ALL. Upper panel: In a B-ALL case, the MPO showed dim positive nonspecific binding using MPO antibody conjugated with fluorescein (FITC) (left); the MPO was essentially negative using another antibody conjugated with allophycocyanin (APC) (right). Lower panel: In a T-ALL case, the blasts (red) showed dim nonspecific MPO (FITC) staining (left), but it is dimmer than the granulocytes (blue). The dot plot on the right revealed that the blasts showed heterogeneous expression of cytoplasmic CD3, but reaching the same intensity as the normal T-cells (green cluster on the top).

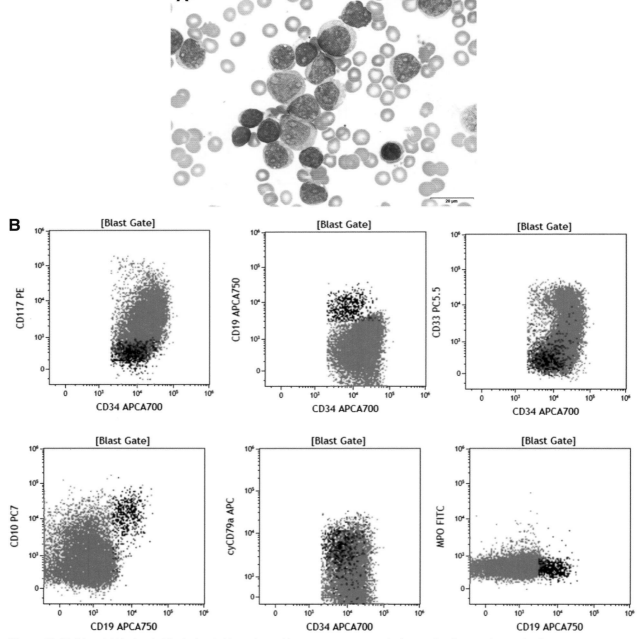

Figure 15.17 B/myeloid leukemia. The leukemic blasts showed heterogeneity in acute leukemia of ambiguous lineage by flow cytometry.

a. A bone marrow aspirate showed mostly myeloid blasts with a few lymphoblasts (Wright-Giemsa, 1,000x).

b. There are minute B lymphoblasts (black) expressing CD19, CD10, CD79a, TdT (c), and CD34 but negative for CD33 and CD117, and a larger blast population (red), expressing CD34, CD117, CD33, and dim CD79a but negative for MPO.

c. The population in (b) was further separated based on TdT expression. A TdT positive subpopulation was shown to express CD10 (subpopulation) (light blue).

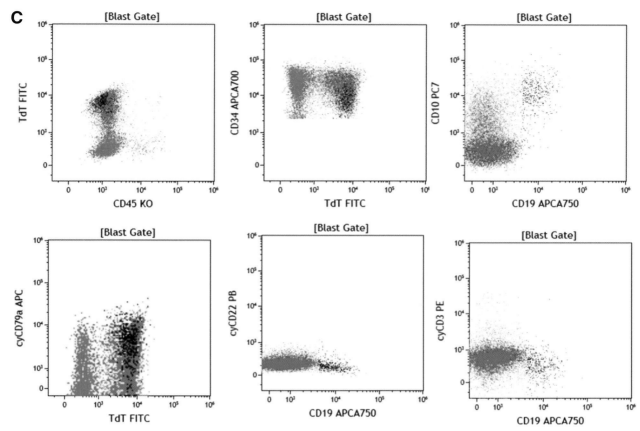

Figure 15.17 (cont.)

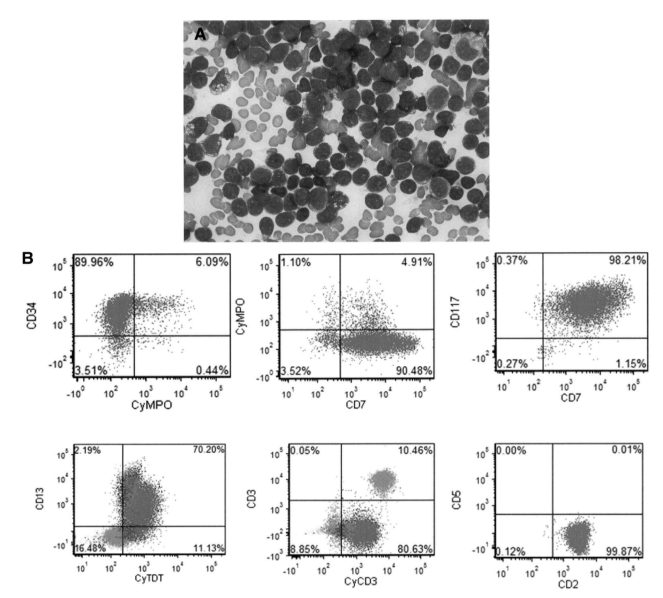

Figure 15.18 T/myeloid leukemia.

a. The bone marrow aspirate showed sheets of small immature mononuclear cells (T-lymphoblasts). The blasts have an irregular nuclear contour, relative condensed chromatin, inconspicuous nucleoli, and minimal cytoplasm. Admixed are a few larger immature cells with a few cytoplasmic azurophilic granules (Wright-Giemsa, 1,000x).

b. Flow cytometry shows a predominance of a T-lymphoblastic population (red) expressing CD2, cCD3, CD13, CD34, CD117, and TdT but lacking CD5. A minor population of myeloid blasts expresses cytoplasmic MPO and CD34. Also note the normal T-cell population in the sample (larger green population).

Table 15.6 Revised ELN non-AML classification and risk stratification by genetics [11]

Risk Category	Genetic Abnormalities
Favorable	t(8;21) (q22; q22.1); *RUNX1-RUNX1T1*
	Inv (16) (p13.1q22) or t(16;16) (p13.1; q22); *CBFb-MYH11*
	Biallelic mutated *CEBPA* (need to rule on germline mutation)
	Mutated *NPM1* without *FLT-3 ITD* or with *FLT-3 ITD*[low (<0.5)]
Intermediate	Mutated *NPM1* and *FLT-3 ITD*[high (>0.5)]
	Wild type *NPM1* without FLT-3 ITD or with *FLT-3 ITD*[low] (without adverse-risk genetic lesions)
	t(9;11) (p21.3; q23.3); *MLLT3-KMT2A* (takes precedence over rare, concurrent adverse-risk gene mutation)
	Cytogenetic abnormalities not classified as favorable or adverse
Adverse	t(6;9) (p23; q34.1); *DEK-NUP214*
	t(v;11q23.3); *KMT2A* rearranged
	t(9;22) (q34.1; q11.2); *BCR-ABL1*
	Inv (3) (q21.3; q26.2) or t(3;3) (q21.3; q26.2); *GATA2, MECOM(EVI1)*
	-5 or del(5q); -7; -17/abn (17p)
	Complex karyotype; monosomy karyotype
	Wild type *NPM1* and *FLT-3 ITD*[high (>0.5)]
	Mutated *RUNX1* or Mutated *ASXL1* (should not be considered "Adverse" if they co-occur with favorable subtype)
	Mutated *p53* (associated with complex and monosomy karyotype)

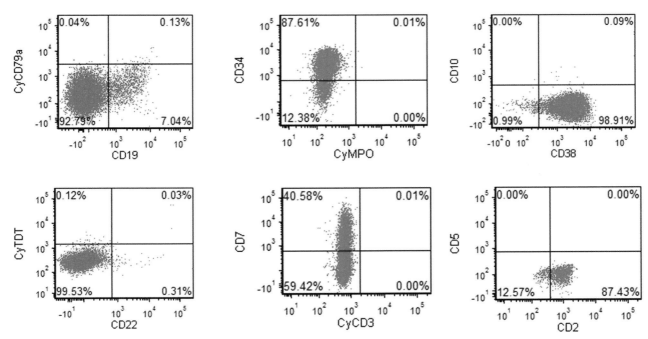

Figure 15.19 Flow analysis showed an acute leukemia without evidence of lineage differentiation. There are no lineage specific markers such as cytoplasmic CD3, MPO, or cCD79a.

Chapter 16

Myeloproliferative Neoplasms

Tracy I. George, Karen M. Chisholm

Myeloproliferative neoplasms (MPNs) are clonal hematopoietic stem cell disorders characterized by a proliferation of one or more of the myeloid lineages [1]. These components include erythroid cells, megakaryocytes, and granulocytes, the latter of which include eosinophils. In many cases, these MPNs are associated with acquired clonal genetic abnormalities involving cytoplasmic or receptor protein tyrosine kinases.

MPNs are very rare in pediatric patients. The most common disorder in this demographic is *BCR-ABL1* positive chronic myeloid leukemia, while the rest of the neoplasms are exceedingly rare. The *BCR-ABL1* negative disorders include polycythemia vera, primary myelofibrosis, essential thrombocythemia, chronic neutrophilic leukemia, chronic eosinophilic leukemia, not otherwise specified (NOS), and myeloproliferative neoplasm, unclassifiable. The bone marrow manifestations of most of the aforementioned disorders are discussed in this chapter; chronic eosinophilic leukemia NOS along with its counterpart myeloid/lymphoid neoplasms with eosinophilia and rearrangement of *PDGFRA*, *PDGFRB*, or *FGFR1*, or with *PCM1-JAK2* are discussed in Chapter 21.

Chronic Myeloid Leukemia, *BCR-ABL1* Positive

In chronic myeloid leukemia (CML) (Figure 16.1), granulocytes are the predominant proliferative lineage in the marrow. By definition, a fusion of the *BCR* and *ABL1* genes forms the Philadelphia (Ph) chromosome, t(9;22) (q34.1;q11.2) in all cases. Not only is this translocation identified in the myeloid lineage, but it can also be found in lymphoid and endothelial cells. In pediatrics, most cases present in chronic phase.

While chronic phase is defined as typically ≤2% blasts in the peripheral blood and <5% in bone marrow, the diagnosis of accelerated phase is made by having one or more of the following features per the 2016 World Health Organization (WHO) classifications [2]:

(1) persistent or increasing WBC ($>10 \times 10^9$/L) unresponsive to therapy
(2) persistent or increasing splenomegaly unresponsive to therapy
(3) persistent thrombocytosis ($>1,000 \times 10^9$/L) unresponsive to therapy
(4) persistent thrombocytopenia ($<100 \times 10^9$/L) unrelated to therapy
(5) ≥20% basophils in blood
(6) 10–19% blasts in blood and/or marrow
(7) additional clonal chromosomal abnormalities in the Ph cells at diagnosis
(8) new clonal chromosomal abnormality in Ph cells during therapy

Additionally, three provisional criteria can aid in the diagnosis of accelerated phase: (1) hematologic resistance (or failure to achieve complete hematologic response) to the first tyrosine kinase inhibitor (TKI); (2) any hematological, cytogenetic, or molecular indications of resistance to two sequential TKIs; and/or (3) occurrence of ≥2 mutations in the *BCR-ABL1* fusion gene during TKI therapy [2]. Finally, blast phase is defined as ≥20% blasts in the peripheral blood or bone marrow, or an extramedullary proliferation of blasts [2].

Essential Thrombocythemia

Essential thrombocythemia (ET) (Figure 16.2) is the most common of the non-CML MPNs in the pediatric age range, though with an incidence of less than 1 per 100,000 patients per year [3]. The predominant lineage of proliferation is megakaryocytes. According to the 2016 WHO classification, the diagnosis of ET requires all of the major criteria or the first three major criteria plus one minor criterion [4]:

Major Criteria
1. Platelet count ≥450 × 10^9/L
2. Bone marrow biopsy with: (a) proliferation of predominantly megakaryocyte lineage with increased

numbers of enlarged megakaryocytes with hyperlobulated nuclei; (b) no significant increase or left shift in granulocytes or erythrocytes; (c) minimal reticulin fibrosis (≤MF-1)
3. WHO criteria for CML, PV, PMF, and other MPNs not met
4. *JAK2*, *CALR*, or *MPL* mutation

Minor Criteria
1. Presence of clonal marker
2. No evidence of a reactive thrombocytosis

Of note, in a recent study of pediatric ET using these criteria, Kucine and colleagues recommended that the platelet count be ≥450 × 10^9/L for at least 3 months [5]. ET is an acquired condition and must be differentiated from hereditary thrombocytosis/familial thrombocythemia (often with mutations in *MPL* or *TPO*) and reactive thrombocytosis. The rate of *JAK2*, *CALR*, and *MPL* acquired gene mutations is less in pediatric than in adult populations, with *JAK2* V617F mutations identified in 31–48% of cases, *CALR* mutations in 10%, *MPL* mutations in 2% of ET, and the remaining pediatric patients not having any mutations in these three genes [3, 6, 7].

Polycythemia Vera

Polycythemia vera (PV) (Figure 16.3) is an MPN with proliferation primarily of the erythroid lineage. According to the 2016 WHO classification, the diagnosis of PV requires all of the following major criteria or the first two major criteria plus the one minor criterion [8]:

Major Criteria
1. Hemoglobin >16.5 g/dL in men or >16.0 g/dL in women OR hematocrit >49% in men or >48% in women OR increased red blood cell mass (>25% above mean normal predicted value)
2. Bone marrow biopsy with: (a) hypercellularity; (b) panmyelosis with prominent erythroid, granulocytic, and megakaryocytic proliferation; and (c) pleomorphic, mature megakaryocytes
3. *JAK2* V617F or *JAK2* exon 12 mutation

Minor Criterion
1. Subnormal serum erythropoietin level

Hereditary and secondary causes of erythrocytosis should be excluded. Some studies have reported that the WHO criteria for PV diagnosis are not entirely inclusive of children given different age-specific normal ranges, and a revision to hemoglobin or hematocrit >97.5th percentile for age/gender or red blood cell count >97.5th percentile for age/gender without evidence of thalassemia trait has been suggested [5]. Additionally, only 25% of pediatric cases have low serum erythropoietin levels [9]. Teofili and colleagues also showed that the presence of clonal hematopoiesis can be considered a specific marker of MPN in pediatric patients [9].

In PV, the peripheral blood smear shows increased red blood cells, usually normochromic and normocytic. Additionally, platelets may be increased while white blood cells may be normal to mildly increased [3, 7, 10, 11]. Unlike in adults, the rate of *JAK2* V617F mutations in pediatrics has been reported to be quite low at 24–37%, with *JAK2* exon 12 mutations estimated at 0–3% and the rest of the cases (up to 73%) being negative for *JAK2* mutations [3, 7, 9].

Two phases of PV are noted, a polycythemic phase and a post-polycythemia myelofibrosis phase. The latter is diagnosed by documented history of PV and bone marrow fibrosis grade 2–3 on a 0–3 scale or grade 3–4 on a 0–4 scale [8]. Two additional criteria are required among the following: (a) anemia or sustained loss of requirement of phlebotomy or cytoreductive treatment for erythrocytosis; (b) leukoerythroblastosis; (c) increasing splenomegaly >5cm from baseline or the development of new palpable splenomegaly; and (d) development of ≥2 constitutional symptoms: >10% weight loss in 6 months, night sweats, and/or unexplained fever of >37.5 degrees Celsius [8].

Primary Myelofibrosis

Primary myelofibrosis (PMF) (Figure 16.4) demonstrates a proliferation of abnormal megakaryocytes and granulocytes associated with fibrosis. Both a prefibrotic/early stage and an overt fibrotic stage are defined by the 2016 WHO criteria, the diagnosis requiring all three major and more than one minor criterion (confirmed on two consecutive determinations) [12]:

Prefibrotic/early stage

Major Criteria
1. Bone marrow with (a) megakaryocytic proliferation and atypia; (b) reticulin fibrosis MF-0 or MF-1; and (c) increased bone marrow cellularity, granulocytic proliferation, and (often) decreased erythropoiesis
2. WHO criteria for CML, PV, ET, MDS, and other MPNs not met

---

3. *JAK2*, *CALR*, or *MPL* mutation or presence of another clonal marker or absence of reactive myelofibrosis

Minor Criteria
1. Anemia not attributed to comorbid condition
2. Leukocytosis $\geq 11 \times 10^9$/L
3. Palpable splenomegaly
4. Lactate dehydrogenase level above the upper limit of reference range

The overt fibrotic stage has the same major criteria except the bone marrow should have MF-2 or MF-3 fibrosis. The minor criteria are the same with the addition of leukoerythroblastosis. Reactive and neoplastic causes of marrow fibrosis must be excluded for this diagnosis.

While early-stage PMF can show a mild anemia, leukocytosis, and thrombocytosis, the overt fibrotic stage has a leukoerythroblastic smear with immature granulocytes and nucleated red blood cells, as well as dacrocytes. Extramedullary hematopoiesis is typical with splenomegaly.

In contrast to adults, pediatric cases often lack mutations in *JAK2*, *CALR*, or *MPL*. In one study, 17 children with PMF all lacked *JAK2* V617F and *MPL* W515K/L mutations [13]. In another study, 7 of 14 children with PMF had heterozygous *CALR* mutations while none had *JAK2* V617F or *MPL* W515L/K mutations [14].

Chronic Neutrophilic Leukemia

Chronic neutrophilic leukemia (CNL) is a very rare MPN, with only three pediatric cases reported in the literature [15–17]. The diagnosis requires five criteria [18]:

1. Peripheral blood:
   White blood cell (WBC) count $\geq 25 \times 10^9$/L
   Band and segmented neutrophils $\geq 80\%$ of WBC
   Promyelocytes, myelocytes, and metamyelocytes <10% of WBC
   Only rare myeloblasts
   Monocyte count $<1 \times 10^9$/L
   No granulocytic dysplasia
2. Bone marrow:
   Hypercellular
   Increased neutrophil percentage and number
   Normal neutrophil maturation
   Myeloblasts <5% of nucleated cells
3. WHO criteria for CML, PV, ET, and PMF not met

4. No rearrangement of *PDGFRA*, *PDGFRB*, or *FGFR1*, and no *PCM1-JAK2* fusion
5. Activating *CSF3R* mutation (such as T618I)
   or
   Persistent neutrophilia (≥ 3 months), splenomegaly, and no identifiable cause of reactive neutrophilia

The peripheral blood demonstrates a leukocytosis with a predominance of segmented and band neutrophils and a lack of blasts and dysplasia. Toxic granulation may be present. Red blood cells can be mild to moderately decreased and platelets can be normal or mildly decreased in number. Bone marrow evaluation shows a hypercellular marrow with neutrophilic proliferation. In addition to the neutrophil proliferation, erythroid precursors and megakaryocytes may be increased, though also without dysplasia. Yet the myeloid-to-erythroid (M:E) ratio is usually markedly increased at ≥ 20:1. Fibrosis is usually not present. Cytogenetic evaluation often reveals a normal karyotype.

Myeloproliferative Neoplasm, Unclassifiable

Myeloproliferative neoplasm, unclassifiable (MPN-U) (Figure 16.5) is the correct term to employ when a case has features of an MPN, including clinical, peripheral blood, bone marrow, and molecular findings, but does not meet the diagnostic criteria for any of the aforementioned MPNs [19]. Specifically, the diagnosis of MPN-U requires that three criteria are met:

1. MPN features are present
2. WHO criteria for any other MPN, MDS, or MDS/MPN not met
3. *JAK2*, *CALR*, or *MPL* mutation
   Or
   Presence of another clonal marker
   Or
   Absence of a cause of reactive fibrosis

In pediatrics, the diagnosis of MPN-U is often recommended when the disease is in a very early stage such that the differences between PV and ET are difficult to distinguish [5]. In both of these disorders, there can be peripheral blood thrombocytosis and a hypercellular marrow with a megakaryocytic proliferation. MPN-U can also be employed when there is advanced-stage MPN with significant myelofibrosis, when there is transformation with increased dysplasia and/or blasts obscuring the underlying disorder, or when a coexisting neoplastic or inflammatory disorder obscures the underlying disorder [19].

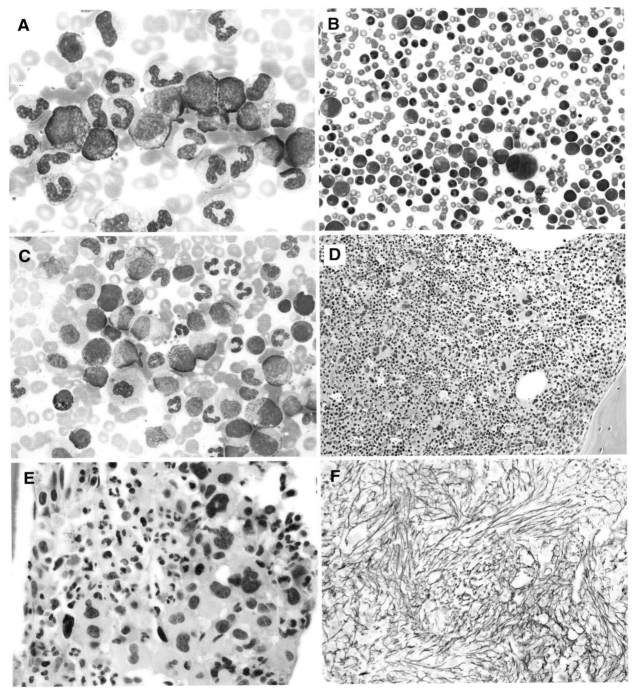

Figure 16.1 Chronic myeloid leukemia.

a. This 17-year-old male presented with marked splenomegaly and WBC count of 551.2 x 10⁹/L, consisting of mature and immature granulocytes with only 2% blasts. Peripheral blood smear shows leukocytosis with all stages of granulocyte maturation present, but with increases in neutrophils and myelocytes. Absolute eosinophilia, basophilia, and/or monocytosis may also be present. Platelets may be normal to increased in number (Wright-Giemsa stain, peripheral blood, 1,000x).

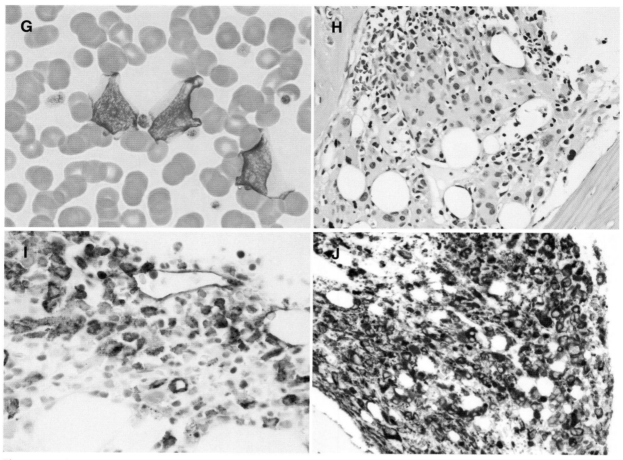

Figure 16.1 (cont.)

b. This 16-year-old male presented with 1 month of blurry vision, intermittent headaches, and a WBC count of 337.1 x 10^9/L, consisting of mature and immature granulocytes with 1% blasts. Bone marrow aspirate demonstrated a relative myeloid hyperplasia with full-spectrum maturation as well as scattered dwarf megakaryocytes characterized as smaller-sized megakaryocytes with hypolobated nuclei (Wright-Giemsa stain, bone marrow aspirate, 400x).

c. Sea blue histiocytes or lipid-laden histiocytes in patients with CML are due to a high turnover state in the marrow that leads to a high lipid content. They are not specific to a diagnosis of CML (Wright-Giemsa stain, bone marrow aspirate, 100x).

d. This 16-year-old female presented with two months of lower back pain, fatigue, and splenomegaly. Her peripheral blood demonstrated a WBC count of 38.3 x 10^9/L with left-shifted granulocytes. Typical of chronic-phase CML, her bone marrow was hypercellular for age with myeloid and megakaryocytic hyperplasia (H&E, bone marrow biopsy, 200x).

e. The bone marrow biopsy from this 10-year-old male presenting with a neutrophilic leukocytosis shows sheets of tightly clustered megakaryocytes with many small hypolobate forms (so-called dwarf megakaryocytes) and micromegakaryocytes (H&E, bone marrow biopsy, 100x).

f. The extensive megakaryocytic proliferation in Figure 16.1e was accompanied by marked reticulin fibrosis (MF-3). Moderate to marked reticulin fibrosis is observed in approximately 30% of CML cases (reticulin, bone marrow biopsy, 40x).

g. This 18-year-old male with a known diagnosis of CML and trisomy 8 presented with 66% circulating myeloblasts 3 months after a hypocellular marrow. The peripheral blood smear shows three large blasts with abundant lightly basophilic cytoplasm, smooth chromatin, and prominent nucleoli (Wright-Giemsa, peripheral blood, 200x).

h. The bone marrow biopsy from the patient in Figure 16.1g was hypercellular with aggregates of atypical small hypolobate megakaryocytes and blasts (H&E, bone marrow biopsy, 50x).

i, j. Immunohistochemical stain for CD34 (Figure 16.1i) highlights the many myeloblasts occupying 60% of marrow elements, while a CD61 immunostain (Figure 16.1j) marks numerous megakaryocytes and megakaryoblasts (i. CD34, biopsy, 50x) (j. CD61, biopsy, 40x).

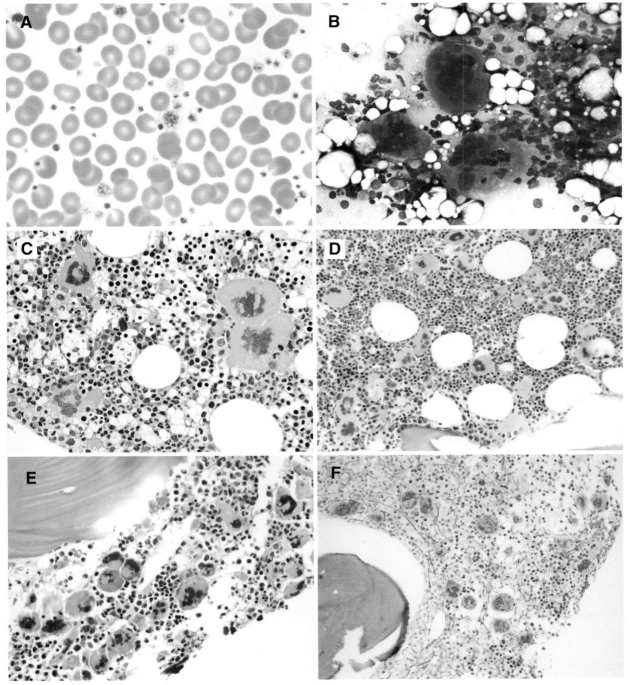

Figure 16.2 Essential thrombocythemia.

a. The peripheral blood smear from this 16-year-old female shows a marked thrombocytosis of 1,443 x 10⁹/L with frequent large and giant platelets, a subset of which appears hypogranular. She initially presented with swelling, pain, and bruising of her left foot, without injury or trauma, and excessive bruising in the previous eight months. A *JAK2* V617F mutation was present with a variant allele fraction of 40% (Wright-Giemsa, peripheral blood, 200x).

b. This 14-year-old female presented with 2 months of chest pain and was found to have a significant thrombocytosis of 1,146 x 10⁹/L. A *JAK2* V617F mutation was detected. Bone marrow aspirate revealed increased megakaryocytes that were large with hyperlobulated nuclei (Wright-Giemsa stain, bone marrow aspirate, 400X magnification).

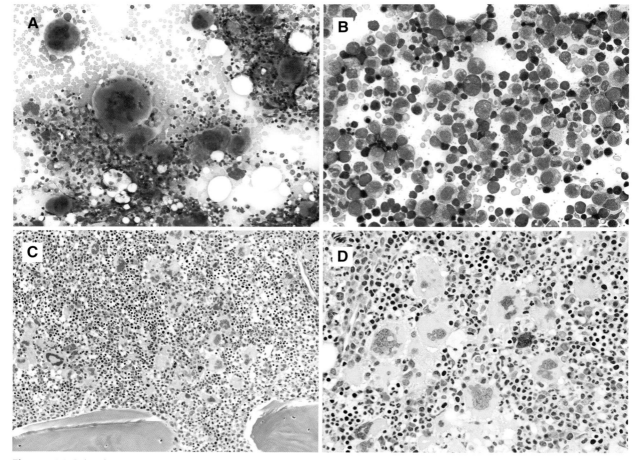

Figure 16.3 Polycythemia vera.

a. This 14-year-old female with periodic headaches was incidentally found to have a white blood count of 13.9 x 10^9/L, hemoglobin of 15.2 g/dL, hematocrit of 51.8%, and platelet count of 2,483 x 10^9/L. A *JAK2* V617F mutation was detected and her serum erythropoietin was low at 1.3 mIU/mL. Her bone marrow aspirate demonstrated increased megakaryocytes of different sizes (Wright-Giemsa stain, bone marrow aspirate, 200x magnification).

b. On higher power, her myeloid and erythroid precursors demonstrated full-spectrum maturation with an intact M:E ratio (Wright-Giemsa stain, bone marrow aspirate, 400X magnification).

c. Bone marrow core biopsy demonstrated a hypercellular marrow with panmyelosis, including many pleomorphic megakaryocytes in a background rich in erythroid and myeloid precursors. In PV, often the erythroid and megakaryocyte hyperplasias can be most prominent. The megakaryocytes are dispersed or form loose clusters throughout the marrow (H&E, bone marrow biopsy, 200x).

d. This panmyeloisis is also evident on higher-power magnification. Megakaryocytes can often demonstrate hypersegmented nuclei (H&E, bone marrow biopsy, 400x).

Caption for Figure 16.2 (cont.)

c. Bone marrow core biopsy from patient in Figure 16.2b demonstrated a mildly hypercellular marrow at 70–75% cellularity with increased megakaryocytes having hyperlobulated nuclei with stag-hornlike features. Background erythropoiesis and myelopoiesis were intact without significant hyperplasia (H&E, bone marrow biopsy, 400x).

d. The bone marrow biopsy is normocellular for age with a normal M:E ratio, but a striking atypical megakaryocytic hyperplasia of enlarged mature megakaryocytes. This previously healthy 16-year-old female was incidentally found to have a marked thrombocytosis. Molecular genetic testing on blood detected a *CALR* exon 9 mutation that was not one of the common type 1 or 2 mutations but did result in a frameshift (H&E, bone marrow biopsy, 40x).

e. This biopsy from a 14-year-old female presenting with severe thrombocytosis shows a proliferation of enlarged hyperlobulated and hyperchromatic megakaryocytes in a background of normal granulopoiesis and erythropoiesis. Molecular testing revealed a 52 base pair deletion in the *CALR* gene consistent with a type 1 or type 1-like mutation (H&E, bone marrow biopsy, 40x).

f. The corresponding reticulin stain in this patient from Figure 16.1e demonstrates an absence of significant reticulin fibrosis, as is typical in patients with ET (reticulin, bone marrow biopsy, 40x).

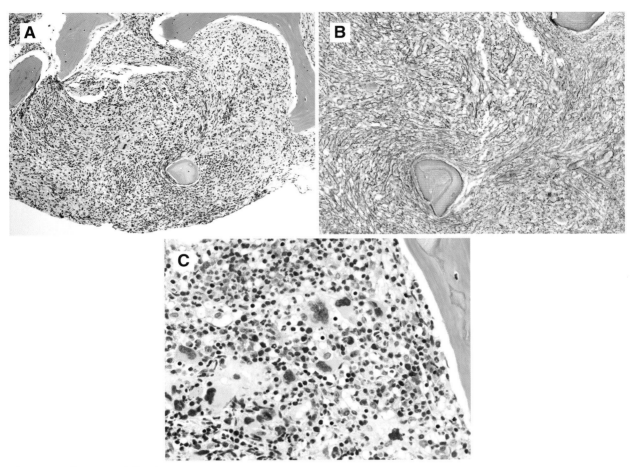

Figure 16.4 Primary myelofibrosis.

a. This 16-year-old female presented with long-standing anemia that required transfusions, thrombocytopenia, and hepatosplenomegaly. Typical of PMF, her bone marrow aspirate was aparticulate and hemodilute. Her bone marrow core biopsy demonstrated a streaming quality to the cells with increased and clustered megakaryocytes with hyperchromatic nuclei (H&E, bone marrow biopsy, 100x).

b. Reticulin stain from the core biopsy in Figure 16.4a showed increased reticulin fibrosis (MF-2) (reticulin, bone marrow biopsy, 200x).

c. This 7-year-old female was found to have pancytopenia with a peripheral blood smear showing leukoerythroblastosis as well as 1+ dacrocytes. Her bone marrow aspirate was hemodilute and aparticulate, but her bone marrow core biopsy was hypercellular for age with clusters of atypical megakaryocytes, some with hyperchromatic nuclei and others with plump lobation and cloudlike nuclei (H&E, bone marrow biopsy, 400x).

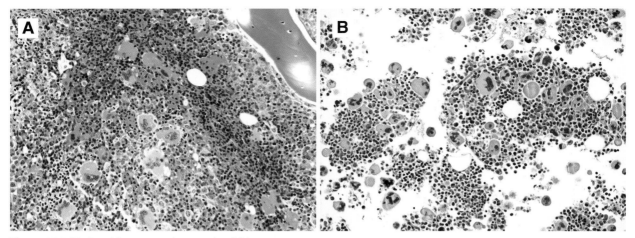

Figure 16.5 Myeloproliferative neoplasm, unclassifiable

a. This 15-year-old female presented with abdominal pain and splenomegaly and was found to have a markedly elevated platelet count of 2,152 x 10^9/L with normal hemoglobin, hematocrit, and WBC count. Molecular testing identified the *JAK2* V617F mutation. Bone marrow aspirate and core biopsy demonstrated a hypercellular marrow with panmyelosis and a mild increase in reticulin fibrosis (MF-1). While the hypercellular marrow with panmyelosis was more consistent with a PV, her peripheral counts were more consistent with an ET, so she was diagnosed with MPN-U (H&E, bone marrow biopsy, 200x).

b. This 19-year-old male was incidentally found to have a leukocytosis without significant left shift (WBC count of 28 x 10^9/L), elevated hemoglobin (18.9 g/dL), and thrombocytosis (983 x 10^9/L). Bone marrow aspirate and particle section demonstrated a hypercellular marrow (95% cellularity) with panmyelosis and atypical megakaryocytes of varying sizes. A *JAK2* V617F mutation was identified. PV may present in this manner, as can the early cellular phase of PMF, with ET less likely; as such this early presentation was best categorized as an MPN-U (H&E, bone marrow particle section, 200x).

References

1. Arber DA, Orazi A, Hasserjian RP, Brunning RD, Le Beau MM, Porwit A, et al. Introduction and overview of the classification of myeloid neoplasms. In Swerdlow SH, Campo E, Harris NL, Jaffe ES, Pileri SA, Stein H, et al., eds. WHO classification of tumours of haematopoietic and lymphoid tissues. Lyon: IARC Press; 2017:16–27.

2. Vardiman JW, Melo JV, Baccarani M, Radich JP, Kvasnicka HM. Chronic myeloid leukaemia, BCR-ABL1-positive. In Swerdlow SH, Campo E, Harris NL, Jaffe ES, Pileri SA, Stein H, et al., eds. WHO classification of tumours of haematopoietic and lymphoid tissues. Lyon: IARC Press; 2017:30–6.

3. Ianotto JC, Curto-Garcia N, Lauermanova M, Radia D, Kiladjian JJ, Harrison CN. Characteristics and outcomes of patients with essential thrombocythemia or polycythemia vera diagnosed before 20 years of age: A systematic review. Haematologica. 2019; 104(8): 1580–8.

4. Thiele J, Kvasnicka HM, Orazi A, Gianelli U, Tefferi A, Gisslinger H, et al. Essential thrombocythaemia. In Swerdlow SH, Campo E, Harris NL, Jaffe ES, Pileri SA, Stein H, et al., eds. WHO classification of tumours of haematopoietic and lymphoid tissues. Lyon: IARC Press; 2017:50–3.

5. Kucine N, Al-Kawaaz M, Hajje D, Bussel J, Orazi A. Difficulty distinguishing essential thrombocythaemia from polycythaemia vera in children with JAK2 V617F-positive myeloproliferative neoplasms. Br J Haematol. 2019; 185(1): 136–9.

6. Giona F, Teofili L, Capodimonti S, Laurino M, Martini M, Marzella D, et al. CALR mutations in patients with essential thrombocythemia diagnosed in childhood and adolescence. Blood. 2014; 123(23): 3677–9.

7. Giona F, Teofili L, Moleti ML, Martini M, Palumbo G, Amendola A, et al. Thrombocythemia and polycythemia in patients younger than 20 years at diagnosis: Clinical and biologic features, treatment, and long-term outcome. Blood. 2012; 119(10): 2219–27.

8. Thiele J, Kvasnicka HM, Orazi A, Tefferi A, Birgegard G, Barbui T. Polycythaemia vera. In Swerdlow SH, Campo E, Harris NL, Jaffe ES, Pileri SA, Stein H, et al., eds. WHO classification of tumours of haematopoietic and lymphoid tissues. Lyon: IARC Press; 2017:39–43.

9. Teofili L, Giona F, Martini M, Cenci T, Guidi F, Torti L, et al. The revised WHO diagnostic criteria for Ph-negative myeloproliferative diseases are not appropriate for the diagnostic screening of childhood polycythemia vera and essential thrombocythemia. Blood. 2007; 110(9): 3384–6.

10. Karow A, Nienhold R, Lundberg P, Peroni E, Putti MC, Randi ML, et al. Mutational profile of childhood myeloproliferative neoplasms. Leukemia. 2015; 29(12): 2407–9.

11. Teofili L, Giona F, Martini M, Cenci T, Guidi F, Torti L, et al. Markers of myeloproliferative diseases in childhood polycythemia vera and essential thrombocythemia. J Clin Oncol. 2007; **25**(9): 1048–53.

12. Thiele J, Kvasnicka HM, Orazi A, Gianelli U, Barbui T, Barosi G, et al. Primary myelofibrosis. In Swerdlow SH, Campo E, Harris NL, Jaffe ES, Pileri SA, Stein H, et al., eds. WHO classification of tumours of haematopoietic and lymphoid tissues. Lyon: IARC Press; 2017:44–50.

13. DeLario MR, Sheehan AM, Ataya R, Bertuch AA, Vega C, 2nd, Webb CR, et al. Clinical, histopathologic, and genetic features of pediatric primary myelofibrosis: An entity different from adults. Am J Hematol. 2012; **87**(5): 461–4.

14. An W, Wan Y, Guo Y, Chen X, Ren Y, Zhang J, et al. CALR mutation screening in pediatric primary myelofibrosis. Pediatr Blood Cancer. 2014; **61**(12): 2256–62.

15. Druhan LJ, McMahon DP, Steuerwald N, Price AE, Lance A, Gerber JM, et al. Chronic neutrophilic leukemia in a child with a CSF3 R T618I germ line mutation. Blood. 2016; **128**(16): 2097–9.

16. Hasle H. Incidence of essential thrombocythaemia in children. Br J Haematol. 2000; **110**(3): 751.

17. Uygun V, Daloglu H, Ozturkmen S, Karasu G, Avci Z, Yesilipek A. Chronic neutrophilic leukemia, an extremely rare cause of neutrophilia in childhood: Cure with hematopoietic stem cell transplantation. Pediatr Transplant. 2018; **22**(5): e13199.

18. Bain BJ, Brunning RD, Orazi A, Thiele J. Chronic neutrophilic leukaemia. In Swerdlow SH, Campo E, Harris NL, Jaffe ES, Pileri SA, Stein H, et al., eds. WHO classification of tumours of haematopoietic and lymphoid tissues. Lyon: IARC Press; 2017:37–8.

19. Kvasnicka HM, Thiele J, Orazi A, Horny H-P, Bain BJ. Myeloproliferative neoplasm, unclassifiable. In Swerdlow SH, Campo E, Harris NL, Jaffe ES, Pileri SA, Stein H, et al., eds. WHO classification of tumours of haematopoietic and lymphoid tissues. Lyon: IARC Press; 2017:57–9.

Myelodysplastic/Myeloproliferative Neoplasms

Kristian T. Schafernak, Rachel A. Mariani, Nicole Arva, Jeffrey Jacobsen, Katherine R. Calvo

Myelodysplastic/myeloproliferative neoplasm (MDS/MPNs) constitute a group of clonal hematopoietic disorders with hybrid features; those of a myeloproliferative neoplasm (MPN) include bone marrow hypercellularity due to proliferation of one or more of the myeloid (as opposed to lymphoid) lineages with effective hematopoiesis, leading to a peripheral "cytosis" or "cytoses." At the same time, these disorders show variable morphologic or functional dysplasia with ineffective hematopoiesis, resulting in cytopenia(s), findings more characteristic of myelodysplastic syndrome (MDS). The blast percentage is always less than 20, though sometimes transformation to acute myeloid leukemia (AML) occurs.

The revised fourth edition of the World Health Organization's (WHO) *Classification of Tumours of Haematopoietic and Lymphoid Tissues* recognizes five specific MDS/MPN entities: chronic myelomonocytic leukemia (CMML); atypical chronic myeloid leukemia, *BCR-ABL1*-negative; juvenile myelomonocytic leukemia (JMML); MDS/MPN with ring sideroblasts and thrombocytosis; and MDS/MPN, unclassifiable (MDS/MPN-U) [1]. Only three of these occur with any frequency in pediatric hematopathology: CMML, JMML, and MDS/MPN-U, with JMML the most common and the only entity exclusive to this age group. The recently described rat sarcoma virus (RAS)–associated autoimmune leukoproliferative disorder (RALD) overlaps with both JMML and autoimmune lymphoproliferative syndrome (ALPS) and is also discussed in this chapter.

Juvenile Myelomonocytic Leukemia

Juvenile myelomonocytic leukemia (JMML) is a leukemia that occurs from infancy to early adolescence. The majority of patients are age 3 years or younger, with boys more frequently affected than girls. Patients typically have leukocytosis with absolute monocytosis and left shift in the neutrophil series, including occasional blasts. Morphologic dysplasia is not always obvious even after an exhaustive search. The marrow is hypercellular with a myeloid hyperplasia but typically far fewer monocytes than in the blood. Hepatosplenomegaly is extremely common and lymph nodes, tonsils, skin, and the respiratory tract can also be involved.

The current diagnostic criteria for JMML, now incorporating splenomegaly and molecular genetics [1], represent an improvement over the diagnostic criteria outlined in the fourth (2008) edition of the WHO blue book [2].

Of JMML cases, 80–90% are due to alterations in one of five genes (*PTPN11*, *NRAS*, *KRAS*, *CBL*, and *NF1*), all encoding proteins involved in the granulocyte-monocyte colony-stimulating factor (GM-CSF) receptor signaling pathway, leading downstream to uncontrolled activation of the RAS/MAPK pathway. Table 17.1 lists the genetic subtypes of JMML and clinical behavior. For mutations with a high variant allele frequency of >35%, it is critical to know if the mutation is somatic or germline for clinical management. Germline mutation may be suggested by physical stigmata such as those of neurofibromatosis type 1 (multiple café au lait macules, Lisch nodules/iris hamartomas or neurofibromas, or 1 plexiform neurofibroma, freckling in the axillary or inguinal regions, optic glioma, or a distinctive osseous lesion such as sphenoid dysplasia or tibial pseudarthrosis seen in neurofibromatosis type 1 (NF1) [3]. Children with NF1 face a 200–500x increased risk of developing a myeloid malignancy (mainly in the form of JMML). In addition, patients with JMML and germline *NF1* mutations are typically managed more aggressively than those with germline mutations in the other genes associated with JMML.

Noonan syndrome is associated with germline mutations in *PTPN11* (most common, seen in about 50% of patients), *KRAS* (< 2%), and *NRAS* (frequency unknown), among other genes like *SOS1* and *RAF1* [4]. It is critical to recognize Noonan syndrome since as many as 10% of infants with it develop a transient JMML-like myeloproliferative disorder that is benign/non-clonal in 90% of cases and does not require HSCT, though 10% acquire

Table 17.1 JMML genetic subtypes and salient features

PTPN11 somatic heterozygous gain-of-function mutation	~35–38%	Fatal without hematopoietic stem cell transplant (HSCT) with high relapse rate; mutations in sporadic JMML show stronger gain-of-function effects than in Noonan syndrome/myeloproliferative disorder, which may explain why the latter is transient
PTPN11 germline mutation		Noonan syndrome/myeloproliferative disorder occurs in infancy and is non-clonal with spontaneous resolution in 90% of cases; 10% acquire secondary cytogenetic abnormality and progress to JMML
NRAS somatic heterozygous point mutation mostly in codons 12, 13, or 61	~17–18%	Aggressive, requires urgent HSCT; high relapse rate (especially in older children with high hemoglobin F [HbF]) but indolent in infants or those with G12S mutation (normal or only slightly elevated HbF)
KRAS somatic heterozygous point mutation mostly in codons 12, 13, or 61	~14%	Aggressive, requires HSCT; mostly seen in infants, often with monosomy 7, low relapse rate
CBL1	~10–18%	Somatic mutations: aggressive Germline mutations (missense alterations in exons 8 and 9 or splice-site mutation): can be accompanied by developmental delay, cryptorchidism; often indolent with spontaneous regression of leukemia but later may develop multiorgan vasculitis; HSCT can be considered for immune reconstitution, though mixed chimerism occurs often
NF1 biallelic inactivation by uniparental disomy or compound heterozygous mutations, occasionally somatic interstitial deletions	~5–15%	Fatal without HSCT; older age at diagnosis; higher platelet count and bone marrow blast percentage
Unknown	~10–20%	

References: [1, 8, 10].

clonal chromosome abnormalities and develop JMML. Physical examination findings in newborns and infants with Noonan syndrome are well documented [5]. Facial abnormalities can be difficult to recognize in the neonatal period, but a history of congenital heart defect, with pulmonary valve stenosis the most common, and cryptorchidism in boys may be helpful clues [6].

RAS-associated autoimmune leukoproliferative disorder (RALD) typically presents in the same age range as JMML, resulting from somatic mutations in codons 12 or 13 in NRAS or KRAS [7]. These patients have monocytosis. Lymphadenopathy and splenomegaly are very common. They typically have autoimmune cytopenias and autoantibodies such as antinuclear, anti-cardiolipin, and lupus anticoagulant antibodies. The NRAS or KRAS mutations are found in all RALD patients in both myeloid and lymphoid cells, leading to reduced expression of a pro-apoptotic protein called BCL2-Interacting Mediator of cell death (BIM), suggesting that RALD, like ALPS, results from a defect in apoptosis, though TCRαβ+CD4-CD8- (double negative) T-cells are not increased in the blood. These children do not have circulating blasts or cytogenetic abnormalities and typically follow an indolent course, but they should probably be followed closely since RALD is a relatively new diagnosis and because transformation to more aggressive JMML has been documented [8, 9].

Pediatric CMML is very rare and, like JMML, has exclusionary criteria: AML, the four classic MPNs, and myeloid/lymphoid neoplasms with eosinophilia and PDGFRA, PDGFRB, or FGFR1 rearrangement and PCM1-JAK2 fusion. In contrast to JMML, it requires > 10% monocytes. In the absence of cytogenetic or molecular abnormalities or morphologic dysplasia, the absolute monocytosis should be persistent to exclude secondary causes.

Pediatric MDS/MPN-U is also very rare, with mixed myeloproliferative and myelodysplastic features at onset, but does not meet the criteria for AML, MPN, or any other MDS/MPN. The WHO criteria indicate that this neoplasm does not meet the criteria for an MDS [1]; MDS/MPN-U often resembles an MDS with thrombocytosis (platelet count $\geq 450 \times 10^9$/L associated with bone marrow megakaryocytic proliferation) and/or leukocytosis (WBC count of $\geq 13 \times 10^9$/L) and no history of recent cytotoxic or growth factor therapy that could explain these features, and no PDGFRA, PDGFRB, or FGFR1 rearrangement and no PCM1-JAK2 fusion.

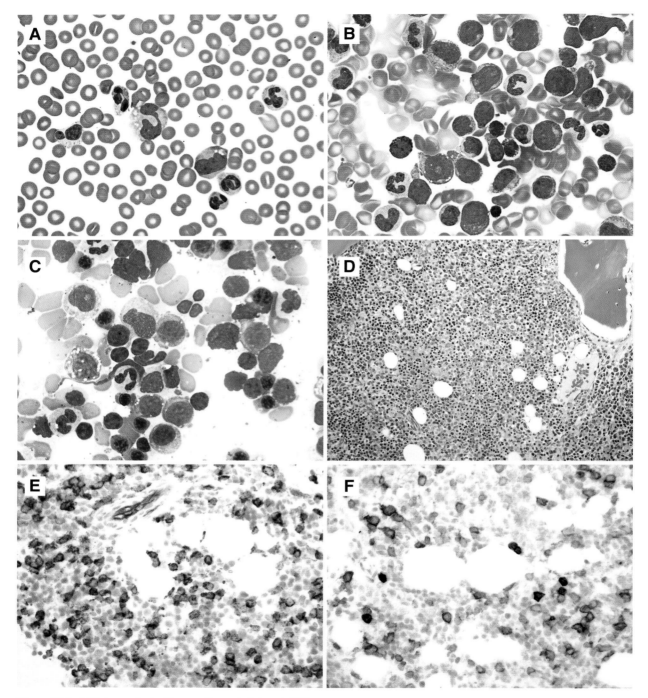

Figure 17.1 JMML in a patient with neurofibromatosis type 1 (NF1).

This 7-year-old girl with NF1 was diagnosed with JMML after gradually worsening leukocytosis with absolute monocytosis and rare circulating blasts, accompanied by thrombocytopenia; additionally, she had hepatosplenomegaly and an elevated HbF fraction for age at 15.8% [normal, <2%]. Her peripheral blood smear is depicted in Figure A (Wright-Giemsa stain, 400x), while her bone marrow aspirate (Figure B, Wright-Giemsa stain, 400x) showed 15% blasts, 8% basophils, 2% monocytes, and a chromosome 5 abnormality. She underwent allogeneic HSCT but was found to have relapsed on her day +100 bone marrow examination (Figure C, bone marrow aspirate, Wright-Giemsa stain, 400x; D, core biopsy, H&E, 100x; E, IHC, CD34; F, 400x; IHC, CD117, 400x).

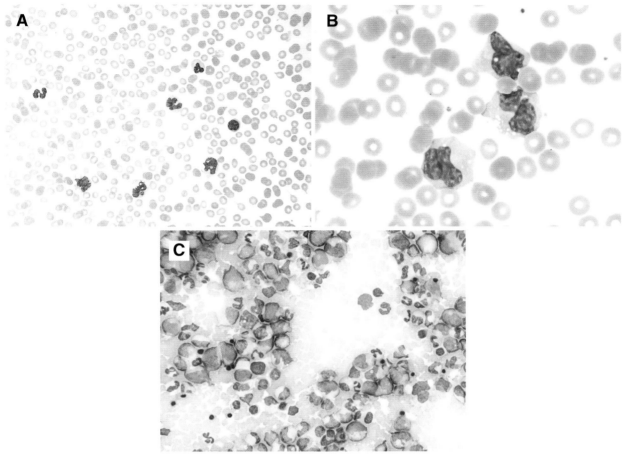

Figure 17.2 JMML with *CBL* mutation.

This child had a germline *CBL* mutation. The peripheral blood (A, Wright-Giemsa stain, 100x, and B, Wright-Giemsa stain 1,000x) shows absolute monocytosis. The monocytes are atypical with vacuolated cytoplasm and abnormal nuclear lobation. The bone marrow aspirate (C, H&E, 100x) smears show granulocytic hyperplasia. While such patients often experience spontaneous regression of their JMML, unlike those with somatic/non-syndromic *CBL* mutations in whom it follows a more aggressive clinical course, they may face constitutional abnormalities such as impaired growth, developmental delay and cryptorchidism, and multiorgan vasculitides later in life.

References

1. Swerdlow SH, Campo E, Harris NL, Jaffe ES, Pileri SA, Stein H, et al., eds. WHO classification of tumours of haematopoietic and lymphoid tissues. Lyon: IARC Press; 2017.

2. Swerdlow SH, Campo E, Harris NL, Jaffe ES, Pileri SA, Stein H, et al., eds. WHO classification of tumours of haematopoietic and lymphoid tissues. Lyon: IARC Press; 2008.

3. Friedman JM. Neurofibromatosis 1. Adam MP, Ardinger HH, Pagon RA, et al., eds. GeneReviews® [Internet]. Seattle (WA): University of Washington, Seattle; 1993–2022. www.ncbi.nlm.nih.gov/books/NBK1109" www.ncbi.nlm.nih.gov/books/NBK1109.

4. Denayer E, Peeters H, Sevenants L, Derbent M, Fryns JP, Legius E. NRAS mutations in Noonan syndrome. Mol Syndromol. 2012; **3**: 34–8.

5. Bhambhani V, Muenke M. Noonan syndrome. Am Fam Physician. 2014; **89**: 37–43.

6. Digilio MC, Marino B. Clinical manifestations of Noonan syndrome. Images Paediatr Cardiol. 2001; **3**: 19–30.

7. Calvo KR, Price S, Braylan RC, Oliveira JB, Lenardo M, Fleisher TA, et al. JMML and RALD (RAS-associated autoimmune leukoproliferative disorder): Common genetic etiology yet clinically distinct entities. Blood. 2015; **125**: 2753–8.

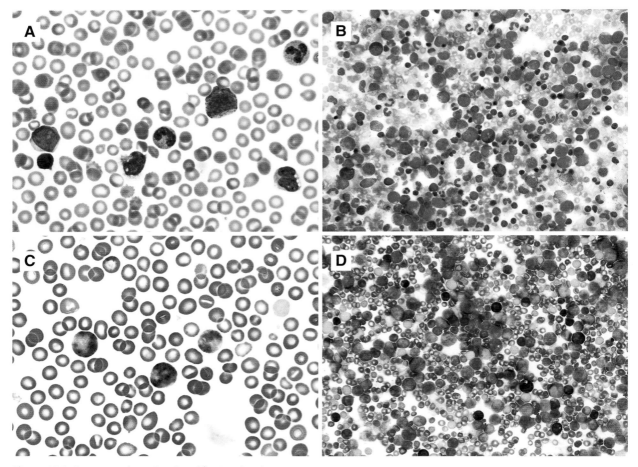

Figure 17.3 Noonan syndrome/myeloproliferative disorder.

This infant, an 11-week-old boy born at 40 weeks' gestation, was referred for evaluation for JMML. During the neonatal period, he was found to have a ventricular septal defect and thrombocytopenia. He developed leukocytosis with a few circulating blasts prior to referral. Facial abnormalities include large anterior fontanel with split sutures, low-set ears, widely spaced eyes, and a sacral dimple with tuft. The peripheral blood smear (A, Wright-Giemsa stain, 400x) showed marked thrombocytopenia and leukocytosis with 4% circulating blasts, a shift to immaturity in the neutrophil series, and an absolute monocytosis of 9.0 x 10⁹/L [0.15–1.95]. The bone marrow aspirate (B, Wright-Giemsa stain, 100x) was cellular, with a myeloid hyperplasia and 9% blasts. Myeloperoxidase (MPO) activity is demonstrated by enzyme cytochemistry in peripheral blood (C, Wright-Giemsa stain, 400x) and bone marrow (D, Wright-Giemsa stain, 400x) granulocytes, while alpha-naphthyl butyrate esterase (ANBE) activity is shown in peripheral blood (E) and bone marrow (F) monocytes. The core biopsy (G, H&E, 100x; H, H&E, 400x) was hypercellular at 100% with myeloid hyperplasia. Genetic testing was done and revealed a c.218C>T (p. Thr73Ile) mutation in exon 3 of *PTPN11*; although it can arise somatically, this is the most common germline mutation in patients with Noonan syndrome/myeloproliferative disorder.

8. Ganapathi KA, Schafernak KT, Rao VK, Calvo KR. Pediatric myelodysplastic/myeloproliferative neoplasms and related diseases. J Hematopathol. 2015; **8**: 159–67.

9. Lanzarotti N, Bruneau J, Trinquand A, Stoltzenberg MC, Neven B, Fregeac J, et al. RAS-associated lymphoproliferative disease evolves into severe juvenile myelo-monocytic leukemia. Blood. 2014; **123**: 1960–3.

10. Niemeyer CM, Flotho C. Juvenile myelomonocytic leukemia: Who's the driver at the wheel? Blood. 2019; **133**: 1060–70.

11. Röttgers S, Gombert M, Teigler-Schlegel A, Busch K, Gamerdinger U, Slany R, et al. ALK fusion genes in children with atypical myeloproliferative leukemia. Leukemia. 2010; **24**: 1197–200.

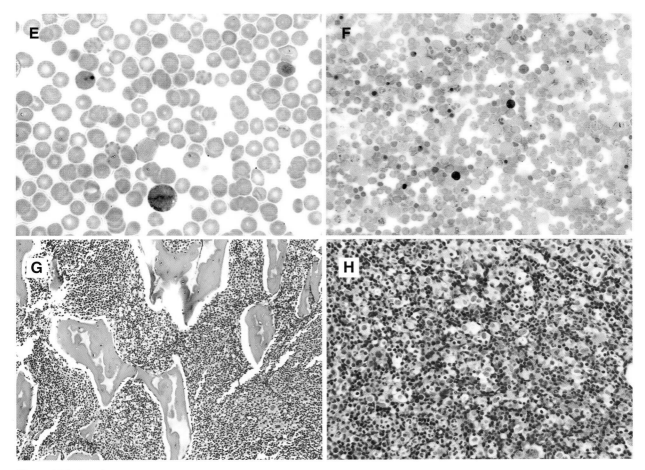

Figure 17.3 (cont.)

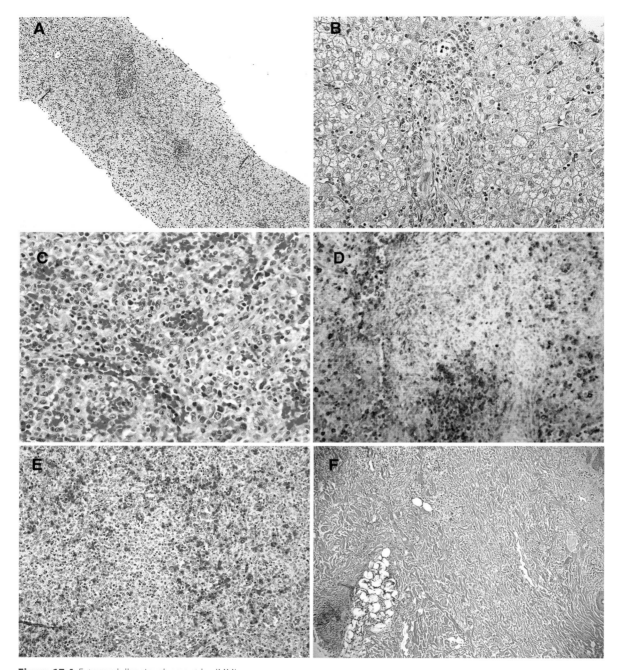

Figure 17.4 Extramedullary involvement by JMML.

The liver and spleen are virtually always involved in JMML, which also commonly involves lymph nodes, tonsils, the skin, the respiratory tract, and the gastrointestinal tract. A (H&E) and B (H&E) are images of a liver biopsy from a JMML patient. The periportal and sinusoids are infiltrated by myelomonocytic cells. C to E are images of spleen from a 22-month-old with JMML, who was status-post cord blood transplant and presented in relapse with splenomegaly (352 g; normal, 33 g). There was diffuse red pulp infiltration by a myelomonocytic proliferation (C, H&E; D, myeloperoxidase, IHC E, Leder chloracetate esterase stain). F to I are from a skin biopsy from another patient with JMML. F (H&E) demonstrates superficial and deep dermal and perivascular infiltrates. G (H&E) shows the infiltrates are mostly monocytoid cells with folded nuclear contours. H (IHC, lysozyme). I (IHC, myeloperoxidase).

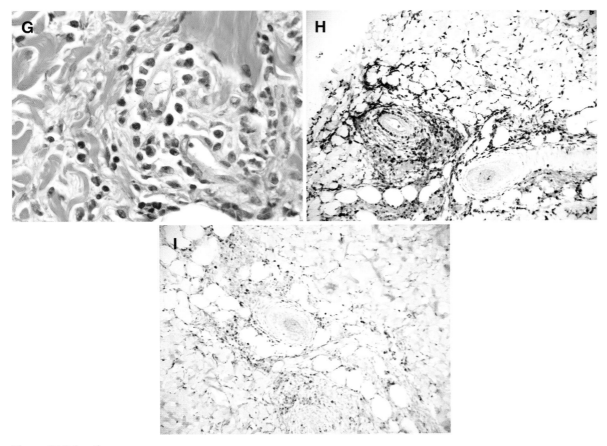

Figure 17.4 (cont.)

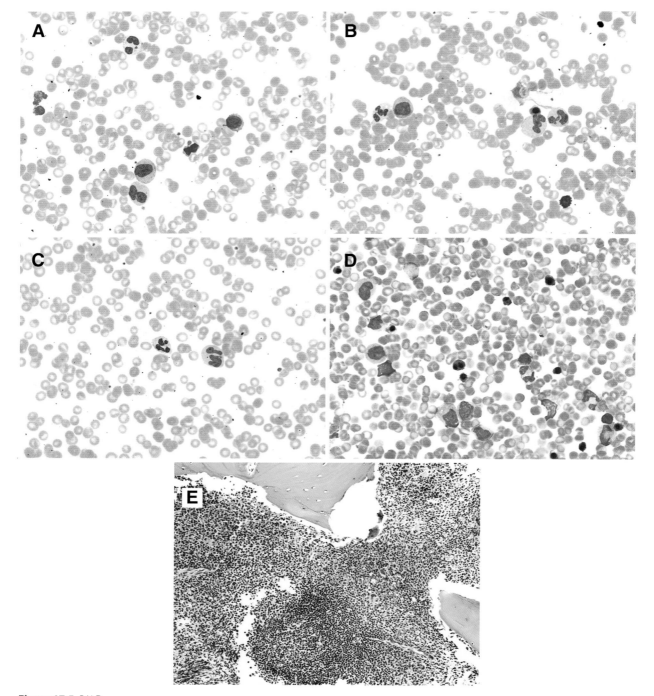

Figure 17.5 RALD.

A 19-month-old girl presented with normocytic anemia, thrombocytopenia, and splenomegaly. There was an absolute monocytosis of 3.3 x 10^9/L [0.2–1.4 x 10^9/L] and slight left shift without circulating blasts. Peripheral blood showed a monocyte with absolute nuclear segmentation. The neutrophil showed Döhle bodies and decreased cytoplasmic granules (A–C, Wright-Giemsa stain, 400x). The bone marrow aspirate (D, Wright-Giemsa stain, 400x) similarly displayed an increase in monocytes; the bone marrow biopsy (E, H&E, 100x) revealed cellularity approaching 100% and a large and rather well-circumscribed non-paratrabecular lymphoid aggregate, not a common finding in pediatric marrows.

Next-generation sequencing demonstrated a mutation in *KRAS* [c.37G>T, p.Gly13Cys (NM_004985.4)] with a variant allele frequency of 32.2% likely representing a somatic rather than germline variant. Although the patient met the criteria for JMML, flow cytometry immunophenotyping of the peripheral blood (F) proved quite useful. There were several myelomonocytic populations, including (A) 1.4% immature granulocytes, 0.6% eosinophils, and a trivial 0.05% CD34-positive blasts (latter not shown). Phenotypically normal neutrophils (9.8% of leukocytes) were bright positive for CD16 and moderate positive for CD24, CD33, and CD66c without significant CD14.

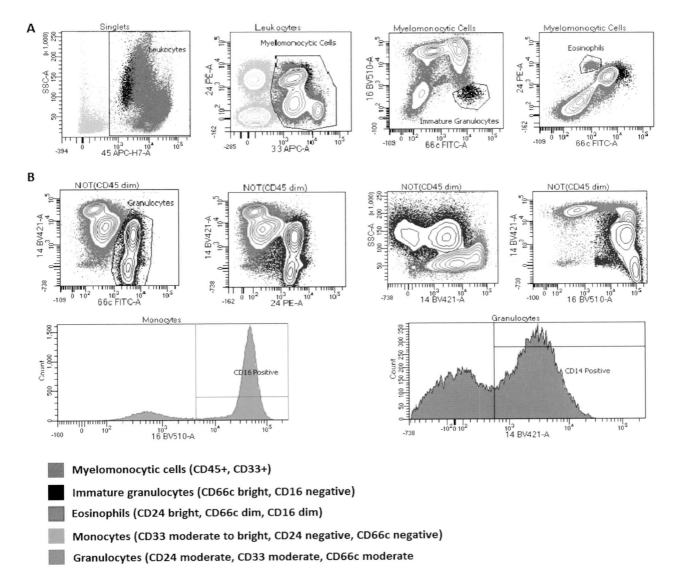

Myelomonocytic cells (CD45+, CD33+)

Immature granulocytes (CD66c bright, CD16 negative)

Eosinophils (CD24 bright, CD66c dim, CD16 dim)

Monocytes (CD33 moderate to bright, CD24 negative, CD66c negative)

Granulocytes (CD24 moderate, CD33 moderate, CD66c moderate

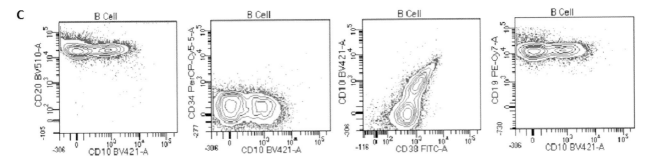

Figure 17.6 Phenotypically normal monocytes (6.7% of leukocytes) were bright positive for CD14 and CD33 without CD24, CD66c, or significant CD16. Just as there were cells intermediate between granulocytes and monocytes on morphology, (B) there were cells that were dual positive for CD14 and CD16 and that could not be resolved as either granulocytes or monocytes based on CD45 or CD33 expression or scattered light intensity characteristics, but they could be defined as CD14-positive granulocytes or CD16-positive monocytes based on CD24 and CD66c. Although not reported in JMML, in 82% of cases of RALD, monocytes show a CD16-positive activated phenotype and, in 64% of cases, atypical dim CD14 expression is observed on granulocytes [8]. These subtle immunophenotypic features, taken together with (C) the presence of circulating transitional B cells (40.1% of B cells and 3.6% of leukocytes, with dim to moderate CD10, bright CD20, and moderate CD38 expression), absence of circulating blasts or cytogenetic abnormality, and germinal center formation in the marrow, suggested a diagnosis of RALD.

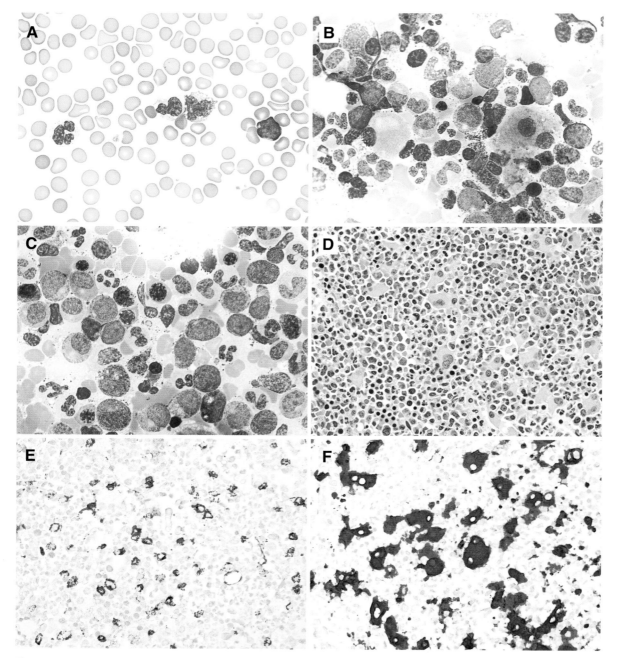

Figure 17.7 CMML.

A 15-year-old reportedly healthy boy with a family history of MDS/AML and CMML, known to be *GATA2* mutation positive, presented for family screening. His WBC count was greater than 15 x 10⁹/L (A, Wright-Giemsa stain, 100x), with absolute monocytosis and circulating blasts.
B is bone marrow aspirate smear shows predominance of myeloid cells, increased eosinophils and basophils, and two micromegakaryocytes. C shows increased blasts and many immature eosinophils. Flow cytometry immunophenotyping performed on the aspirate revealed 7% abnormal myeloblasts, absent B-cell precursors, and a marked decrease in mature B-cells and NK cells. The core biopsy was hypercellular (D, H&E) with many dysplastic megakaryocytes with monolobated nuclei and forming loose clusters. There are increased blasts (E, CD34, IHC). F shows increased megakaryocytes (CD61, IHC). Monosomy 7 was seen in all 20 metaphase cells, and a pathogenic mutation in *ASXL1* was identified by next-generation sequencing.

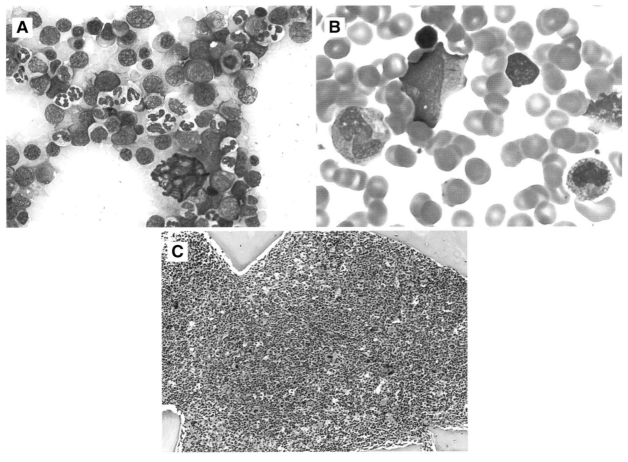

Figure 17.8 MDS/MPN-U.

This 7-year-old presented with 2- to 3-week history of fatigue, worsening headache, and vomiting and was found to have leukocytosis with 7% blasts with Auer rods and absolute monocytosis with 7% monocytes, profound macrocytic anemia, and moderate thrombocytopenia. Bone marrow aspirate revealed megaloblastoid erythropoiesis (A, Wright-Giemsa stain, 400x) and 3% blasts with Auer rod (B, Wright Giemsa stain, 1,000x). The core biopsy showed markedly hypercellular marrow with 100% cellularity (C, H&E, 100x). Megakaryocytes are inconspicuous, but careful examination showed the scattered hypolobated form. The combined myelodysplastic and myeloproliferative features and absence of a history of recent cytotoxic or growth factor therapy, *PDGRFA*, *PRGFRB*, or *FGFR1* rearrangement or *PCM1-JAK2* fusion, did not meet the CMML criteria (<10% monocytes), so MDS/MPN-U was the more appropriate diagnosis.

Chapter 18

Childhood Myelodysplastic Syndrome

Alina Dulau-Florea, Nisha Patel, Kristian T. Schafernak, Katherine R. Calvo

Introduction

Myelodysplastic syndrome (MDS) is a heterogeneous group of clonal disorders characterized by ineffective hematopoiesis causing cytopenias, dysplastic morphology, and risk for progression to acute myeloid leukemia (AML) [1]. Sporadic MDS is typically a disease of the elderly, whereas, in the pediatric population, the annual incidence is very low with one to two cases per million [2]. Pediatric MDS constitutes less than 5% of childhood hematologic malignancies [3].

Childhood MDS can present either as a primary disease in a previously healthy child or secondary to chemotherapy or radiation therapy, inherited bone marrow failure syndromes, or acquired severe aplastic anemia. The clinical manifestations are related to the type and degree of cytopenias: easy fatigability as a consequence of anemia, infectious complications due to neutropenia, and hemorrhagic tendencies due to thrombocytopenia. In contrast to MDS in adults, isolated anemia is uncommon, whereas neutropenia and thrombocytopenia are frequently present [1]. Asymptomatic cases have also been described.

Recent advances in next-generation sequencing (NGS) have helped in recognizing that many pediatric MDS are associated with underlying germline predisposition syndromes such as those caused by mutations in *GATA2*, *ETV6*, *ANKRD26*, *RUNX1*, *SAMD9/SAMD9L*, and other genes. Myeloid neoplasms with germline predisposition are described in Chapter 19.

Evaluation of suspected MDS in a child or adolescent with persistent, unexplained cytopenia starts with a thorough family history, physical exam, complete blood count with differential, and assessment of cell morphology. A chromosome fragility test and telomere length measurement are performed to rule out an inherited bone marrow failure disorder. Clues suggestive of MDS, particularly if more than one feature is present include circulating blasts, persistent megaloblastosis despite a normal vitamin B12 concentration, dysplastic morphology of any of the three hematopoietic cell lineages (erythroid, myeloid, and megakaryocytics), and chromosomal abnormalities. A family history of myeloid malignancies, other organ involvement, and/or unusual physical characteristics suggests a germline predisposition syndrome [4]. Therefore, a comprehensive assessment of clinical, laboratory, and genetic features is essential for an accurate diagnosis.

Genetic Profile of Pediatric Myelodysplastic Syndrome

Conventional cytogenetic analysis by chromosome banding of the bone marrow aspirate is usually performed after a standard 48-hour culture. A normal karyotype is present in approximately 60% of cases [5]. If abnormal, copy number changes are more common than balanced rearrangements, similar to MDS in adults. Monosomy 7 is the most frequent cytogenetic abnormality in childhood MDS, followed by trisomy 8 [5]. A complex karyotype, with up to or more than three chromosomal abnormalities of which at least one is a structural aberration, is the strongest prognostic factor for poor outcome [6]. While deletion 5q, deletion 20q, and loss of chromosome Y are more common cytogenetic abnormalities in adults, they are rare to absent in childhood MDS.

Next-generation sequencing results on primary pediatric MDS cases revealed that somatic mutations in myeloid genes are seen in approximately 13% of refractory cytopenia of childhood (RCC) cases and 68% of MDS with excess blasts (MDS-EB) [7]. Somatic mutations are also more common in patients with monosomy 7 compared to other karyotypes. Mutations in RNA splicing factors are nearly absent whereas mutations in genes involved in chromatin modification, DNA methylation,

This work was supported by the National Institutes of Health, Division of Intramural Research in the NIH Clinical Center.

signaling, and transcription are seen at frequencies similar to adult MDS [7]. In one study, the most commonly mutated genes were *SETBP1, ASXL1, RUNX1, PTPN11,* and *NRAS* [7]. Less common mutations were in *KRAS, EZH2, NF1,* and *NPM1*. Mutations that are frequently detected in adult MDS or in age-related clonal hematopoiesis, such as *TET2, DNMT3A,* and spliceosome mutations, were not seen [8]. Overall, approximately 80% of young patients with MDS have at least one cytogenetic or molecular genetic aberration, similar to adult MDS [7].

Myelodysplastic syndrome survival and risk of transformation to AML in adults depends on multiple factors, including percentage of bone marrow blasts, type of cytogenetic abnormality, and number and type of molecular genetic abnormalities. A study analyzing the value of the International Prognostic Scoring System (IPSS) in children with de novo MDS found that a bone marrow blast percentage under 5% and platelet count more than $100 \times 10^9/L$ were significantly associated with superior survival in this population, and those with advanced MDS had a poorer outcome [8]. Other studies have shown that monosomy 7 or multilineage dysplasia confers a higher risk of disease progression [9]. Coexisting clonal events, including somatic mutations, karyotypic abnormalities, and germline mutations in *GATA2* or *RUNX1* genes, are known to constitute cooperative mechanisms leading to leukemic transformation [7].

According to the 2017 World Health Organization (WHO) classification of myeloid neoplasms, pediatric MDS include two entities: refractory cytopenia of childhood (RCC), a low-grade MDS, and myelodysplastic syndrome with excess blasts (MDS-EB), a more advanced disease [9].

Refractory Cytopenia of Childhood

Refractory cytopenia of childhood, a provisional MDS entity in the 2017 WHO classification, is the most common MDS subtype in children and adolescents. It is a low-grade MDS characterized by persistent cytopenias, less than 2% blasts in the peripheral blood, less than 5% bone marrow blasts, and dysplastic morphology. A threshold of at least 10% dysplastic cells in at least one lineage is required to define dysplasia. Lesser degrees of dysplasia are accepted if they are present in two or three lineages [9]. The peripheral blood smear reveals red cell anisopoikilocytosis and macrocytosis. Neutrophils may show hypolobated (pseudo-Pelger-Huet) nuclei and/or cytoplasmic hypogranularity. Platelets show anisocytosis and giant platelets may be noted. Whether RCC with multilineage dysplasia is clinically different from RCC with unilineage dysplasia remains controversial [10].

Currently, MDS with multilineage dysplasia in childhood is considered as RCC. Evaluation of the BM core biopsy reveals that in about 80% of RCC, the marrow is hypocellular for age and may mimic acquired severe aplastic anemia (SAA) or an inherited bone marrow failure (BMF) syndrome [9, 11]. Therefore, a thorough morphologic evaluation is required to distinguish these entities (Table 18.1). Erythroid islands often have a patchy distribution and can be abnormally localized in paratrabecular areas where granulocytic precursors are normally found. Erythroid precursors show impaired maturation with left shift and increased mitotic figures. In aspirate smears, features of dyserythropoiesis include abnormal nuclear lobulation, multinuclearity, nuclear bridging, and megaloblastic changes. Granulopoiesis is usually decreased and often left-shifted. An inverted myeloid-to-erythroid (M:E) ratio is common. Assessment of dysplasia in mature neutrophils is easier in the peripheral blood, where hypolobation of the nuclei (pseudo-Pelger-Huet cells) and/or cytoplasmic hypogranularity are easy to observe. Megakaryocytes are usually decreased in number, abnormally localized to paratrabecular areas, and show dysplastic features such as hypolobation of nuclei or abnormally small size with mononuclearity ("micromegakaryocytes") or dissociated nuclear lobes. Identification is made easier by immunohistochemical stains for CD61 or CD42b. Of note, absence of megakaryocytes does not rule out RCC [12].

Estimation of myeloblasts as a percentage of nucleated cells in the bone marrow biopsy can be performed by a CD34 immunohistochemical stain. In RCC, CD34-positive precursors are not increased (less than 5% of BM cells) and are scattered singly without clustering. Caution is needed when assessing a CD34 stain since endothelial cells and early normal B-cell precursors ("hematogones") are also CD34-positive. Multiparameter flow cytometric analysis can help in differentiating myeloblasts (CD13+, CD34+) from early B-cell progenitors/hematogones (CD34+, CD19+), and in fact, a decreased percentage of progenitor B-cells within the CD34+ compartment is commonly seen in MDS [12]. Blasts percentage is also evaluated in the bone marrow aspirate with a 500-cell differential count.

Table 18.1 highlights clinical and histologic characteristics of pediatric MDS subtypes in comparison with acquired (severe) aplastic anemia, a benign disease that can mimic MDS. In addition to AA, the differential diagnosis of RCC is broad and includes many conditions that present with dysplastic morphologic features mimicking MDS (Table 18.2) [9, 10]. Secondary changes mimicking myelodysplasia are reversible. Because cytogenetic abnormalities are sometimes

Table 18.1 Clinical and laboratory characteristics of patients with childhood MDS (refractory cytopenia of childhood and MDS-EB) in comparison with patients with severe aplastic anemia (SAA)

Characteristic	Severe Aplastic Anemia (SAA)	Refractory Cytopenia of Childhood (RCC)	Myelodysplastic Syndrome with Excess Blasts (MDS-EB)
Bone marrow biopsy	Hypocellular Blasts: <5% *Erythroid precursors*: absent or single small focus with <10 cells, normal localization, intact maturation *Granulopoiesis*: absent or markedly decreased, intact maturation *Megakaryocytes*: absent or rare, normal localization, and no micromegakaryocytes	Hypocellular: 80% of cases Blasts: <5%, no clusters *Erythroid precursors*: clusters, abnormal localization, left-shifted maturation, increased mitoses *Granulopoiesis*: left-shifted *Megakaryocytes*: micromegakaryocytes, abnormal localization	Normo-/hyper-/hypocellular Blasts: 5–19%, clusters *Erythroid precursors*: abnormal localization; left-shifted maturation increased mitoses *Granulopoiesis*: intermingled with erythroid elements (loss of normal architecture), left-shifted *Megakaryocytes*: dysplastic, abnormal localization
Bone marrow aspirate	*Erythroid precursors*: Absent or small focus, no dysplasia, no megaloblastoid changes *Granulocytes*: decreased, no dysplastic changes, <5% blasts *Megakaryocytes*: absent or very few, no dysplasia	*Erythroid precursors*: dysplastic (nuclear budding/binucleation) or megaloblastoid changes *Granulocytes*: dysplastic changes (hypogranularity, hyposegmentation), <5% blasts *Megakaryocytes*: micromegakaryocytes +/− other dysplastic changes	*Erythroid precursors*: dysplastic (nuclear budding/binucleation) or megaloblastoid changes *Granulocytes*: dysplastic changes (hypogranularity, hyposegmentation), 5–19% blasts *Megakaryocytes*: micromegakaryocytes +/− other dysplastic changes
Peripheral blood	<2% blasts Pancytopenia: frequent Red cells: reduced, Neutrophils: reduced, no dysplasia	<2% blasts Sustained cytopenias (neutropenia, thrombocytopenia; anemia less common) * Red cells: macrocytic, anisopoikilocytosis Neutrophils: reduced, +/− hyposegmented nuclei, hypogranular cytoplasm	2–19% blasts Pancytopenia Red cells: macrocytic, anisopoikilocytosis Neutrophils: reduced, +/− hyposegmented nuclei, hypogranularity
Cytogenetics	Normal karyotype; common; Cytogenetic abnormalities: rare, transient	Normal karyotype: 40% Monosomy 7, del 7q: relatively more common	Normal karyotype: rare Monosomy 7, del 7q: relatively more common
Spliceosomal gene mutations	N/A	Uncommon (<2%)	Uncommon (<2%)
Hypermethylation	N/A	Common (>50%)	Common (>50%)

* Isolated anemia with Hb < 10 g/dl is uncommon in RCC [9].
Adapted with modifications from [2, 13, 15].

present in inherited BMF syndromes like Fanconi anemia and Shwachman-Diamond syndrome, and even in acquired AA (although in this latter condition they tend to be transient), proof of clonality of the hematopoietic cells does not by itself warrant a diagnosis of MDS.

Myelodysplastic Syndrome with Excess Blasts

Myelodysplastic syndrome with excess blasts (MDS-EB) is a higher-grade MDS that can occur in children and is morphologically indistinguishable from its adult counterpart. It is characterized by 2–19% circulating and 5–19% bone marrow blasts, in addition to persistent cytopenia(s) and dysplastic changes. In contrast to adult MDS, there are no data on the prognostic relevance of distinguishing MDS-EB-1 and MDS-EB-2 in children and, despite the excess blasts, children maintain relatively stable peripheral blood counts for weeks or months [9]. Also, some cases with blast percentage between 20 and 29%, which would be diagnosed as AML, have a slower progression in children and behave more akin to MDS,

Table 18.2 Disorders that present with atypical morphologic features that may mimic RCC

Nutritional deficiencies: Vitamin B12, folate, vitamin E, vitamin D, copper

Toxins and drugs

Infections: Cytomegalovirus, herpes virus, parvovirus B19, HIV, hepatitis C, tuberculosis

Metabolic disorders: Mevalonate kinase deficiency

Autoimmune disorders: Systemic lupus erythematosus, juvenile rheumatoid arthritis, polyarteritis nodosa, immune thrombocytopenic purpura

Autoimmune lymphoproliferative syndrome: FAS deficiency

Pearson syndrome: Mitochondrial DNA deletion

Inherited BM failure disorders: Fanconi anemia, Dyskeratosis congenita, Shwachman-Diamond syndrome, others

Chronic hemolytic anemia

Post transplantation of solid organs (alteration of marrow microenvironment, T-cell dysfunction)

Aplastic anemia in hematologic recovery after immunosuppressive treatment

Adapted from [9] and [16].

and are thus categorized by the French-American-British (FAB) classification as refractory anemia with excess blasts in transformation (RAEB-t) [9].

Therapy-Related and Secondary Myelodysplastic Syndrome in Childhood

Therapy-related myelodysplastic syndrome (t-MDS) occurs several months to years after exposure to chemotherapy and/or radiotherapy for solid tumors (neuroblastoma, Ewing sarcoma) or hematologic malignancies (acute lymphoblastic leukemia, Burkitt lymphoma, or Hodgkin lymphoma). Cytogenetic abnormalities include monosomy 7/deletion 7q, deletion 5q, deletion 17p or dic(5;17)(q11.1-q13.3;p11.1-13) with *TP53* loss of function, translocation t(3;21)(q26.2;q22.1), or a complex karyotype[15]. t-MDS also has a high incidence of *TP53* mutations, which can be either somatic or germline [13]. Secondary MDS may develop in the evolution of acquired severe aplastic anemia, and is usually preceded by genetic abnormalities such as monosomy 7/deletion 7q and somatic mutations in *ASXL1* and *DNMT3A* [14].

References

1. Hasserjian RP OA, Brunning RD, Germing U, Le Beau MM, Porwit A, et al. Myelodysplastic syndromes: Overview. In Swerdlow SH, Campo E, Harris NL, et al., eds. World Health Organization classification of tumours of haematopoietic and lymphoid tissues. Revised 4th ed. Lyon: IARC Press; 2017:97–106.

2. Hasle H. Myelodysplastic and myeloproliferative disorders of childhood. Hematology Am Soc Hematol Educ Program. 2016; **2016**(1): 598–604.

3. Niemeyer CM, Baumann I. Classification of childhood aplastic anemia and myelodysplastic syndrome. Hematology Am Soc Hematol Educ Program. 2011; **2011**: 84–9.

4. Babushok DV, Bessler M, Olson TS. Genetic predisposition to myelodysplastic syndrome and acute myeloid leukemia in children and young adults. Leuk Lymphoma. 2016; **57**(3): 520–36.

5. Kardos G, Baumann I, Passmore SJ, Locatelli F, Hasle H, Schultz KR, et al. Refractory anemia in childhood: A retrospective analysis of 67 patients with particular reference to monosomy 7. Blood. 2003; **102**(6): 1997–2003.

6. Göhring G, Michalova K, Beverloo HB, Betts D, Harbott J, Haas OA, et al. Complex karyotype newly defined: The strongest prognostic factor in advanced childhood myelodysplastic syndrome. Blood. 2010; **116**(19): 3766–9.

7. Pastor V, Hirabayashi S, Karow A, Wehrle J, Kozyra EJ, Nienhold R, et al. Mutational landscape in children with myelodysplastic syndromes is distinct from adults: Specific somatic drivers and novel germline variants. Leukemia. 2017; **31**(3): 759–62.

8. Hasle H, Baumann I, Bergsträsser E, Fenu S, Fischer A, Kardos G, et al. The International Prognostic Scoring System (IPSS) for childhood myelodysplastic syndrome (MDS) and juvenile myelomonocytic leukemia (JMML). Leukemia. 2004; **18**(12): 2008–14.

9. Baumann I NC, Bennett JM. Childhood myelodysplastic syndrome. In Swerdlow SH, Campo E, Harris NL, et al., eds. World Health Organization classification of tumours of

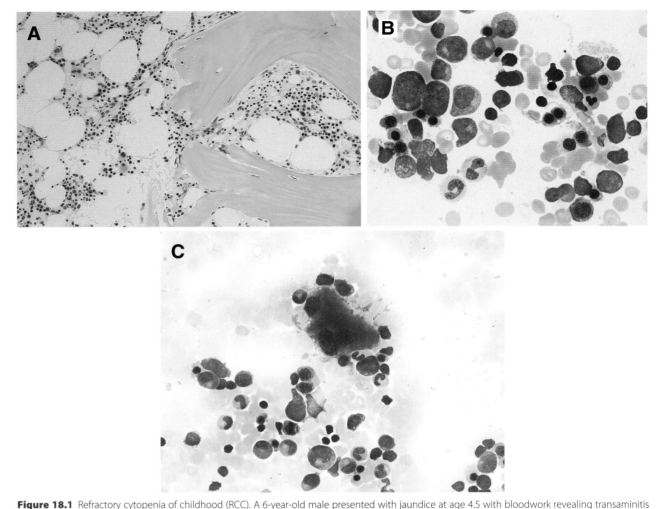

Figure 18.1 Refractory cytopenia of childhood (RCC). A 6-year-old male presented with jaundice at age 4.5 with bloodwork revealing transaminitis and elevated bilirubin. Infectious workup was negative and liver biopsy was suggestive of autoimmune hepatitis. His liver enzymes normalized 6 months after treatment with prednisone. Although the initial complete blood count was within normal limits, he became progressively pancytopenic following a rotavirus infection. Bone marrow examination was performed at this time point, showing decreased cellularity (A, 200x) and erythroid-predominant hematopoiesis and a few dysplastic megakaryocytes. Bone marrow aspirate (B, 200X) shows occasional blasts, dysplastic erythroid precursors, and dysplastic megakaryocytes (C).

Cytogenetic analysis revealed monosomy 7 in 10 out of 20 metaphases. Genetic studies for bone marrow failure and familial AML/MDS were negative. Danazol was initiated, which led to improvement of anemia (hemoglobin, 9–10 g/dL) and thrombocytopenia (20–22×10^9 platelets/L), though the absolute neutrophil count remained very low (0.2×10^9/L). Matched unrelated donor stem cell transplant was planned because, despite being a full HLA match, his sister's telomere length was at the lower end of normal.

haematopoietic and lymphoid tissues. Revised 4th ed. Lyon, IARC Press; 2017:116–20.

10. Iwafuchi H, Ito M. Differences in the bone marrow histology between childhood myelodysplastic syndrome with multilineage dysplasia and refractory cytopenia of childhood without multilineage dysplasia. Histopathology. 2019; **74**(2): 239–47.

11. Niemeyer CM, Baumann I. Myelodysplastic syndrome in children and adolescents. Semin Hematol. 2008; **45**(1): 60–70.

12. Olcay L, Yetgin S. Disorders mimicking myelodysplastic syndrome and difficulties in its diagnosis. In Fuchs O., ed. Myelodysplastic syndromes. London, IntechOpen; 2016:43–94.

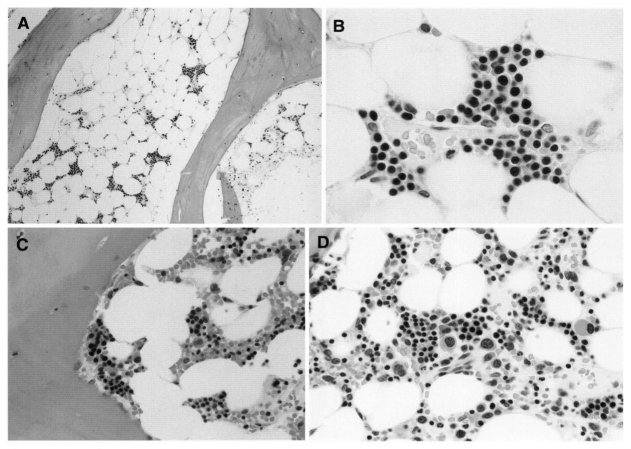

Figure 18.2 Secondary MDS: RCC.

This secondary MDS developed in a 7-year-old female with a history of aplastic anemia. At age 3 years, she presented with excessive bruising and complete blood count showed anemia and thrombocytopenia. The bone marrow biopsy was markedly hypocellular (<10%) with trilineage hypoplasia and no dysplasia. Workups for BMF were all negative. She was followed by observation only, but ultimately developed pancytopenia. Treatment with immunosuppression and subsequent erythropoietin led to temporary improvement, but 4 years after initial presentation, her blood counts again declined. The bone marrow was hypocellular for age (A, 200x) with erythroid-predominant hematopoiesis (B, 500X) and some erythroid islands abnormally localized to the paratrabecular region, a feature of dyserythropoiesis (C, 500x). Granulopoiesis was decreased, left-shifted, and intermingled with erythroid elements and dysplastic megakaryocytes, with loss of the normal marrow architecture (D, 500x). CD61 immunohistochemistry demonstrated small, monolobate megakaryocytes (E, 500x), while CD34 immunostain revealed mildly increased blasts (F, 500x). The aspirate contained 5% blasts (G, 1,000x) and dysplastic megakaryocytes with monolobated small megakaryocytes (H, 1,000x). Cytogenetic analysis revealed an abnormal karyotype: 46,XX,der(5)t(1;5)(q11;q11.2[3]/46,XX[17].

13. Wong TN, Ramsingh G, Young AL, Miller CA, Touma W, Welch JS, et al. Role of TP53 mutations in the origin and evolution of therapy-related acute myeloid leukaemia. Nature. 2015; **518**(7540): 552–5.

14. Yoshizato T, Dumitriu B, Hosokawa K, Makishima H, Yoshida K, Townsley D, et al. Somatic mutations and clonal hematopoiesis in aplastic anemia. N Engl J Med. 2015; **373**(1): 35–47.

15. Baumann I, Führer M, Behrendt S, Campr V, Csomor J, Furlan I, et al. Morphological differentiation of severe aplastic anaemia from hypocellular refractory cytopenia of childhood: Reproducibility of histopathological diagnostic criteria. Histopathology. 2012; **61**(1): 10–17.

16. Olney HJ LBM. Meylodysplastic syndromes. In Heim S, Mitelman F, eds. Cancer cytogenetics. 4th ed. Hoboken, NJ, Wiley Blackwell; 2015:126–52.

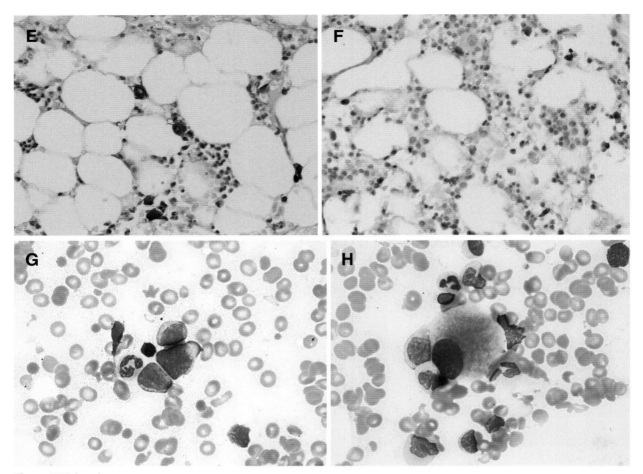

Figure 18.2 (cont.)

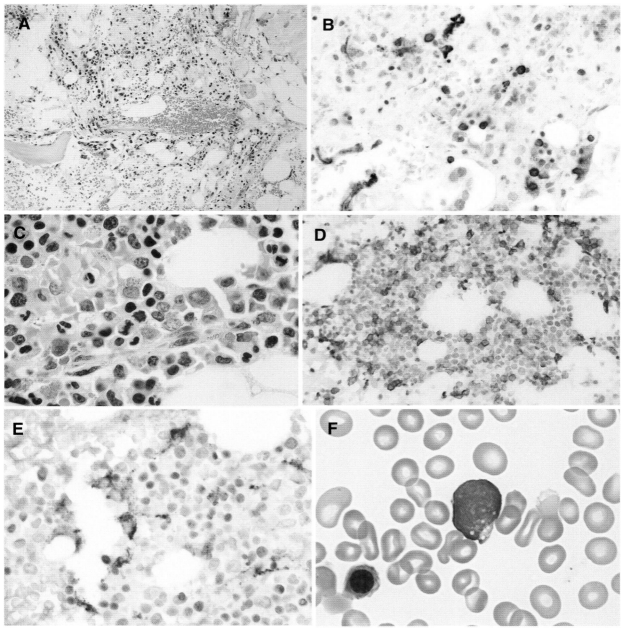

Figure 18.3 Secondary MDS: Myelodysplastic syndrome with excess blasts (MDS-EB). This is a 19-year-old male with history of fatigue, "black spots" (burst vessels) in his eyes, and easy bruising, which started at age 18. Complete blood count at that time showed a hemoglobin of 6.5 g/dL, absolute neutrophil count of 0.4 K/μL and platelets 7 K/μL, reticulocyte count less than 10 K/μL, and markedly hypocellular (5–10% cellular) bone marrow with trilineage hypoplasia without dysplasia. Cytogenetic analysis was normal. Since there are no matched related donors, he was treated with horse ATG and cyclosporine. Although there was some improvement in counts and reduction in frequency of transfusions, he remained transfusion dependent with weekly red cells and platelets transfusion and required growth factor to maintain his white blood cell count. Subsequent treatment with eltrombopag (a small molecule agonist of the c-MPL receptor) was also unsuccessful, and bone marrow examination performed at 3-month assessment after eltrombopag revealed monosomy 7. The marrow was variably hypocellular (A, 200x) with increased immature precursors highlighted by CD34 immunostain (B, 500x). Moreover, the clot section contained clusters of immature precursors (C, 200x), highlighted by CD34 immunostain (D, 500x). Factor VIII-related antigen immunostain demonstrated megakaryocytic dysplasia with several small, hypolobate forms (E, 500x). The bone marrow aspirate was hemodilute and unsuitable for a differential count but showed occasional blasts (F, 1,000x) dysplastic erythroid precursors with nuclear budding (G, 1,000x), and dysplastic neutrophils with hyposegmented nuclei (H, 1000X).

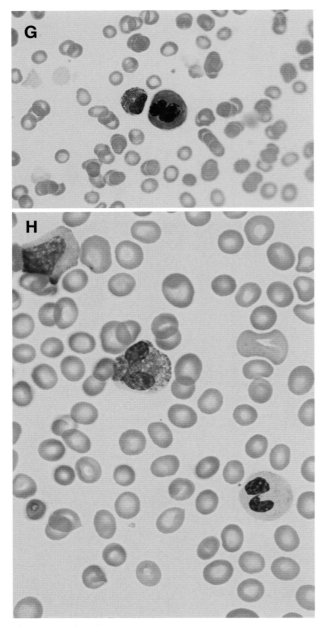

Figure 18.3 (cont.)

Chapter 19

Germline Predisposition to Myeloid Neoplasia

Katherine R. Calvo, Nisha Patel, Alina Dulau-Florea, Kristian T. Schafernak

Introduction

There is increasing recognition of the role inherited and de novo germline mutations play in the development of myeloid neoplasia [1], particularly in children, adolescents, and young/middle-aged adults [2, 3]. Germline mutation inheritance may be autosomal dominant with variable penetrance, X-linked, or autosomal recessive. Family history of neoplasia or cytopenia may be helpful in identifying potential cases with germline predisposition. However, variability in disease penetrance within family members harboring the same mutation may mask early recognition of familial disease. Additionally, patients harboring de novo germline mutations may have no family history of disease. The World Health Organization's (WHO) 2016 classification of tumors of the hematopoietic and lymphoid tissues recognizes three major classifications of myeloid neoplasms with germline predispositions: myeloid neoplasms without preexisting disorder or organ dysfunction, myeloid neoplasms with preexisting platelet disorders, and myeloid neoplasms with other organ dysfunctions (including inherited bone marrow failure syndromes) [1]. In this chapter, we address genes associated with germline predisposition to myeloid neoplasia (Table 19.1), including *CEBPA*, *DDX41*, *RUNX1*, *ANKRD26*, *ETV6*, GATA2, and those associated with telomere disease and classic bone marrow failure (BMF) syndromes (Table 19.2). Newly identified genes predisposing to BMF and myelodysplastic syndrome (MDS) are also addressed, including *SAMD9*, *SAMD9L*, and *MECOM*. Juvenile myelomonocytic leukemia associated with neurofibromatosis, Noonan syndrome, or Noonan syndrome-like disorders is addressed in Chapter 17.

Recognition of neoplasia associated with germline mutations is critical for appropriate patient management, particularly when screening potential related donors for hematopoietic stem cell transplantation (HSCT). Multiple studies have shown donor-derived MDS and acute myeloid leukemia (AML) have been acquired after HSCT when relatives harboring the same germline mutation have been used as donors (*GATA2*, *RUNX1*, *CEBPA*, etc.). For many diseases with germline mutations (e.g., Fanconi anemia and GATA2 deficiency), optimal conditioning regimens may vary due to excessive toxicity of standard chemotherapy or high risk of infection due to underlying immunodeficiency.

Identification of germline mutations also has significant implications for family members, underscoring the importance of genetic counseling [2]. Patients with germline mutations in *RUNX1*, *ANKRD26*, *ETV6*, and other genes may have dysmegakaryopoiesis at baseline as a feature of the disease even in the presence of mild or minimal thrombocytopenia. For this reason, pathologists are cautioned against overdiagnosing MDS in the setting of isolated thrombocytopenia and dysmegakaryopoiesis. Transformation to MDS/AML is associated with hypercellularity, multilineage dysplasia, increased blasts, abnormal karyotype [4], and/or additional (somatic) molecular genetic defects.

Use of next-generation-sequencing-targeted panels and whole exome sequencing can be helpful in identifying patients with germline mutations. Optimal specimens for germline mutation testing include cultured fibroblasts from a skin biopsy, hair follicles, or nail clippings (Table 19.3). A pathogenic mutation with a high variant allele frequency (VAF) (30–50%) may suggest germline mutation, but it does not exclude a somatic mutation with a high VAF. If germline mutation is suspected, confirmation of the germline mutation can be made using DNA from a germline source. Alternatively, a biologically related parent or sibling harboring the same mutation

This work was supported by the National Institutes of Health, Division of Intramural Research in the NIH Clinical Center.

Table 19.1 Myeloid neoplasm with germline predisposition (and other select syndromes)

	Age of Presentation	Inheritance	Gene(s)	Associated Hematologic Neoplasms	Clinical Presentation	Select Non-hematologic Abnormalities	Common Karyotype Abnormalities	Ancillary Diagnostic Tests	Approximate Risk of MDS/AML
AML with germline *CEBPA* mutation	Median age: 24.5 years (range: 2–50 years)	AD	*CEBPA* (19p13.1)	AML	AML without preceding cytopenia(s)	None	Normal	GS	100%
Myeloid neoplasms with germline *DDX41* mutation	Median age: 62 years (range: 40–85 years)	AD	*DDX41* (5q35.3)	MDS/AML, CMML (*HL and NHL have been reported*)	Leukopenia with or without other cytopenia(s)	None	Normal	GS	Not clearly established
Myeloid neoplasms with germline *RUNX1* mutation	Median age: 33 years	AD	*RUNX1* (21q22.12)	MDS/AML, CMML, T-ALL (*B-cell neoplasms have also been reported*)	Thrombocytopenia and bleeding tendencies	None	Both clonal and non-clonal karyotypes can be seen	– GS – Impaired platelet aggregation studies and storage pool deficiencies	30–40%
Myeloid neoplasms with germline *ANKRD26* mutation	Not clearly established	AD	*ANKRD26* (10p12.1)	AML, MDS, CMML, CLL, CML	Thrombocytopenia and bleeding tendencies	None	Not clearly established	– GS, – Platelets can have alpha granule deficiency	30-fold risk of a myeloid neoplasm
Myeloid neoplasms with germline *ETV6* mutation	Not clearly established	AD	*ETV6* (12p13.2)	MDS, AML, CMML, B-ALL, and PCM	Thrombocytopenia and bleeding tendencies	Colorectal adenocarcinoma, skin cancer, myopathy, GERD	Not clearly established	– GS – Impaired platelet aggregation studies	Not clearly established
Myeloid neoplasms with germline *GATA2* mutation	Median age: 20 years (range 4–78 years)	AD	*GATA2* (3q21.3)	MDS, AML, and CMML	Deficiencies of dendritic cells, B-cells, B-cell precursors, NK cells, and monocytes	Infections (mycobacterial, fungal, viral), warts, lymphedema, deafness, and PAP	Monosomy 7, Trisomy 8, der (1;7) (q10; p10)	GS	Estimated 50–75% develop myeloid neoplasia
SAMD9 and *SAMD9L* mutations	*SAMD9*: Infants *SAMD9L*: Infants to adults	AD	*SAMD9* and *SAMD9L* (7q212)	MDS, AML	Transient or permanent cytopenia(s)	**SAMD9:** infection, growth restriction, adrenal hypoplasia, genital phenotypes, and enteropathy **SAMDL:** Cerebellar hypoplasia	Aberrations in chromosome 7 (can be transient)	GS	Not clearly established
Myeloid proliferations associated with Down syndrome (TAM) (ML-DS)	**(TAM) –** Usually within first 3 months of life **(ML-DS) –** Usually occurs before 5 years of age	Typically Constitutional A subset can have trisomy 21 mosaicism	*GATA1* (Xp11.23)	**(TAM)** Transient increase in blasts (self-resolving) **(ML-DS)** AML	**(TAM) –** Can include thrombocytopenia, leukocytosis and/or hepatosplenomegaly **(ML-DS) –** Most cases have prior history of TAM	– Constitutional abnormalities associated with Down syndrome – Can be phenotypically normal in trisomy 21 mosaicism	Trisomy 21 **(ML-DS):** trisomy 8 is also common	GS	**(TAM)** 1–20% develop AML by 5 years of age. **(ML-DS)** - Approximately 150-fold increase of AML

AD, autosomal dominant; AML, acute myeloid leukemia; B-ALL, B-lymphoblastic leukemia/lymphoma; CMML, chronic myelomonocytic leukemia; GERD, gastroesophageal reflux disease; HL, Hodgkin lymphoma; MDS, myelodysplastic syndrome; ML-DS, AML associated with Down syndrome; NHL, non-Hodgkin lymphoma; PAP, pulmonary alveolar proteinosis; PCM, plasma cell myeloma; T-ALL, T-lymphoblastic leukemia/lymphoma; TAM, transient abnormal myelopoiesis; SAMD9, sterile a-motif domain-containing protein 9; SAMD9L, sterile a-motif domain-containing protein 9-like; GS, gene sequencing.

Note: Juvenile myelomonocytic leukemia associated with neurofibromatosis, Noonan syndrome, or Noonan-like syndrome is addressed in Chapter 17.

Table 19.2 Select inherited bone marrow failure syndromes

	Age of Presentation	Inheritance	Gene(s)	Associated Hematologic Neoplasms	Clinical Presentation	Select Non-hematologic Abnormalities	Common Karyotype Abnormalities	Ancillary Diagnostic Tests	Approximate risk of MDS/AML
Li-Fraumeni syndrome	Leukemia: Median age of 12 years	AD	TP53	ALL, MDS/AML, CML	Early onset of cancer, multiple cancers, family history of cancer	Soft tissue sarcoma, osteosarcoma, breast cancer, CNS tumors, and adrenocortical carcinoma	Hypodiploidy in B-ALL Complex karyotype AML	GS	2–4% for leukemia
Fanconi anemia	BMF usually occurs between 5 and 10 years of age)	AR, XLR	FANCA, FANCB, FANCC, BRCA2, FANCD2, FANCE, FANCF, FANCG, FANCI, BRIP1, FANCL, FANCM, PAMLB2, RAD51C, SLX4	MDS, AML, ALL (Rare)	Cytopenia(s); macrocytosis	Short stature, café au lait spots, abnormal thumbs, absent radii, microcephaly, micro-ophthalmia, and renal anomalies	+1q, +3q, +13q; 7q-, 20q-; Monosomy 7	– Chromosomal fragility test – GS	– 6,000-fold (MDS) – 700-fold (AML)
Shwachman-Diamond syndrome	Infants to young adults	AR	SBDS	MDS, AML	Cytopenia(s); (classically neutropenia)	Exocrine pancreatic insufficiency and skeletal abnormalities	7q- Isochromosome 7q (Monosomy 7), 20q-	GS	Risk for AML- 15–30%
Diamond-Blackfan anemia	Early infancy (median age 2 months)	AD, XLR	RPS19, RPS17, RPS24, RPL35A, RPL5, RPL11, RPS7, RPS26, RPS10, GATA1	MDS, AML	Macrocytic anemia with reticulocytopenia	Craniofacial abnormalities, thumb deformities, renal and heart defects. Also have increased risk of colon carcinoma, osteosarcoma, and urogenital malignancies	Usually normal karyotype	– GS – Elevated erythrocyte adenosine deaminase – Elevated fetal hemoglobin	5–20%
Telomere biology disorders including dyskeratosis congenita and syndromes due to TERC and TERT mutations	Variable but usually second or third decade	XLR, AD, AR	DKC1, TERC, TERT, RTEL1, TINF2, TERT, CTC1, WRAPS3, NHP2, NOP10	MDS, AML	– Variable cytopenia(s)	Depends on subgroup. Can include pulmonary fibrosis, retinopathy, cerebellar hypoplasia, nail dystrophy; skin pigmentation changes, oral leukoplakia, and squamous cell cancer	Not clearly established	– GS – Telomere length analysis	2–30%
Severe congenital neutropenia	Usually first months of life, but can present in early childhood	AD, AR, XLR	ELANE, CSF3 R, GFI1, HAX1, G6PC3, JAGN1, WAS	MDS, AML	Severe neutropenia with recurrent infections	Most lack physical abnormalities, but can include osteopenia, stunted growth, and cardiac defects.	Not clearly established	– GS	– Variable amongst subtypes; approximately 10–30%
MECOM in myeloid malignancies	– Pancytopenia in first two years of life. – MDS has so far been reported in older adults	AD	MECOM/EVI1	MDS, MDS/MPN	Thrombocytopenia/pancytopenia with or without other congenital abnormalities	Limb dysmorphisms (i.e, radioulnar synostosis) and hearing impairment	Not clearly established	– GS	– Not clearly established

AD, autosomal dominant; AML, acute myeloid leukemia; AR, autosomal recessive; B-ALL, B-lymphoblastic leukemia/lymphoma; BMF, bone marrow failure; CNS, central nervous syndrome; GS: gene sequencing; MDS, myelodysplastic syndrome; MECOM, MDS1 and EVI1 complex locus; MPN, myeloproliferative neoplasms; XLR, X-linked recessive; GS: gene sequencing.

Table 19.3 Specimen types for germline mutation testing

Tissue Type	Suitability for Germline Testing
Skin fibroblast culture	Gold standard as germline source
Nail clippings and hair follicles	Can be used as germline source
Peripheral blood and bone marrow	Not ideal sources of germline DNA as they can contain somatic mutations in hematopoietic cells
Saliva and buccal swabs	Often contaminated with peripheral blood and not ideal for germline testing

would also be supportive of the germline nature of the mutation.

Acute Myeloid Leukemia with Germline *CEBPA* Mutation

CEBPA is located on chromosome 19p13.1 and encodes a core-binding transcription factor that is critical for myeloid maturation. In 2004, Smith and colleagues reported germline mutations primarily in the 5' region associated with familial AML [5]. The development of AML is associated with a second acquired mutation in the 3' region of the wild-type *CEBPA* allele. Approximately 7–11% of CEBPA-mutated AMLs have been found to have a germline mutation, thus identification of AML with biallelic *CEBPA* mutations should raise consideration for possible germline *CEBPA* mutation [6, 7]. The median age of AML onset is reported as 25 years with a range of 2 to 50 years [8]. Patients typically present with AML without a preceding period of myelodysplasia or cytopenia. Morphologic and immunophenotypic features are similar to sporadic AML with *CEBPA* mutation, including AML with or without maturation (Figure 19.1), presence of Auer rods, aberrant expression of CD7, and normal karyotype. AML with germline *CEBPA* mutation has an overall good prognosis, but may relapse with new AML clones representing a new leukemia.

Myeloid Neoplasms with Germline *DDX41* Mutation

DDX41 is located on chromosome 5q35 and encodes a DEAD box RNA helicase. Germline mutations in *DDX41* were first reported in families with MDS/AML in 2015 [9]. In contrast to the majority of genes discussed in this

chapter, the development of hematologic malignancy typically occurs in late adulthood (median age of 62 years) and not in the pediatric or young adult age groups. Patients with germline *DDX41* mutation who develop MDS/AML frequently present with hypocellular bone marrows with prominent dyserythropoiesis. Lymphoid malignancies are also reported [10]. Penetrance is not fully established.

Myeloid Neoplasms with Germline *RUNX1* Mutation

RUNX1 (previously known as *CBFA2* or *AML1*) is located on chromosome 21q22 and encodes a subunit of the core-binding transcription factor that regulates expression of several genes that are critical for hematopoiesis and that is particularly important for megakaryocytic maturation and proplatelet formation. *RUNX1* is one of the most frequently involved genes in chromosomal translocations in acute leukemia. Germline mutations in *RUNX1* were first described in families with familial platelet disorder with propensity for acute myeloid leukemia (FDP/AML) [4]. This disorder was characterized by thrombocytopenia and abnormal platelet function with an increased risk of developing MDS/AML or, less frequently, T-lymphoblastic leukemia. *RUNX1* mutations have an autosomal dominant inheritance pattern with incomplete penetrance and lead to haploinsufficiency. Patients may present with variable bleeding tendencies at a young age. The risk of developing MDS/AML is estimated at 30–40% with a median age of onset of 33 years with a wide age range, including very young pediatric ages [11]. The bone marrow may be hypocellular or normocellular for age with small hypolobated megakaryocytes with eccentric nuclear lobes at baseline before development of MDS [12]. Transformation to MDS is typically associated with hypercellularity, multilineage dysplasia, increased blasts, or acquisition of cytogenetic abnormalities [13] (Figure 19.2).

Myeloid Neoplasms with Germline *ANKRD26* Mutation

ANKRD26 is located on chromosome 10p12.1 and is important for regulation of signaling through the TPO/MPL pathway. In 2011, germline heterozygous mutations in the 5'UTR of the gene were identified in families with familial thrombocytopenia who had increased risk of MDS/AML [14]. Affected patients typically have moderate thrombocytopenia with mild or absent bleeding. Platelets are normal in size and

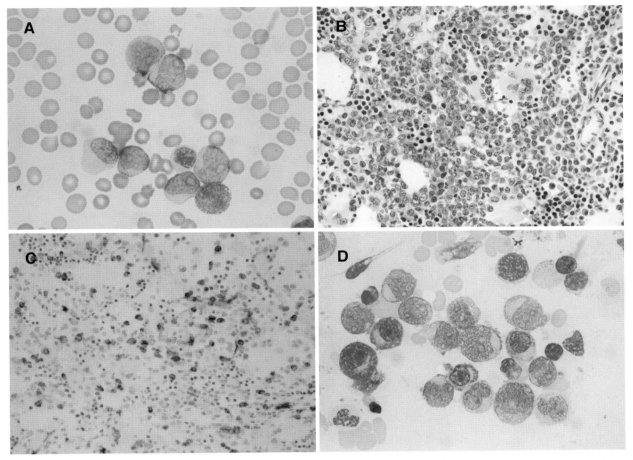

Figure 19.1 CEBPA. 19-year-old male with history of bruising, chest pain, and night sweats. Complete blood count showed marked leukocytosis composed primarily of large blasts with high N:C ratio, prominent nucleoli, and dispersed chromatin on peripheral smear (A, Wright-Giemsa, 1,000x). Bone marrow core biopsy was hypercellular (B, H&E stain, 400x) with increased immature precursors, highlighted by immunohistochemistry for CD34 (C, IHC, 400x). The aspirate showed 43% myeloblasts (D, Wright-Giemsa, 1,000x). Molecular studies identified biallelic pathogenic mutations in *CEBPA* involving the N terminus and C terminus with VAFs of 50% and 56%, and a pathogenic mutation in *NRAS*. Buccal swab analysis identified the N-terminus mutation (interpreted as germline); the C terminus *CEBPA* mutation and the *NRAS* mutation were not present in the buccal swab specimen. Images provided by Dr. Rena Xian.

may have reduced alpha granules. Studies have shown the germline *ANKRD26* mutations are gain-of-function mutations resulting in increased TPO/MPL signaling and defective proplatelet formation. Baseline bone marrows typically show increased megakaryocytes, including small forms with hypolobated nuclei and micromegakaryocytes [1]. As in the case of *RUNX1* familial platelet disorder, pathologists are cautioned against diagnosing MDS in the setting of isolated thrombocytopenia and dysmegakaryopoiesis (Figure 19.3). Transformation to MDS is typically associated with additional cytopenias, multilineage dysplasia, or cytogenetic abnormalities.

Myeloid Neoplasms with Germline *ETV6* Mutation

ETV6 encodes a transcription factor in the ETS family and is located on chromosome 12p13.2. In 2015, multiple families with thrombocytopenia and increased incidence of B-lymphoblastic leukemia (B-ALL), MDS/AML, CMML, plasma cell myeloma, and other cancers were

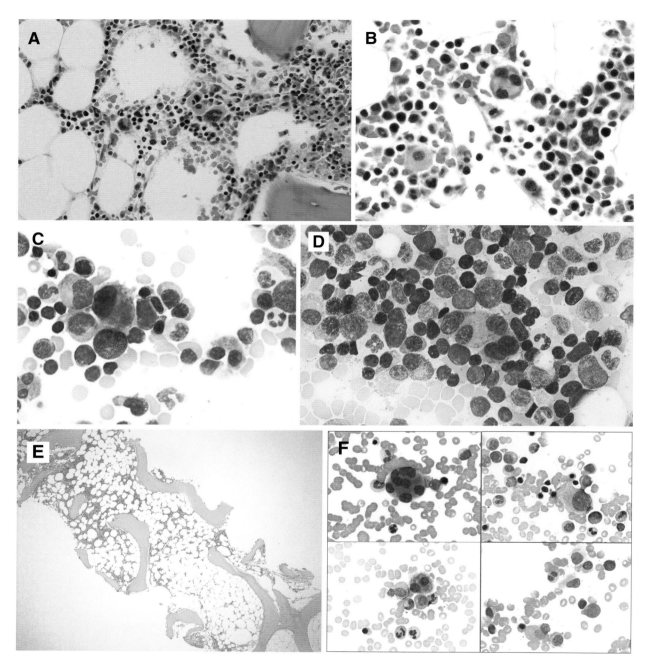

Figure 19.2 RUNX1. A–D. 4-year-old male with a history of easy bruising and moderately thrombocytopenia since infancy was previously diagnosed with ITP and did not respond to steroids. Family history of thrombocytopenia led mother and son to be tested, and they were found to have germline mutations in *RUNX1*. The bone marrow biopsy showed a hypocellular marrow with frequent megakaryocytes (A, H&E, 500x) and a subset with hypolobated nuclei or separated nuclear lobes (B–D, Wright-Giemsa, 1,000x). E–F. A 15-year-old male with a history of thrombocytopenia and germline *RUNX1* mutation developed progressive pancytopenia. The bone marrow core biopsy showed a hypocellular marrow (E, H&E, 40x). The aspirate showed numerous dysplastic megakaryocytes with separated nuclear lobes and mononuclear forms in addition to dysmyelopoiesis, including few pseudo-pelgeroid forms (F, 1,000x, bottom right panel). Cytogenetic analysis revealed del(5q). The patient was diagnosed with MDS with germline *RUNX1* mutation. Second case provided by Dr. Karen Chisholm.

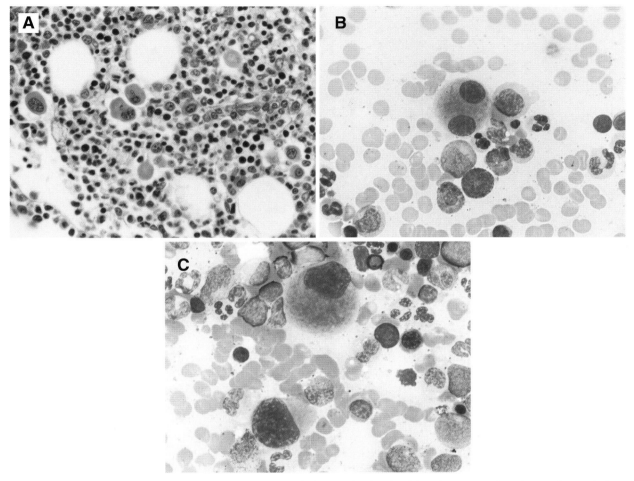

Figure 19.3 *ANKRD26.* Images from the marrow of a 19-year-old male diagnosed with isolated thrombocytopenia from the age of 4 years in the range of 30–40 K/mcL. His father was diagnosed with ITP at 9 years of age, which never resolved. One sibling was diagnosed with a hematologic malignancy. The family was found to harbor a germline mutation in *ANKRD26*. The core biopsy is cellular with frequent small hypolobated megakaryocytes (A, H&E, 500x). The marrow aspirate showed atypical megakaryocytes with separated nuclear lobes (B, Wright-Giemsa, 1,000x) and monolobated forms (C, Wright-Giemsa, 1,000x). Images provided by Dr. Mark Fleming.

reported who were found to harbor germline mutations in *ETV6* [15]. The germline mutations were autosomal dominant and shown to have a dominant negative mechanism that impaired binding of wild-type ETV6 to DNA, resulting in impaired transcriptional repression and reduced expression of platelet-associated genes. There is high penetrance of thrombocytopenia with or without anemia and neutropenia. The risk of neoplasia is not yet clearly defined. The bone marrow typically shows evidence of dysmegakaryopoiesis at baseline with small hypolobated megakaryocytes with or without dyserythropoiesis

(Figure 19.4). Non-hematologic associations have also been reported and include colorectal adenocarcinoma, skin cancer, myopathy, and GERD [16].

Myeloid Neoplasms with Germline *GATA2* Mutation

GATA2 encodes a transcription factor that is critical for regulation of hematopoiesis and is located on chromosome 3q21.3. Germline heterozygous mutations result in haploinsufficiency with a spectrum of phenotypic presentations

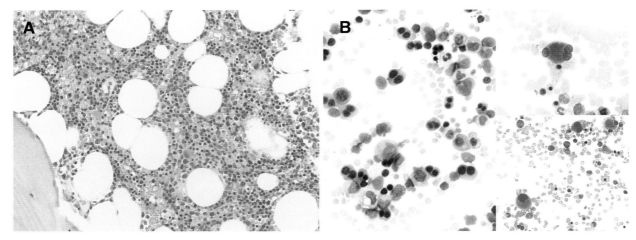

Figure 19.4 *ETV6*. Images from a 17-year-old female with history of easy bruising and thrombocytopenia from infancy. Her platelets dropped as low as 5–10 K/mcL and she developed severe menorrhagia in adolescence, requiring menstrual suppression with oral contraceptives. Family history included thrombocytopenia and B-lymphoblastic leukemia (sister) and colon cancer in 40s (mother). The patient developed progressive pancytopenia. The marrow was mildly hypocellular for age (A, 500x) with evidence of dyserythropoiesis (B, left panel 500x), megakaryocytic atypia/dysplasia (right panel), and 7% blasts. The patient was diagnosed with MDS-EB 1. Cytogenetic analysis revealed an abnormal karyotype with t(X;5) (p11.2; q22) in 8/20 metaphases. A germline mutation in *ETV6* was identified in the patient and family members. Images provided by Drs. Keith Loeb and Akiko Shimamura.

now referred to as GATA2 deficiency. Familial cases show autosomal dominant inheritance; however, de novo germline mutations are also common. Patients can present with loss of monocytes, B-cells, NK cells, and dendritic cells with severe immunodeficiency and susceptibility to *Mycobacterium avium* complex (MAC), severe and disseminated infections of human papillomavirus (HPV), cytomegalovirus and/or Epstein-Barr virus (EBV), and other opportunistic infections [17]. Other systemic manifestations may include lymphedema, deafness, pulmonary alveolar proteinosis, and hemophagocytic lymphohistiocytosis. There is a profound predisposition to the development of MDS, AML, chronic myelomonocytic leukemia (CMML), or BMF (Figure 19.5). Pediatric patients in particular may present with MDS or AML without systemic manifestations of immunodeficiency or significant loss of immune cell populations. In one large European pediatric/adolescent study of more than 400 MDS cases [18], 35% of cases with monosomy 7 had germline *GATA2* mutations and 75% of adolescent MDS patients with monosomy 7 were shown to have germline *GATA2* mutations. Unlike the adult cases of GATA2 deficiency, which often show monocytopenia, many pediatric cases present with adequate or increased monocytes. In one European study of pediatric GATA2 deficiency, the most common feature

according to bone marrow flow cytometric analysis was the loss of B-cell precursors [19]. Despite the loss of B-cells and precursors, nearly all cases have preservation of plasma cells. Likewise, despite loss of monocytes, tissue macrophages and histiocytes are abundant. A subset of adolescent and adult cases may develop monocytosis, CMML, or MDS/MPN.

Healthy mutation-positive children in families with GATA2 deficiency benefit from close monitoring for progressive cytopenias and surveillance for disease progression. Due to the increased susceptibility to viral infections, HPV vaccination is recommended.

Li-Fraumeni Syndrome

Li-Fraumeni syndrome (LFS) is a cancer-predisposing condition resulting from germline heterozygous *TP53* mutations and is inherited in an autosomal dominant manner [20]. Individuals with this mutation are predisposed to multiple solid tumors as well as hematologic malignancies. The most common hematologic neoplasm in LFS is B-lymphoblastic leukemia (discussed further in Chapter 20). Myeloid neoplasms are also common in LFS (Figure 19.6). Myeloid neoplasms often arise in the setting of prior therapy and usually harbor complex karyotypic abnormalities. Hints for suspecting LFS are early

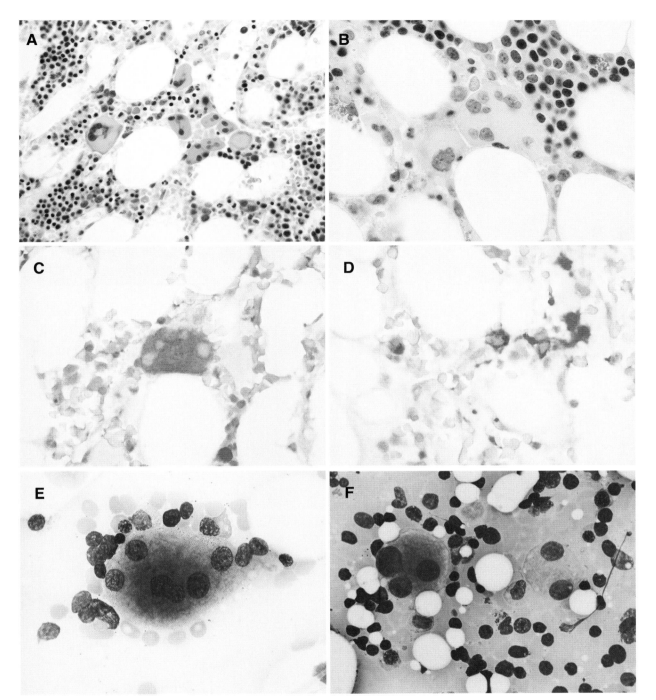

Figure 19.5 GATA2. GATA2 deficiency in children and adolescents can present with marrow features of hypoplastic MDS. The megakaryocytes formed clusters (A, H&E, 500x), and dysmegakaryocytes with separated nuclear lobes (B, 1,000x). CD61 highlights atypical/dysplastic megakaryocytes with separated nuclear lobes (C, CD61 1,000x) and micromegakaryocytes (D, CD61, 1,000x) on the core biopsy. Atypical megakaryocytes are also found on aspirate smears (E–G). Myeloid dysplasia may be present. Figure 19.5H shows a binucleated myeloid precursor (Wright-Giemsa, 1,000x). Erythroid dysplasia (Figure 19.5I, 1,000x) may also be seen with nuclear budding or binucleation. A subset of patients may precede with aplastic anemia, as seen in this marrow from a 17-year-old male who presented with severe pancytopenia and a markedly hypocellular marrow with trilineage hypoplasia and evidence (Figure 19.5J, H&E, 200x). The patient was treated with steroids without significant improvement. One year later, the patient progressed to MDS-EB1 with monosomy 7 and subsequently transformed to AML (Figure 19.5K, core biopsy, H&E, 500x) with increased CD34 positive blasts (Figure 19.5L, IHC, 500x). dysplastic megakaryocytes (Figure 19.5m, aspirate 1000x), and over 30% blasts with high N:C ratio, dispersed chromatin, prominent nucleoli, and some with granules (Figure 19.5n, aspirate, 1000x); hypogranular granulocytes can be seen in the background. Some patients may present with markedly atypical marrows as seen in this case from a 12 year old male with history of pancytopenia, disseminated MAC infections, and warts. The bone marrow showed marked cellular depletion with appearance of stromal damage (Figure 19.5o, 100x), atypical megakaryocytes (Figure 19.5p, 1000x), and marked fibrosis demonstrated on reticulin stain (Figure 19.5q, 500x) and trichrome stain (Figure 19.5r, 500x). Cytogenetic analysis revealed monosomy 7 and a germline GATA2 mutation was found in the patient and his brother who also had MDS.

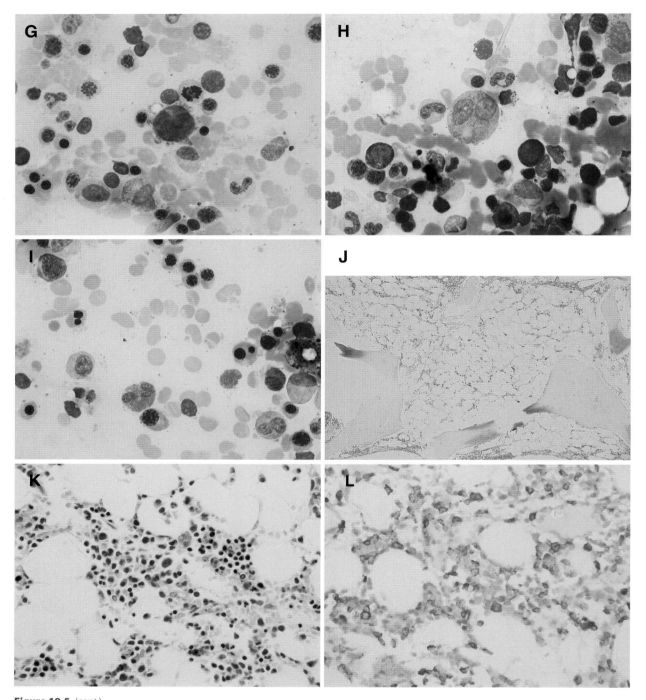

Figure 19.5 (cont.)

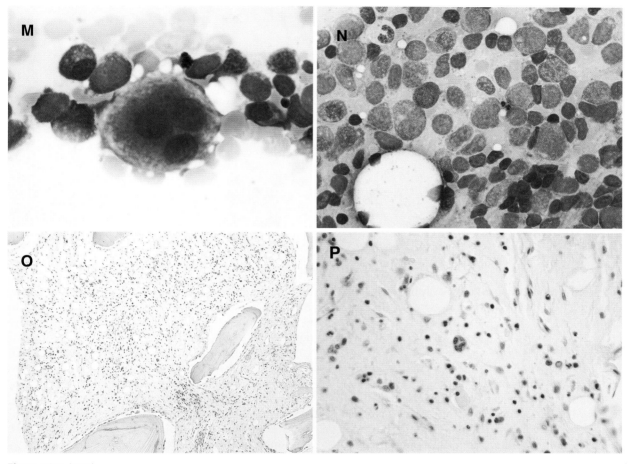

Figure 19.5 (cont.)

onset of cancers, multiple cancers throughout life, and family history of cancers. Surveillance programs and screening tests for early detection of tumors are important.

Telomere Biology Disorders Including Dyskeratosis Congenital and Syndromes Due to TERC and TERT Mutations

Dyskeratosis congenita and telomeropathies are inherited BMF syndromes caused by germline mutations in genes involved in telomere formation or stabilization [21]. Telomeres are nucleotide repeats and protein complexes located at chromosome ends and are essential for chromosome stability. Telomeres shorten with each cell division due to incomplete replication of the 3' ends of DNA and, in this manner, they prevent senescent cells from multiplying and further dividing. Telomeropathies are characterized by mucocutaneous features (skin pigmentation, nail dysplasia, oral leukoplakia), pulmonary fibrosis, liver disease, esophageal stenosis, solid malignancies, and bone marrow failure [22]. Telomere biology genes include *DKC1* (encoding dyskerin) and *TERT* (encoding telomerase reverse transcriptase), and its RNA component, *TERC*. Additional pathologic variants causing dyskeratosis congenita can occur in components of the shelterin complex, *TINF2*, *ACD*, *POT1*, in the DNA helicase *RTEL1*, and the telomere protein-encoding genes *NAF1* and *STN1*. Telomere length analysis in total leukocytes and/or in leukocyte subsets by flow-FISH and gene sequencing are helpful in establishing the diagnosis. Patients may develop cytopenias with red cell

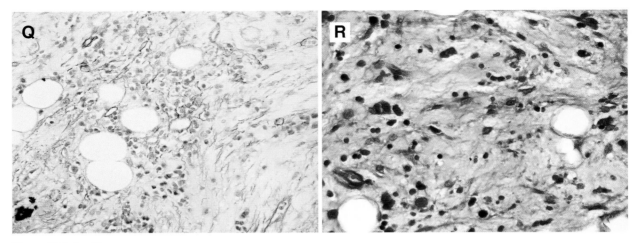

Figure 19.5 (cont.)

macrocytosis. The bone marrow is typically hypocellular for age (Figure 19.7) with varying degrees of trilineage hypoplasia.

Fanconi Anemia

Fanconi anemia (FA) is a heterogeneous disorder characterized by BMF, predisposition to solid tumors and myeloid malignancies, and hypersensitivity to DNA cross-linking agents [23]. Additionally, congenital anomalies including café-au-lait spots, short stature, skeletal malformations (abnormal thumbs, absent radii), cardiac or renal abnormalities, and metabolic defects are common but may be absent or subtle. Genetic defects in any of over 15 *FANC* genes *can* lead to the classical triad of chromosome fragility, malformations, and BMF. The proteins *FANC* genes encode play important roles in DNA repair and cell cycle control, detoxification of reactive oxygen species, energy metabolism, and cytokine homeostasis. Bone marrow failure frequently presents early, between 5 and 10 years of age, with hypocellular bone marrow and panhypoplasia. Associated features at the BMF stage are increased fetal hemoglobin (HbF) and macrocytosis. Over time, patients may gradually evolve to MDS/AML (Figure 19.8). Compared to the general population, the risk of AML in FA patients is increased 700-fold, and that of MDS is increased 6,000-fold. For these reasons, surveillance of hematopoietic function and monitoring for morphologic changes and clonal evolution are done immediately after diagnosis. Sometimes patients are found to have Fanconi anemia only after they have been diagnosed with a malignancy.

The diagnosis of FA is confirmed by chromosomal fragility test, performed on peripheral blood lymphocytes or skin fibroblasts. When exposed to DNA-cross-linking agents, chromosomes undergo excessive breakage. Gene sequencing for relevant mutations establishes the specific molecular defect. MDS/AML developed in the setting of FA often harbors cytogenetic abnormalities, including gains of 1q, 3q, monosomy 7, or del(7q), del(20q), del (11q), or rearrangements of *RUNX1*.

Hematopoietic stem cell transplant is the best therapeutic option, preferably performed after progression of cytopenia and before acquisition of poor risk abnormalities or development of AML. Patients with Fanconi anemia can develop serious and sometimes fatal reactions to DNA-damaging agents and often require reduced-intensity regimens.

Shwachman-Diamond Syndrome

Shwachman-Diamond syndrome (SDS) is a rare autosomal recessive congenital disorder resulting from abnormal ribosomal biogenesis caused by mutations in the *SBDS* gene located at chromosome 7q11 [24]. *SBDS* also prevents genomic instability during mitosis.

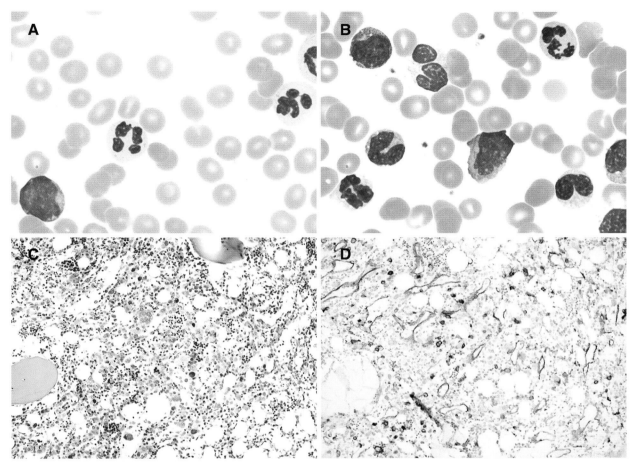

Figure 19.6 *TP53.* A–B. A 17-year-old girl developed a therapy-related MDS 22 months after beginning therapy for Ewing sarcoma involving her ribs. The blood smear (A, 200x) showed leukocytosis with 60% circulating blasts, dysplastic neutrophils with abnormal nuclear segmentation, and hypogranular cytoplasm (B, Wright-Giemsa 1,000x) Bone marrow examination (C, Wright-Giemsa, 1,000x) showed the blasts containing two slender Auer rods. Cytogenetics demonstrated t(11;19) (q23; p13.1) with *KMT2A* rearrangement. She was ultimately found to have Li-Fraumeni syndrome. D–F (all 100x). This 19-year-old man with Li-Fraumeni syndrome and osteosarcoma diagnosed 36 months earlier developed a therapy-related MDS with an excess of blasts. The blasts were megakaryocytic, negative for CD34 (E) but positive for CD117 (E) and CD61 (F). Chromosome analysis showed complex karyotype.

Patients may present in infancy or young adulthood with cytopenia and exocrine pancreatic insufficiency. Other non-hematologic manifestations include short stature and skeletal abnormalities. Of all cytopenia, neutropenia is the most common and is associated with frequent infections. Thrombocytopenia and macrocytic anemia occur less often.

Bone marrow cellularity in Schwachman-Diamond syndrome can range from hypocellular to hypercellular (Figure 19.9), and cellularity may correlate poorly with the degree of peripheral blood cytopenia. The myeloid lineage is often left-shifted and baseline morphologic atypia in the neutrophil lineage is common, including nuclear hyposegmentation and cytoplasmic hypogranularity. For that reason, it is important to recognize (and not overinterpret) mild morphologic dysplasia. However, baseline erythroid dysplasia is uncommon in SDS and raises concern for MDS, particularly if accompanied by a progressive increase in marrow cellularity [24]. In SDS, acquired cytogenetic abnormalities (such as 7q-, 20q-, isochromosome 7q, and monosomy 7) may appear over time.

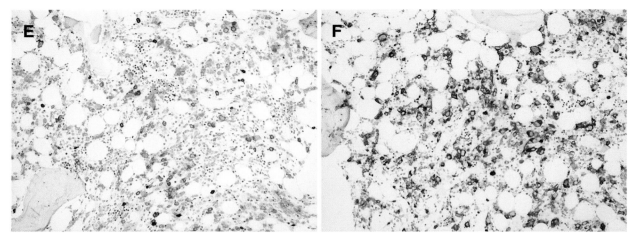

Figure 19.6 (cont.)

Diamond-Blackfan Anemia

Diamond-Blackfan anemia (DBA) is a rare congenital disorder resulting from abnormal ribosomal biogenesis and/or function caused by mutations in any of the following genes: *RPS19* (the most common), *RPS17*, *RPS24*, *RPL35A*, *RPL5*, *RPL11*, *RPS7*, *RPS26*, *RPS10*, *GATA1*, and *TSR2*. The diagnostic criteria for DBA include age less than 1 year, macrocytic anemia with no other significant cytopenia, reticulocytopenia, and normal or near-normal bone marrow cellularity with a paucity of erythroid precursors [25] (Figure 19.10). However, the presence of additional cytopenia does not preclude the diagnosis of DBA if red cell aplasia and other features are present. Supporting major criteria for DBA include gene mutations in the previously described ribosomal protein-encoding genes and positive family history. Minor diagnostic criteria include congenital anomalies (craniofacial, ophthalmologic, thumbs, cardiac, urogenital), elevated levels of fetal hemoglobin (HbF), and elevated erythrocyte adenosine deaminase activity.

Severe Congenital Neutropenia

Severe congenital neutropenia (SCN) is a genetically heterogeneous BMF syndrome [26] characterized by neutrophil counts below 0.5×10^9/L. It clinically presents early in life due to invasive bacterial infections (omphalitis, skin abscesses, pneumonia, or septicemia) and fungal infections, and demonstrates multiple patterns of inheritance, depending on the gene involved. The most commonly mutated gene is *ELANE* (*ELA2*) on 19q13, although, in nearly 40% of SCN cases, the genetic basis is unknown. Other clinical features are uncommon but include neurologic, endocrine, and immunologic abnormalities. Both neutrophil count and function are defective. Bone marrow evaluation shows severely decreased mature granulocytes due to maturation arrest at the promyelocyte or myelocyte stage (Figure 19.11). Morphologically, the neutrophils that do mature show prominent vacuolization and aberrant azurophilic granules. Functional abnormalities include defective migration and bacterial killing and increased propensity to undergo apoptosis. Chromosomal abnormalities, such as monosomy 7 and gain of chromosome 21, as well as acquisition of somatic mutations in *CSF3 R* or *RUNX1*, are frequently detected before transformation to AML [22].

Samd9/Samd9l

In 2016, MIRAGE syndrome was first reported in patients with germline mutations in *SAMD9* manifesting with **M**yelodysplasia with monosomy 7, **I**nfection, growth **R**estriction, **A**drenal hypoplasia, **G**enital phenotypes, and **E**nteropathy [27]. In the same year, a separate group reported germline mutations in a related gene, *SAMD9L*. Mutations in *SAMD9L* are associated with ataxia-pancytopenia syndrome, which includes BMF and MDS with monosomy 7 [28]. Since then, other

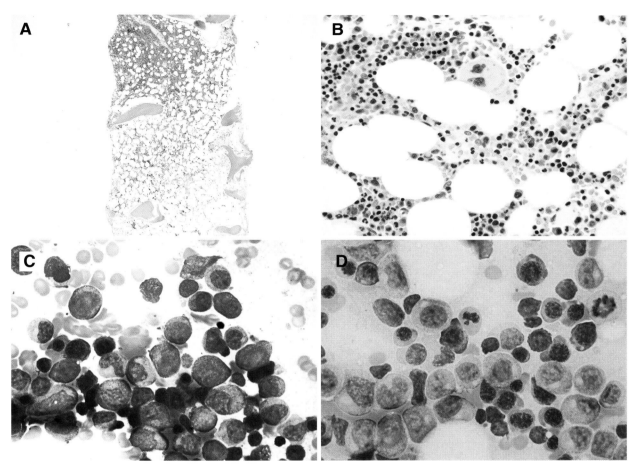

Figure 19.7 Telomeropathies. A–B. A 9-year-old male presented with hepatitis and cytopenias with red blood cell macrocytosis and telomere length less than 1% for age. He was found to have a germline mutation in *TERT*. The marrow was variably hypocellular (A, H&E, 100x) with erythroid predominance and rare atypical megakaryocytes (B, H&E, 500x). Progression to MDS may occur as in this 10 year old male with DKC who developedmonosomy 7, mild increase in blasts and dyserythropoiesis (C, D, 1000x).

groups have identified *SAMD9/SAMD9L* germline mutations in pediatric patients with BMF and MDS with monosomy 7 [29]. *SAMD9* and *SAMD9L* are located on chromosome 7. Mutations are gain-of-function, resulting in decreased proliferation and impaired hematopoiesis. In a process called adaptation through aneuploidy, the allele containing the mutation can be lost, resulting in monosomy 7 and MDS/AML. Bone marrows are often hypocellular for age. In cases with monosomy 7, multilineage dyspoiesis may be evident, indicative of MDS. Some patients develop somatic rescue in the bone marrow via uniparental disomy of chromosome 7, resulting in two wild-type copies of the gene and marrow recovery with normalization of peripheral counts. Other patients may have variable cytopenia and normal karyotype, with low levels of monosomy 7 detected on FISH and minimal or mild evidence of dyspoiesis (Figure 19.12).

MECOM-Associated Syndrome

Germline heterozygous mutations in *MECOM* (*MDS1* and *EVI1* complex locus) have recently been associated with a heterogeneous bone marrow failure syndrome initially

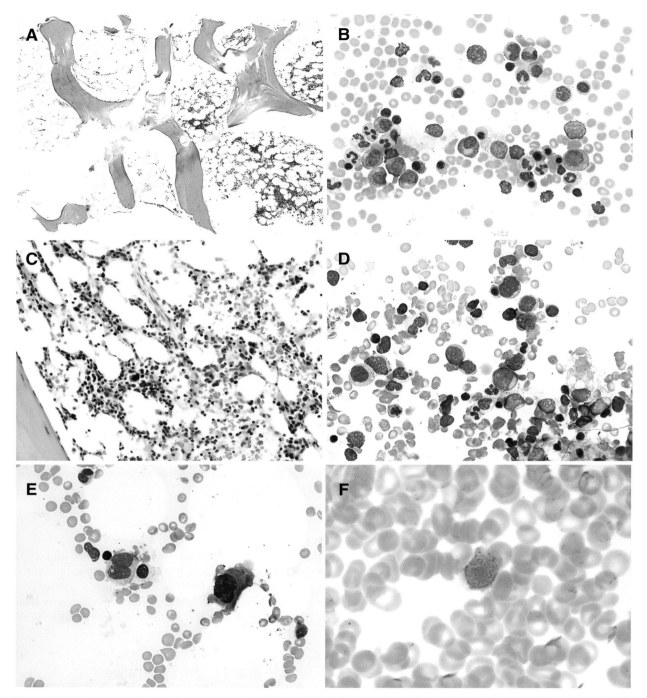

Figure 19.8 Fanconi anemia. Surveillance marrow from a 16-year-old girl with Fanconi anemia, showing patchy hematopoiesis but overall profound hypocellularity for age (A, 40x). Marrow from an 8-year-old boy with fatigue and anemia. His bone marrow was hypocellular for age (C, 200x) but showed increased blasts (D, Wright-Giemsa, 400x), dysplastic megakaryocytes, hyposegmented nuclei, micromegakaryocytes (E, Wright-Giemsa, 400x), and many ring sideroblasts (F, Prussian Blue stain, 1,000x).

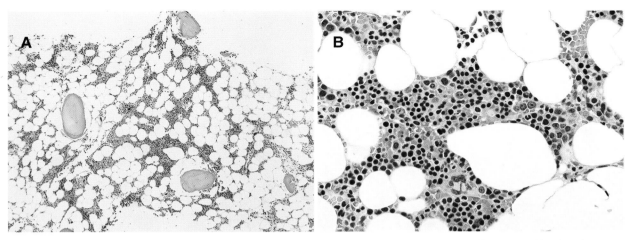

Figure 19.9 Schwachman-Diamond syndrome. Commonly shows a hypocellular marrow for age (A, 40x) as in this 17-year-old male with neutropenia, mild thrombocytopenia, and macrocytosis in the peripheral blood. The marrow shows erythroid predominance with myeloid hypoplasia (B, 500x).

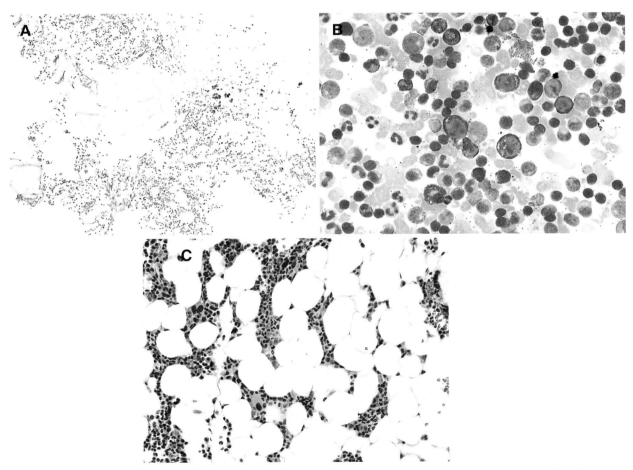

Figure 19.10 Diamond-Blackfan anemia. Images from the marrow of a 7-year-old girl with DBA. CD71 is used to highlight erythroid precursors and shows marked erythroid hypoplasia with only a few positive cells (A, IHC, 100x). The bone marrow aspirate shows erythroid hypoplasia with few basophilic normoblasts and virtually no orthochromic normoblasts or more mature erythroid precursors (B, 1000x). Occasionally, sparse fine cytoplasmic vacuoles are present in the erythroid progenitors. Often, one sees a hypocellular marrow with erythroid hypoplasia and iron overload as a consequence of repeated red cell transfusions (C, 200x)

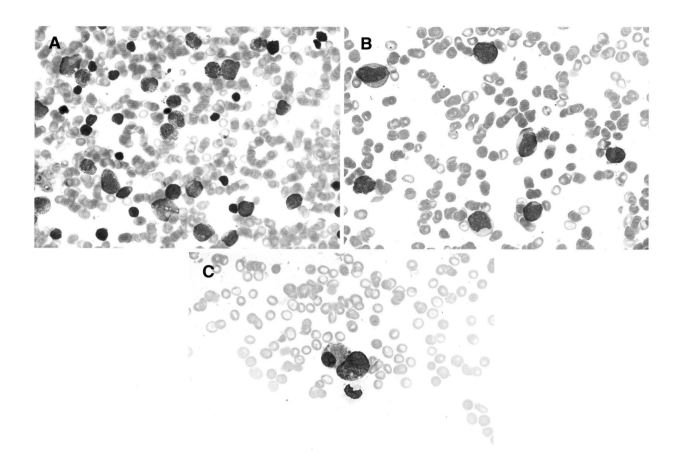

Figure 19.11 Severe congenital neutropenia. Bone marrow images from a 12-week-old boy with neutropenia showing a maturation arrest in the neutrophil series (A, 400x) characterized by occasional myeloblasts and promyelocytes without granulocytic maturation despite full maturation in the eosinophil and basophil series. The patient was found to have SCN with a germline mutation in *ELANE*.

A second patient, while receiving long-term therapy with granulocyte-colony stimulating factor, developed MDS that later transformed into AML. Note the increased bone marrow myeloblasts (B, Wright-Giemsa, 500x) and a micromegakaryocyte (C, 500x); abnormal cytogenetics included a *EVI1* rearrangement.

characterized by congenital amegakaryocytic thrombocy-topenia and radioulnar synostosis; however, the clinical spectrum can also include clinodactyly, cardiac and renal malformations, B-cell deficiency, and hearing loss [30]. Penetrance is variable and some patients may only present with bone marrow failure (Figure 19.13). Patients face an increased risk of developing myeloid malignancy, although the level of risk has yet to be defined.

Myeloid Proliferations Associated with Down Syndrome

A variety of hematologic abnormalities occur with frequency in constitutional trisomy 21/Down syndrome (DS) [31–33]. In the neonatal period, neutrophilia is present in up to 80% of cases, with thrombocytopenia observed in up to 66% and polycythemia in up to 34%. A characteristic macrocytosis that is not associated with folate or vitamin B12 deficiency is also sometimes seen. A unique myeloproliferative condition known as transient abnormal myelopoiesis (TAM) can occur in DS characterized by accumulation of immature megakaryoblasts in the fetal liver and peripheral blood, associated with somatic mutations in *GATA1*. It develops in 5–10% of newborns with DS, with a median age at diagnosis of 3–7 days. A subset of patients is asymptomatic and some fetuses with the condition may die in utero. TAM has also rarely been reported in patients in

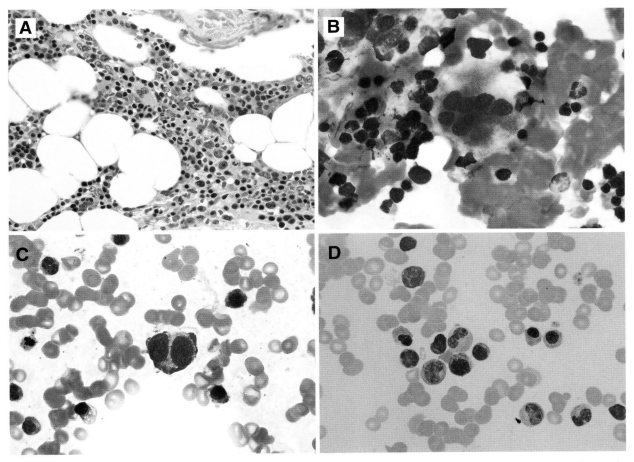

Figure 19.12 *SAMD9L*. Marrow from a 4-year-old girl with pancytopenia and germline mutation in *SAMD9L* shows hypocellularity on the core biopsy (A, H&E, 500x), dysplastic megakaryocytes with separated nuclear lobes on the marrow aspirate (B, Wright-Giemsa, 1,000x), and dyserythropoiesis (C–D, Wright-Giemsa, 1,000x); cytogenetic analysis showed monosomy 7 in 8/12 metaphases. Another patient presented at age 11 months for neutropenia (ANC 500/μL) and thrombocytopenia (74 K platelets/μL). Family history was significant for a sister with MDS and monosomy 7. The peripheral blood smear showed occasional hypolobate and few hypogranular granulocytes. In the marrow (F, 400x), there was also a subset of granulocytes with hypolobate nuclei, hypogranular cytoplasm, or uneven granule distribution. Interestingly, prominent stromal damage was seen in the core biopsy (G, 100x). Cytogenetic analysis and MDS FISH panel were normal. One month later, the marrow showed regenerative features which were reflected in the blood as progressive resolution of his cytopenias. However, two months after that, despite absence of cytopenias, overt dysplasia or increased blasts, and normal cellularity for age (H, 100x), interphase FISH studies were positive for monosomy 7 in 5.5% of nuclei. This boy and his sister were ultimately found to have a germline mutation in *SAMD9L*.

phenotypically normal or slightly dysmorphic neonates with trisomy 21 mosaicism. TAM may be associated with marked leukocytosis with left shift and circulating blasts. Although TAM usually resolves spontaneously without treatment, it is important to recognize to ensure appropriate follow-up since 20–30% subsequently develop myeloid leukemia (ML-DS) that will need to be treated within the first 4 years of life. ML-DS is frequently an acute megakaryoblastic (FAB M7) subtype. Leukemia results after acquisition of additional mutations in *GATA1*-mutant cells, in genes encoding cohesion proteins, epigenetic regulators, and signaling pathways, and/or of chromosomal abnormalities such as +8, dup(1q), del(6q), del(7p), dup(7q), +11, and acquired +21. After the age of 5, acute lymphoblastic leukemia (ALL) predominates (Figure 19.14). The incidence of ALL in patients with DS is 20 times higher than in those without DS. One to two percent of individuals with DS will ultimately develop ALL.

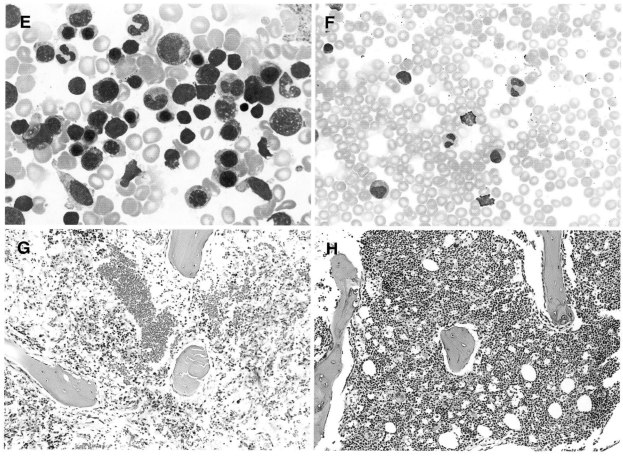

Figure 19.12 (cont.)

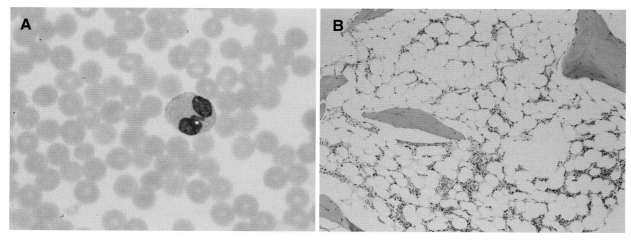

Figure 19.13 *MECOM.* Germline heterozygous mutations in *MECOM* are associated with heterogeneous marrow failure syndrome, often presenting in infancy with amegakaryocytic thrombocytopenia (with or without skeletal abnormalities). A hypocellular bone marrow (A, H&E, 200x) with absence of megakaryocytes was seen in this pediatric case. Courtesy of Dr. Xiayuan Liang.

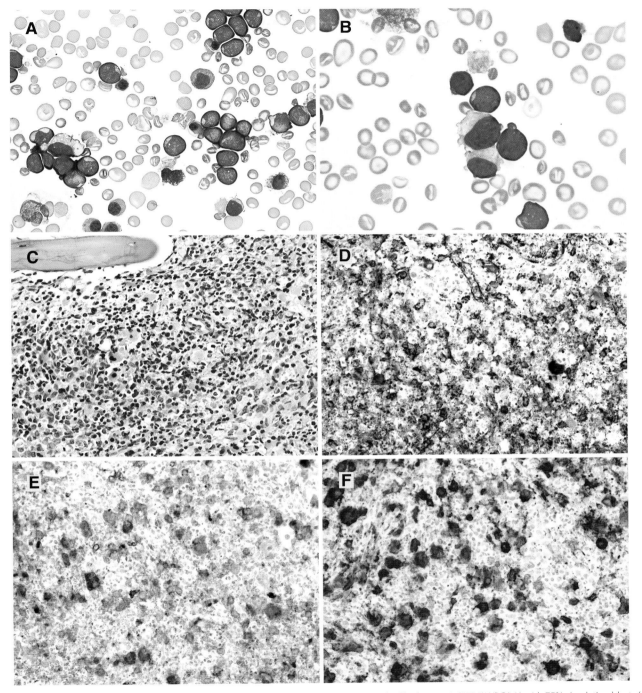

Figure 19.14 Down syndrome. TAM in an infant with constitutional trisomy 21 and marked leukocytosis (272 K WBC/µL) with 75% circulating blasts (A, 500x; B, 1,000x), peripheral blood smear pretreated with albumin) whose phenotype was consistent with megakaryoblasts (positive for CD45 [dim], CD34, CD4 [dim], CD7, CD13, CD33, CD38, CD58, CD41, CD61 [partial], and CD71, with heterogeneous CD56 and HLA-DR expression, and negative for myeloperoxidase and CD15). Images from a 22-month-old female with AML of DS (C, 200x), CD34 (D, 200x) show high background, but blasts and mature megakaryocytes are positive. CD117 (E, 200x) highlights blasts and increased megakaryocytes, which are also positive for CD61 (F, 200x).

References

1. Swerdlow SH, Campo E, Pileri SA, Harris NL, Stein H, Siebert R, et al. The 2016 revision of the World Health Organization classification of lymphoid neoplasms. Blood. 2016; **127**(20): 2375–90.

2. Babushok DV, Bessler M, Olson TS. Genetic predisposition to myelodysplastic syndrome and acute myeloid leukemia in children and young adults. Leuk Lymphoma. 2016; **57**(3): 520–36.

3. Weinberg OK, Kuo F, Calvo KR. Germline predisposition to hematolymphoid neoplasia. Am J Clin Pathol. 2019; **152**(3): 258–76.

4. Song WJ, Sullivan MG, Legare RD, Hutchings S, Tan X, Kufrin D, et al. Haploinsufficiency of CBFA2 causes familial thrombocytopenia with propensity to develop acute myelogenous leukaemia. Nat Genet. 1999; **23**(2): 166–75.

5. Smith ML, Cavenagh JD, Lister TA, Fitzgibbon J. Mutation of CEBPA in familial acute myeloid leukemia. N Engl J Med. 2004; **351**(23): 2403–7.

6. Pabst T, Eyholzer M, Haefliger S, Schardt J, Mueller BU. Somatic CEBPA mutations are a frequent second event in families with germline CEBPA mutations and familial acute myeloid leukemia. J Clin Oncol. 2008; **26**(31): 5088–93.

7. Taskesen E, Bullinger L, Corbacioglu A, Sanders MA, Erpelinck CA, Wouters BJ, et al. Prognostic impact, concurrent genetic mutations, and gene expression features of AML with CEBPA mutations in a cohort of 1182 cytogenetically normal AML patients: Further evidence for CEBPA double mutant AML as a distinctive disease entity. Blood. 2011; **117**(8): 2469–75.

8. Tawana K, Rio-Machin A, Preudhomme C, Fitzgibbon J. Familial CEBPA-mutated acute myeloid leukemia. Semin Hematol. 2017; **54**(2): 87–93.

9. Maciejewski JP, Padgett RA, Brown AL, Müller-Tidow C. DDX41-related myeloid neoplasia. Semin Hematol. 2017; **54**(2): 94–7.

10. Lewinsohn M, Brown AL, Weinel LM, Phung C, Rafidi G, Lee MK, et al. Novel germ line DDX41 mutations define families with a lower age of MDS/AML onset and lymphoid malignancies. Blood. 2016; **127**(8): 1017–23.

11. Schlegelberger B, Heller PG. RUNX1 deficiency (familial platelet disorder with predisposition to myeloid leukemia, FPDMM). Semin Hematol. 2017; **54**(2): 75–80.

12. Chisholm KM, Denton C, Keel S, Geddis AE, Xu M, Appel BE, et al. Bone marrow morphology associated with germline RUNX1 mutations in patients with familial platelet disorder with associated myeloid malignancy. Pediatr Dev Pathol. 2019; **22**(4): 315–28.

13. Kanagal-Shamanna R, Loghavi S, DiNardo CD, Medeiros LJ, Garcia-Manero G, Jabbour E, et al. Bone marrow pathologic abnormalities in familial platelet disorder with propensity for myeloid malignancy and germline RUNX1 mutation. Haematologica. 2017; **102**(10): 1661–70.

14. Pippucci T, Savoia A, Perrotta S, Pujol-Moix N, Noris P, Castegnaro G, et al. Mutations in the 5' UTR of ANKRD26, the ankirin repeat domain 26 gene, cause an autosomal-dominant form of inherited thrombocytopenia, THC2. Am J Hum Genet. 2011; **88**(1): 115–20.

15. Hock H, Shimamura A. ETV6 in hematopoiesis and leukemia predisposition. Semin Hematol. 2017; **54**(2): 98–104.

16. Zhang MY, Churpek JE, Keel SB, Walsh T, Lee MK, Loeb KR, et al. Germline ETV6 mutations in familial thrombocytopenia and hematologic malignancy. Nat Genet. 2015; **47**(2): 180–5.

17. Spinner MA, Sanchez LA, Hsu AP, Shaw PA, Zerbe CS, Calvo KR, et al. GATA2 deficiency: A protean disorder of hematopoiesis, lymphatics, and immunity. Blood. 2014; **123**(6): 809–21.

18. Wlodarski MW, Hirabayashi S, Pastor V, Starý J, Hasle H, Masetti R, et al. Prevalence, clinical characteristics, and prognosis of GATA2-related myelodysplastic syndromes in children and adolescents. Blood. 2016; **127**(11): 1387–97; quiz 518.

19. Nováková M, Žaliová M, Suková M, Wlodarski M, Janda A, Froňková E, et al. Loss of B cells and their precursors is the most constant feature of GATA-2 deficiency in childhood myelodysplastic syndrome. Haematologica. 2016; **101**(6): 707–16.

20. Valdez JM, Nichols KE, Kesserwan C. Li-Fraumeni syndrome: A paradigm for the understanding of hereditary cancer predisposition. Br J Haematol. 2017; **176**(4): 539–52.

21. Dokal I. Dyskeratosis congenita. Hematology Am Soc Hematol Educ Program. 2011; **2011**: 480–6.

22. Savage SA, Bertuch AA. The genetics and clinical manifestations of telomere biology disorders. Genet Med. 2010; **12**(12): 753–64.

23. Alter BP. Fanconi anemia and the development of leukemia. Best Pract Res Clin Haematol. 2014; **27**(3-4): 214–21.

24. Burroughs L, Woolfrey A, Shimamura A. Shwachman-Diamond syndrome: A review of the clinical presentation, molecular pathogenesis, diagnosis, and treatment. Hematol Oncol Clin North Am. 2009; **23**(2): 233–48.

25. Vlachos A, Ball S, Dahl N, Alter BP, Sheth S, Ramenghi U, et al. Diagnosing and treating Diamond Blackfan anaemia: Results of an international clinical consensus conference. Br J Haematol. 2008; **142**(6): 859–76.

26. Skokowa J, Dale DC, Touw IP, Zeidler C, Welte K. Severe congenital neutropenias. Nat Rev Dis Primers. 2017; **3**: 17032.

27. Narumi S, Amano N, Ishii T, Katsumata N, Muroya K, Adachi M, et al. SAMD9 mutations cause a novel multisystem disorder, MIRAGE syndrome, and are associated with loss of chromosome 7. Nat Genet. 2016; **48**(7): 792–7.

28. Chen DH, Below JE, Shimamura A, Keel SB, Matsushita M, Wolff J, et al. Ataxia-pancytopenia syndrome is caused by missense mutations in SAMD9L. Am J Hum Genet. 2016; **98**(6): 1146–58.

29. Davidsson J, Puschmann A, Tedgård U, Bryder D, Nilsson L, Cammenga J. SAMD9 and SAMD9L in inherited predisposition to ataxia, pancytopenia, and myeloid malignancies. Leukemia. 2018; **32**(5): 1106–15.

30. Germeshausen M, Ancliff P, Estrada J, Metzler M, Ponstingl E, Rütschle H, et al. MECOM-associated syndrome: A heterogeneous inherited bone marrow failure syndrome with amegakaryocytic thrombocytopenia. Blood Adv. 2018; **2**(6): 586–96.

31. Ahmed M, Sternberg A, Hall G, Thomas A, Smith O, O'Marcaigh A, et al. Natural history of GATA1 mutations in Down syndrome. Blood. 2004; **103**(7): 2480–9.

32. Khan I, Malinge S, Crispino J. Myeloid leukemia in Down syndrome. Crit Rev Oncog. 2011; **16** (1–2): 25–36.

33. Labuhn M, Perkins K, Matzk S, Varghese L, Garnett C, Papaemmanuil E, et al. Mechanisms of progression of myeloid preleukemia to transformed myeloid leukemia in children with Down syndrome. Cancer Cell. 2019; **36**(2): 123–38.e10.

Chapter 20

Germline Predisposition to Lymphoid Neoplasm

Katherine R. Calvo, Nisha Patel, Alina Dulau-Florea, Kristian T. Schafernak

Introduction

While the number of Chapter germline mutations known to confer predisposition to myeloid malignancy has gained broad recognition, there is also increasing awareness of genes predisposing to lymphoid neoplasia. This chapter addresses select genes associated with germline predisposition to lymphoid neoplasms. Genes covered in this chapter are associated with familial B-lymphoblastic leukemia (B-ALL) [1], general cancer predisposition syndromes, and primary immunodeficiency syndromes (PID) (Table 20.1). Individuals with PID are predisposed to lymphoproliferations as a result of complex interactions between germline genetic defects, viral oncogenes, impaired immunosurveillance, and chronic antigen stimulation [2]. Of note, many of the B-cell lymphoproliferations that occur in the setting of a PID show frequent Epstein-Barr virus (EBV) positivity and tendency to involve extranodal sites.

Identification of patients with germline predisposition is critical for proper patient management, screening related donors for HSCT, and genetic counseling. Given advances in next-generation sequencing and the increased availability of testing, the number of genes associated with germline predisposition to lymphoid neoplasia is likely to increase in the near future.

Acute Lymphoblastic Leukemia with Germline *PAX5* Mutations

PAX5 encodes a transcription factor located on chromosome 9 that is critical for B-cell development. In 2013, inherited mutations in *PAX5* were first described in families with increased incidence of B-lymphoblastic leukemia (B-ALL) [3] with an autosomal dominant inheritance pattern. Leukemic cells characteristically show chromosome 9p deletion, resulting in loss of heterozygosity and retention of the mutant *PAX5* allele at 9p13. Penetrance for developing B-ALL is variable within families harboring the mutation.

The morphologic and immunophenotypic features of B-ALL in these cases overlaps with sporadic B-ALL (Figure 20.1). The *PAX5* gene is mutated in approximately 30% of sporadic B-ALL.

Acute Lymphoblastic Leukemia with Germline *IKZF1* Mutations

IKZF1 encodes the transcription factor IKAROS, which is expressed in lymphoid cells. Somatic mutations in *IKZF1* are associated with B-lymphoblastic leukemia, particularly B-ALL with *BCR-ABL1* and B-ALL, *BCR-ABL1*-like, and confer a poor prognosis. Recently, families were reported with germline mutations in *IKZF1* and common variable immunodeficiency with impaired lymphopoiesis, loss of B-cells, autoimmune manifestations, and increased incidence of B-ALL [4].

Acute Lymphoblastic Leukemia with Germline *ETV6* Mutations

ETV6 encodes a transcriptional repressor in the ETS family of transcription factors and plays a critical role in hematopoiesis (5). *ETV6* is highly expressed in hematopoietic stem cells and the megakaryocytes-erythroid progenitors. Individuals with germline *ETV6* mutations have mild thrombocytopenia and normal or elevated red cell mean corpuscular volume (MCV), and present with mild bleeding tendency and a predisposition for developing B-cell precursor ALL [6] or myeloid malignancies (MDS, AML, described in Chapter 19). Diffuse large B-cell lymphoma (DLBCL) is an infrequent but possible presentation. The age at diagnosis of lymphoid neoplasms varies according to disease type: 3–7 years for B-ALL and 38–45 years for leukemia not otherwise specified. Bone marrows from affected carriers without leukemia often show mild dyserythropoiesis and hypolobulated megakaryocytes [7].

This work was supported by the National Institutes of Health, Division of Intramural Research in the NIH Clinical Center.

Table 20.1 Lymphoid neoplasm with germline predisposition (and other select syndromes)

	Age of Onset/ Diagnosis	Inheritance	Gene(s)	Associated Hematologic Neoplasms	Clinical Presentation	Select Non-hematologic Abnormalities	Ancillary Diagnostic Tests	Risk to for Lymphoid Neoplasm
ALL with germline PAX5 mutation	Infants/young children (1 month–8 years old)	AD	PAX5	B-ALL	B-ALL	No known associations	– Gene sequencing – Cytogenetic/ FISH	ND
Acute lymphoblastic leukemia with germline IKZF1 mutations	Variable; can present in infants to throughout adulthood	AD	IKZF1	– B-ALL – B-cell deficiency – Autoimmune cytopenia(s)	– Asymptomatic – Infections – B-ALL	Autoimmune diseases (ITP, IgA vasculitis, SLE)	– Gene sequencing – Cytogenetic/ FISH analysis	ND
Acute lymphoblastic leukemia with germline ETV6 mutations	Young children: 3–7 years old	AD	ETV6	– B-ALL – Mixed phenotype acute leukemia (MPAL) – DLBCL	– Mild bleeding diathesis: easy bruising, menorrhagia – B-ALL	Not clearly defined (arthritis, skeletal abnormalities, learning disabilities seen in rare cases)	– Gene sequencing – Cytogenetic/ FISH analysis	ND (~30% of carriers develop hematologic malignancies)
Li-Fraumeni syndrome	Leukemia: Median age of 12 years	AD	TP53	– B-ALL (often hypodiploidy) – Also risk of MDS/AML, CML	Early onset of cancer, multiple cancers, family history of cancer	Soft tissue sarcoma, osteosarcoma, breast cancer, CNS tumors, and adrenocortical carcinoma	– Gene sequencing – Cytogenetic/ FISH analysis	2–4% for leukemias
DS-ALL	– Slightly higher age than non-DS ALL and can extend into young adulthood	Typically, constitutional	???	B-ALL	B-ALL	Constitutional abnormalities associated with DS	– Cytogenetic/ FISH analysis	20-fold risk
ALPS	Often in children (but can present in adulthood)	AD	TNFRSF, FASLG, CASP10	– Chronic nonmalignant lymphoproliferation – Increased risk of non-Hodgkin and Hodgkin lymphomas	– Lymphadenopathy and/or splenomegaly – Symptomatic cytopenia(s)	Autoimmune disorders (uveitis, hepatitis, glomerulonephritis, infiltrative, encephalitis, and myelitis)	– Gene sequencing – Assays investigating defective lymphocyte apoptosis – Elevated FASL, IL-10, vitamin B12 levels and IL-18 levels. – DNT cell count – Quantitative serum immunoglobulin levels	HL: 50x higher than the general population NHL: 14-fold increase
Activated PI3Kδ syndrome	Early childhood to adults	AD	PIK3 CD, PIK3R1	– Benign lymphoproliferations – B-cell lymphoma(s) – Immune cytopenia(s)	Lymphadenopathy, hepatosplenomegaly, autoimmune cytopenia(s), infections	Sinopulmonary infections, bronchiectasis, HPV viremia	– Gene sequencing	Reported to have an incidence as high as 13%
CTLA4 haploinsufficiency	Variable infants to throughout adulthood	AD	CTLA4	– Autoimmune cytopenia(s) – T-, B-, and NK-cells lymphopenias – Nonmalignant lymphoproliferation – B-cell lymphoma (EBV positivity is common)	Lymphadenopathy, cytopenia(s), immune dysregulation, and hypogammaglobulinemia	Variable, thyroiditis, diabetes, psoriasis, arthritis, respiratory infections, bronchiectasis, gastric cancer, and enteropathies	Gene sequencing	ND

Table 20.1 (cont.)

	Age of Onset/ Diagnosis	Inheritance	Gene(s)	Associated Hematologic Neoplasms	Clinical Presentation	Select Non-hematologic Abnormalities	Ancillary Diagnostic Tests	Risk to for Lymphoid Neoplasm
SCID	Early after birth	XLR AR	IL-2 R gamma RAG1 RAG2 ADA JAK3 IL-7 R	– Lymphoma not well documented – T-cell LPD in subset of patients after retroviral gene therapy for X-linked SCID – Autoimmune cytopenia	Immunodeficiency Fulminant infectious mononucleosis Severe combined immunodeficiency	Severe recurrent infections, Autoimmune disorders (vitiligo, psoriasis, Guillain-Barre syndrome), Granulomas Failure to thrive	Flow cytometry for study of the T-, B-, and NK-cell repertoire	ND
XLP-1	Often early in childhood to young adulthood	XLR	SH2D1A	– Lymphoma (often EBV+ B-cell NHL)	– Fulminant infectious mononucleosis – HLH – Hypogammaglobinemia – Aplastic anemia – Lymphoma (often extranodal)	– Vasculitis	Gene sequencing	~30%
Ataxia telangiectasia	Early childhood	AR	ATM (11q22.3)	– B-cell lymphomas (NHL and HL), T-cell lymphomas, and leukemia (notably T-ALL and T-PLL)	Progressive cerebellar ataxia, oculocutaneous telangiectasias, thymic aplasia, radiosensitivity, variable immunodeficiency	Cerebellar atrophy, telangiectasia, pulmonary diseases, Increased risk of breast, esophageal, gastric, and liver carcinomas.	Gene sequencing	Cumulative lifetime risk for a malignancy is approximately 25% (in which a majority include hematolymphoid malignancies)
Wiskott-Aldrich syndrome	Often in infancy	XLR	WAS (Xp11.22)	Frequently B-cell NHL	Severe immunodeficiency, microthrombocytopenia, and eczema	Eczema Autoimmune disease, IgA nephropathy Infections (viral, bacterial)	Gene sequencing	~Approximately 20%

AD, autosomal dominant; ALPS, autoimmune lymphoproliferative syndrome; AML, acute myeloid leukemia; B-ALL, B-lymphoblastic leukemia/lymphoma; CML, chronic myeloid leukemia; CNS, central nervous system; CTLA4, cytotoxic T-lymphocyte antigen-4; DNT, double-negative T-cells; DS, Down syndrome; DS-ALL, lymphoid proliferations associated with Down syndrome; EBV, Epstein-Barr virus; FISH, fluorescence in situ hybridization; HL, Hodgkin lymphoma; HLH, hemophagocytic lymphohistiocytosis; HPV, human papillomavirus infection; IKZF1, IKAROS family zinc finger 1; ITP, immune thrombocytopenic purpura; MDS, myelodysplastic syndrome; ND: not clearly defined; nHL, non-Hodgkin lymphoma; PI3Kδ, phosphoinositide 3-kinase-δ; SCID, severe combined immunodeficiency; SLE, systemic lupus erythematosus; T-PLL: T-cell prolymphocytic leukemia; WAS, Wiskott-Aldrich syndrome; XLP-1 X-linked lymphoproliferative syndrome 1; XLR, X-linked recessive.

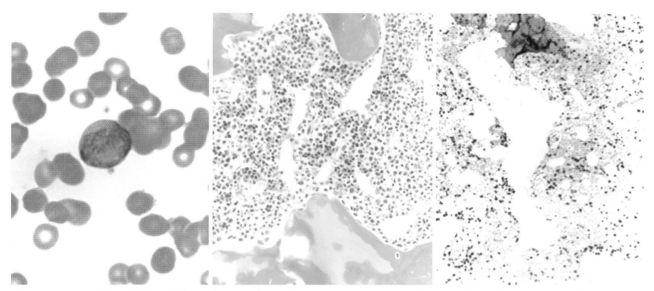

Figure 20.1 Acute B-lymphoblastic leukemia (B-ALL) with germline mutation in *PAX5*. Images from PB and BM of an 18-month-old female who presented with fever and pancytopenia. Family history was significant for three family members with childhood B-ALL; germline *PAX5* mutation was identified. Circulating blast (left, 1,000x), cellular marrow (middle, 200x) with increased TdT-positive cells (right panel, 200x). Contributed by Bachir Alobeid.

Li-Fraumeni Syndrome

Li-Fraumeni syndrome (LFS) is a cancer-predisposing condition resulting from germline heterozygous *TP53* mutations, inherited in an autosomal dominant manner. *TP53*, a tumor suppressor gene (located at chromosome 17p13.1), encodes the TP53 protein, a transcription factor involved in cell cycle regulation, apoptosis, DNA repair, and senescence in response to DNA damage. Individuals with this mutation are predisposed to multiple solid tumors and hematologic malignancies. The most common hematologic neoplasm in LFS is B-ALL. Lymphomas are less common. The age of onset is similar for leukemia (median age 12 years) and lymphoma (median age 13 years) [8]. B-ALL occurring in patients with LFS often exhibits a "low" hypodiploid karyotype in which the leukemic cells contain 32 to 39 chromosomes (Figure 20.2). A low hypodiploid karyotype is important to recognize since the majority of cases harbor loss-of-function mutations in *TP53* and/or *RB1*, with some *TP53* mutations present in the germline suggesting LFS [9]. Myeloid leukemias (AML, CML) and MDS are also common in LFS, often in the setting of prior therapy, and typically have complex karyotypic abnormalities (see Chapter 19).

Hints of LFS are early onset of cancers, multiple cancers throughout life, and family history of cancers. Genetic anticipation in the age of onset of cancer in

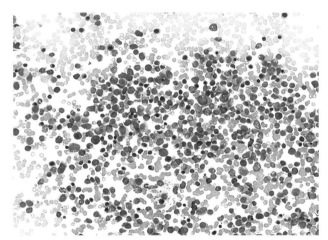

Figure 20.2 LFS. A 14-year-old boy with B-ALL (a, Wright-Giemsa, 200x) and low hypodiploid karyotype: 37, XY, −2, −3, −4, −7, −12, −13, −15, −16, −17[11]/35, sl, −Y, −9[3]/68~72, slx2[cp3]/46, XY [8]. Genetic testing was performed identifying a germline pathogenic mutation in *TP53*, consistent with a diagnosis of LFS.

successive generation has been frequently reported in LFS. Genetic testing and counseling should be done in patients as well as family members, including those being considered as donors for HSCT. Surveillance programs and screening tests for early detection of tumors are important.

233

Down Syndrome

Down syndrome (DS), constitutional trisomy 21, occurs in approximately 1 out of 700 live births. DS predisposes to both lymphoid and myeloid neoplasia. Transient abnormal myelopoiesis (TAM), which commonly occurs in the neonatal period, and MDS/AML in DS are discussed in Chapter 19. After the age of 4 years, the most common malignancy is B-ALL. Children with DS are at 20x increased risk of B-ALL [10] and 1–2% of individuals with DS will ultimately develop B-ALL (Figure 20.3). Rearrangements in *CRLF2* are detected in approximately 50% of ALL cases in DS.

Autoimmune Lymphoproliferative Syndrome

Autoimmune LymphoProliferative Syndrome (ALPS) is a disease of defective lymphocyte apoptosis associated with germline mutations in *FAS*, *FASL*, and *CASP10*. ALPS is characterized by chronic lymphadenopathy, hepatosplenomegaly, and autoimmune cytopenias [11, 12]. Lymphoid tissue typically shows florid follicular hyperplasia with reactive germinal centers and marked paracortical hyperplasia expanded by CD4, CD8 double-negative T-cells, and polyclonal plasmacytosis (Figure 20.4). ALPS patients are at increased risk of developing

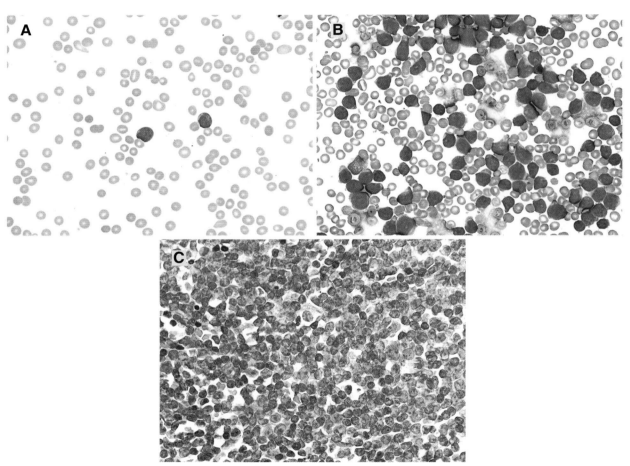

Figure 20.3 DS. This 13-year-old girl with DS was found to have profound anemia and marked thrombocytopenia, accompanied by 55% circulating leukemic B-lymphoblasts (A, Wright-Giemsa, 400x). The vast majority of cells in the bone marrow aspirate (B, Wright-Giemsa, 400x) and biopsy (C, H&E, 400x) were blasts. Comprehensive genetic testing showed B-lymphoblastic leukemia, *BCR-ABL1*-like, with *CRFL2* rearrangement.

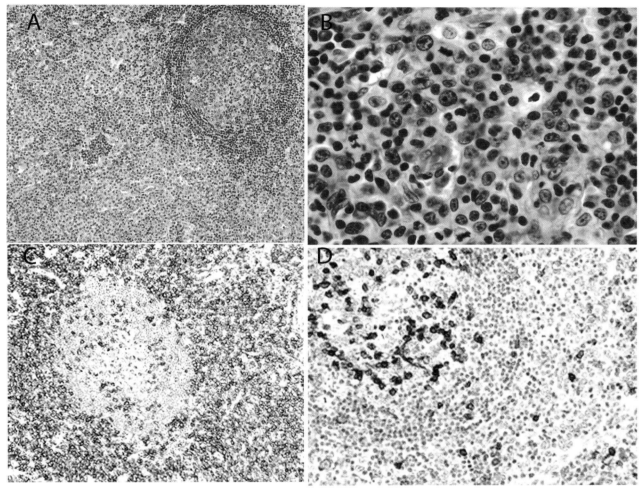

Figure 20.4 Autoimmune lymphoproliferative syndrome (ALPS). A–D. Characteristic features of reactive hyperplasia in a patient with ALPS with *FAS* gene mutation. Lymph node contains reactive germinal centers and expanded paracortex (A, H&E, 200x). Paracortex contains a mixed lymphoid infiltrate consisting of small lymphocytes, immunoblasts, plasma cells, and histiocytes (B, H&E, 400x). Paracortical T-cells are positive for CD3 (C, IHC, 200x) but negative for CD45 RO (D, IHC, 200x), characteristic of naïve T-cells. Contributed by Dr. Elaine Jaffe.

B-cell lymphomas, including Burkitt lymphoma, classical Hodgkin lymphoma (with or without EBV positivity), marginal zone lymphoma, and other B-cell lymphomas (Figure 20.5). Patients may present with lymphocytosis with increased alpha-beta double-negative T-cells (DNT cells) (CD3+/CD4–/CD8–) (Figure 20.6). Serum biomarkers, including vitamin B12, IL10, IL18, sFASL, and IgG, are often elevated. The bone marrow may show evidence of lymphocytosis with increased DNTs and erythroid hyperplasia. T-cell receptor gene rearrangement studies for T-cell clonality are nearly always polytypic. Sinus histiocytosis with massive lymphadenopathy (Rosai-Dorfman disease) is also reported.

Activated PI3Kδ Syndrome due to Gain-of-Function Germline Mutations in *PIK3 CD*

Phosphatidylinositol-3-OH kinases (PI3Ks) are a family of lipid enzymes that encompasses three classes. Class IA PI3Ks are heterodimers composed of a catalytic p110 subunit and a regulatory subunit p85. The catalytic subunit encompasses three isoforms – p110α, p110β, and p110δ – which are encoded by individual genes, *PIK3CA*, *PIK3CB*, and *PIK3 CD*, respectively. The p110δ isoform is preferentially expressed in lymphocytes and plays major roles in

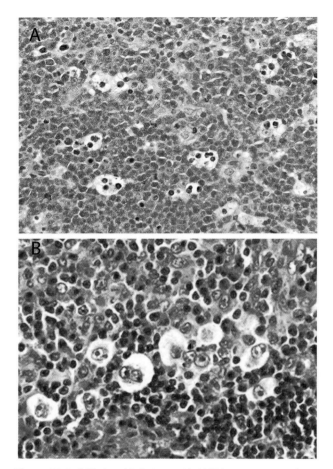

Figure 20.5 ALPS. A and B. Patients with ALPS have an increased incidence of B-cell lymphoma. Two representative examples include Burkitt lymphoma (A, H&E, 400x) and classical Hodgkin lymphoma (B, H&E, 400x). Contributed by Dr. Elaine Jaffe.

lymphocyte development and activation. Autosomal dominant gain-of-function mutations in *PIK3 CD* encoding for the PI(3)K catalytic subunit p110δ cause a combined immunodeficiency syndrome with increased incidence of B-cell lymphomas with EBV positivity [13]. Patients present with recurrent sinopulmonary infections, bronchiectasis, viremia with herpes family viruses (CMV and EBV), lymphoproliferation, and autoimmune cytopenias. Immune phenotype includes naïve CD4+ T-cell lymphopenia, expanded terminally differentiated or exhausted T-cells, increased circulating transitional B-cells, and reduced class-switched memory B-cells. The bone marrow of children with *PIK3 CD* mutations often shows marked hematogone hyperplasia with an atypical B-cell

maturation pattern that is distinctive by flow cytometry analysis (Figure 20.7) [14]. Lymph node biopsies show florid follicular hyperplasia with loss of the germinal center cuff or mantle. Nodular lymphoid hyperplasia may be present in airways and gastrointestinal mucosa.

CTLA4 Haploinsufficiency

Cytotoxic T-lymphocyte antigen-4 (CTLA4) encodes a receptor that is normally expressed on regulatory T-cells. Germline heterozygous mutations in *CTLA4* result in CTLA4 haploinsufficiency, which leads to severe systemic immune dysregulation and a spectrum of autoimmunity and immunodeficiency involving cytopenia, lymphoproliferation with tissue infiltration, lymphadenopathy, EBV infection, recurrent respiratory infections, lymphocytic colitis, type I diabetes, elevated serum IgM, and progressive lymphopenia [15, 16]. Some patients with CTLA4 deficiency present with features that initially suggest ALPS, in particular, autoantibody-mediated cytopenia, lymphadenopathy (Figure 20.8a), and splenomegaly. In pediatric cases, tissue infiltration by lymphocytes may occur in the brain (Figure 20.8b–f), lung (Figure 20.8g–k), gastrointestinal tract, and other tissues. Some patients may develop pancytopenia with markedly hypocellular marrows overlapping with aplastic anemia and bone marrow failure (Figure 20.8l); in these cases, one may see atypical lymphoid aggregates in the marrow composed of T-cells with loss of marrow B-cells (Figure 20.8l–q). Alternatively, more cellular marrows with a marked increase in interstitial T-cells may be seen, or marrow patterns with features of immune thrombocytopenia purpura. There is an increased risk of developing B-cell lymphomas, which may be EBV positive.

Severe Combined Immunodeficiency

Severe combined immunodeficiency (SCID) comprises a heterogeneous group of disorders characterized by abnormal T-cell development, severe T-lymphopenia, and lack of antigen-specific T-cell and B-cell immune responses [17, 18]. Most are autosomal recessive inherited, except for those associated with mutations in interleukin-2 receptor gamma (*IL2RG*), which is X-linked. Based on the immune defects, SCID is divided into several immunological phenotypes. SCID with T-, B+, NK- phenotype is characterized by lack of peripheral blood T-cells, decreased NK-cells, and normal to high number of B-cells, with severely reduced immunoglobulin production. Despite being numerically adequate, B-cells are

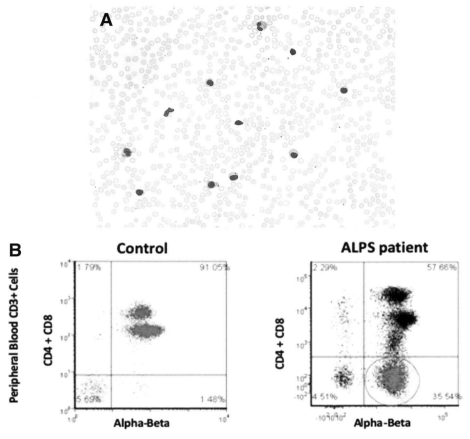

Figure 20.6 ALPS. A and B. 1-year-old girl who presented with leukocytosis with lymphocytosis. A. peripheral blood smear, Wright-Giemsa, 200x), anemia, and inguinal lymphadenopathy. B. Flow cytometry immunophenotyping demonstrated T-cells with 63.2% CD4/CD8-double negative, TCR alpha/beta-positive T-cells [normal: <2.6% of T cells]. *FAS* (*TNFRSF6*) mutation analysis revealed a novel pathogenic splice site mutation.

unable to produce immunoglobulins without T-cell assistance. Diseases belonging to this immunological phenotype include γc deficiency (common gamma chain SCID) due to *IL2RG* mutation and Janus kinase 3 (JAK3) deficiency. A slightly different phenotype is seen in interleukin-7 (IL-7) receptor deficiency, and AR form of SCID with selective lack of T-cells, but normal number of B-lymphocytes and NK-cells.

T-B-NK+ SCID, another immunological phenotype, is characterized by absent or very low T- and B-cells, decreased immunoglobulins, and normal numbers of NK-cells. The most common diseases included here are recombinase-activating (RAG1 and RAG2) deficiency, with their corresponding genetic defects in *RAG1* and *RAG2*, respectively. In complete RAG deficiency, due to null mutations, there is no V(D)J recombination

activity, leading to defective T-cell receptor assembly and signaling. An even more severe phenotype of T-B-NK- SCID is seen in adenosine deaminase (ADA) deficiency, caused by mutations in *ADA*. In ADA deficiency, lymphocytes (and other cell lineages) undergo abnormally increased apoptosis; manifestations include severe immunodeficiency with infections since early life, neurodevelopmental delay, hearing defects, liver dysfunction, pulmonary alveolar proteinosis, skeletal defects, increased risk of tumors (lymphoma, liver cancer), and autoimmune manifestations.

Defective T-cell surveillance to EBV underlies many lymphoid proliferations in primary immune disorders. Lymphomas are described in SCID, mostly of B lineage (Figure 20.9), commonly EBV-associated, due to defective T-cell surveillance to EBV.

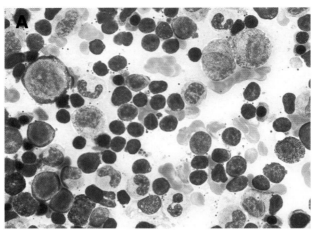

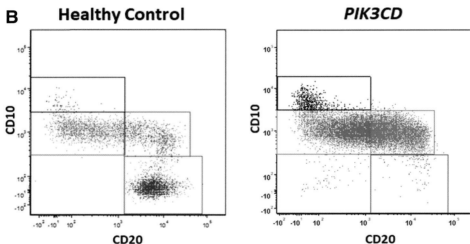

Figure 20.7 Activated PI3Kδ syndrome. Bone marrow aspirate from a 6-year-old male with germline mutation in *PIK3 CD*, showing increased lymphoid cells (A, 1,000x). Flow cytometric analysis of bone marrow CD19+ cells from the patient in comparison to marrow from a healthy child (B). This pattern shows an abundance of early B-cell precursors that mature through the late hematogone or transitional B-cell stage (CD19+/CD10+/CD20+) with a marked decrease to absence of mature B-cells (CD19+/CD20+/CD10−), suggesting impaired B-cell maturation.

X-Linked Lymphoproliferative Syndrome 1

X-linked lymphoproliferative (XLP)-1 syndrome is a rare immunodeficiency disorder caused by mutations in the *SH2D1A* gene [19, 20]. XLP is inherited in an X-linked recessive manner and is frequently associated with EBV-driven diseases. Most females carrying heterozygous mutations are clinically unaffected. Affected males with XLP1 have increased susceptibility to fulminant infectious mononucleosis, hemophagocytic lymphohistiocytosis, lymphoma, and hypogammaglobulinemia. Lymphomas are often of non-Hodgkin B-cell origin and frequently display extranodal presentation [21] (Figure 20.10). XLP1 needs to be considered when Burkitt lymphoma appears to recur after a long period of remission, or when Burkitt lymphoma develops in a male whose family history is significant for Burkitt lymphoma in his male siblings (or male maternal cousins). Other clinical manifestations include aplastic anemia and vasculitis. The underlying disease pathogenesis remains to be fully elucidated. Lack of immune surveillance for EBV may be associated with disease manifestations. However, a subset of symptoms appears to present independent of prior EBV exposure.

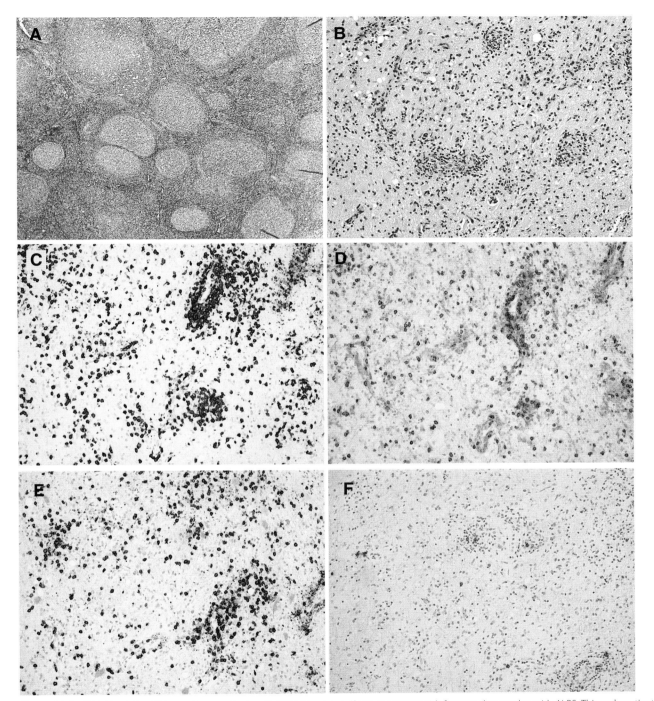

Figure 20.8 CTLA4 haploinsufficiency. Some patients with CTLA4 haploinsufficiency present with features that overlap with ALPS. This male patient with CTLA4 deficiency presented at age 7 years with marked thrombocytopenia and megakaryocytic hyperplasia in the marrow and lymphadenopathy (A, H&E, 20x) that showed preserved architecture with florid follicular hyperplasia, intrafollicular plasmacytoid cells (IgM and IgG variably present) and prominent PD-1 positive interfollicular T-helper cells, with attenuated mantle zones, greatly diminished plasma cells in the medullary cords.

(B–K) A 17-year-old boy with a past medical history of cervical lymphadenopathy 6 years earlier due to EBV infection, hypogammaglobulinemia, thrombocytopenia, asthma, eczema, and eosinophilic esophagitis presented with headaches and transient vertigo and was found to have lesions in the left temporal lobe and cerebellum. Brain biopsy revealed a perivascular and parenchymal lymphoid infiltrate (B, H&E, 100x) in a background of gliosis. The lymphocytes were predominantly T-cells (C, CD3, IHC, 100x), with mixed CD4-positive helper cells (D, IHC, 100x) and CD8-positive cytotoxic/suppressor cells (E, IHC, 100x), with very few B-cells (F, CD20, IHC, 100x). Additional imaging demonstrated innumerable pulmonary nodules with inflammatory infiltrates (G, H&E, 20x; H, H&E, 100x) composed of lymphocytes as well as plasma cells (I, H&E, 400x). T-cells predominated throughout (J, CD3, IHC, 100x), with B-cells scattered singly and also forming small aggregates (K, CD20, IHC, 100x). The findings in both the brain and lungs were compatible with an underlying immune deficiency/dysregulation and he was subsequently diagnosed with CTLA4 deficiency.

(L–O) 16-year-old male with a history of cytopenia, hypogammaglobulinemia, and lymphocytic colitis was evaluated for possible aplastic anemia. Whole-exome sequencing revealed a germline mutation in *CTLA4*. The marrow was markedly hypocellular with atypical lymphoid aggregates (L, H&E, 40x; M, H&E, 500x), composed of T-cells highlighted by CD3 (N, IHC, 40x) and very few B-cells (O, IHC, 40x).

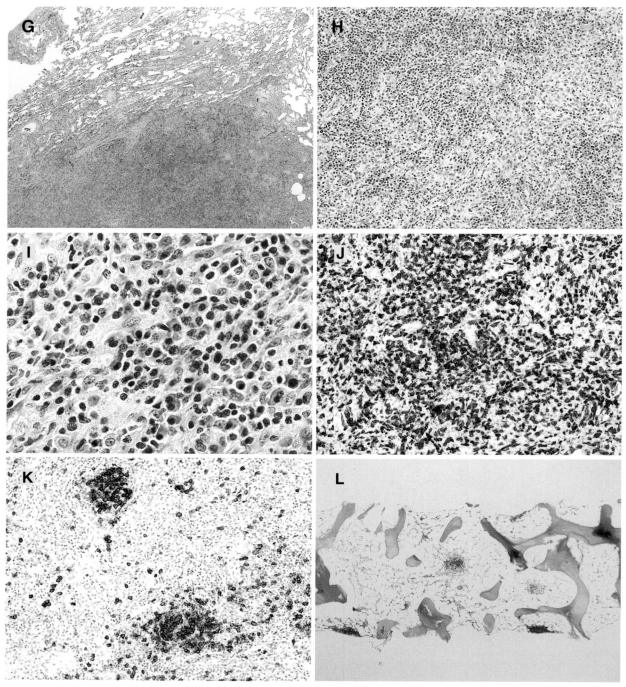

Figure 20.8 (cont.)

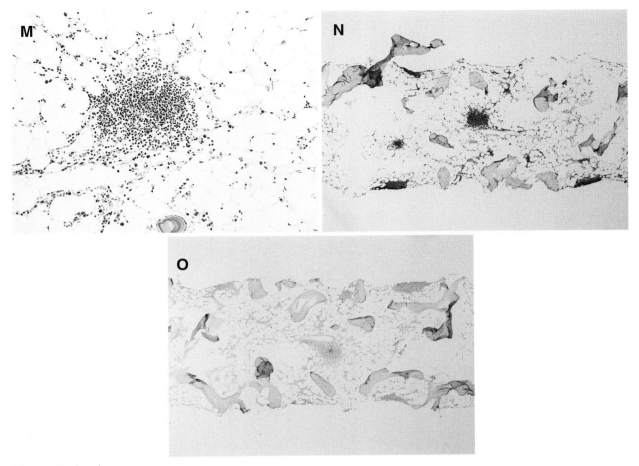

Figure 20.8 (cont.)

Diagnosis tests for XLP1 includes flow cytometry with absence of SAP (the "signaling lymphocytic activation molecule [SLAM]-associated protein) and/or *SH2D1A* mutation analysis. Treatment of XLP1 is generally tailored to the acute disease manifestations. Ultimately, allogeneic HSCT remains the only curative treatment at this time.

Ataxia Telangiectasia

Ataxia telangiectasia (AT) is a rare autosomal recessive disorder caused by inherited biallelic mutations of the ataxia telangiectasia mutated (*ATM*) gene located at chromosome (11q22.3), characterized by defective DNA repair [22]. The clinical presentation of AT is heterogeneous and includes progressive cerebellar ataxia, oculocutaneous telangiectasias, variable immunodeficiency, and increased risk of solid tumor and hematolymphoid malignancies.

Common manifestations of primary immunodeficiency in AT can include B-cell lymphopenia, T-cell lymphopenia, hypogammaglobulinemia, hyper-IgM, and/or selective IgA deficiency. Patients with AT may suffer from frequent infections, including sinopulmonary diseases that may manifest early in life. Additionally, due to the important role of *ATM* in DNA repair mechanisms, patients with AT have an increased sensitivity to ionizing radiation. Lymph node appearance is variable. Follicles/germinal centers can be large and reactive or, in contrast, small, fibrotic, and depleted of B-cells and nonreactive to antigenic stimulation. The most common malignancy in AT patients under the age of 20 are hematolymphoid malignancies whereas adults with AT have increased risk of both hematolymphoid and solid tumors [23]. Hematolymphoid malignancies include leukemias (notably T-ALL and T-cell prolymphocytic leukemia [T-PLL]),

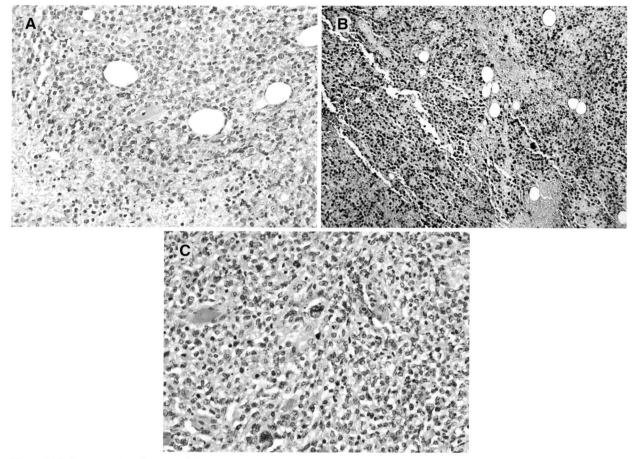

Figure 20.9 Severe combined immunodeficiency (SCID). (A and B) A 14-month-old girl presented with SCID and a history of oral thrush, severe diaper dermatitis, pneumonia, recurrent otitis, seizures, delayed development of gross motor skills and language, and 7 weeks of fever, lymphadenopathy, and night sweats. A cervical lymph node biopsy showed diffuse large B-cell lymphoma (A, H&E, 200x) and EBER FISH positive (B, CISH, 100x). Chromosomal microarray study showed 16p11.2 deletion, which is associated with developmental delay, but is also the gene locus for *CORO1A*. In addition, this patient harbored a missense mutation in the other, non-deleted allele (homozygous mutations), leading to Coronin-1A deficiency and in turn to a profound peripheral T-cell lymphopenia despite the presence of thymic tissue.

B-cell lymphomas (NHL and HL) (Figure 20.11), and T-cell lymphomas. Increased predisposition to solid tumors in adults with AT has been reported to include breast, esophageal, gastric, and liver carcinomas.

Wiskott-Aldrich Syndrome

Wiskott-Aldrich syndrome (WAS) is an X-linked primary immunodeficiency disorder caused by a mutated *WAS* gene, located at chromosome Xp11.23. It is classically characterized with a triad of severe immunodeficiency, thrombocytopenia, and eczema [24]. Thrombocytopenia is nearly universal in patients with WAS, although the severity is variable. A peripheral blood smear will often show decreased platelets that are uniformly small in size. Megakaryocytes in the bone marrow are normal in number and morphology. Due to the thrombocytopenia, patients may often present with variable bleeding tendencies that include petechiae, bruising, and nosebleeds. Patients with WAS often have combined T-cell and B-cell defects. Autoimmune manifestations, IgA nephropathy, and bacterial and viral infections are also common. Histopathologic examination of lymphoid tissues in a few reported studies have shown T-cell depletion in lymph nodes, generalized splenic white pulp depletion, and thymic hypoplasia. Lymphoma is the most common

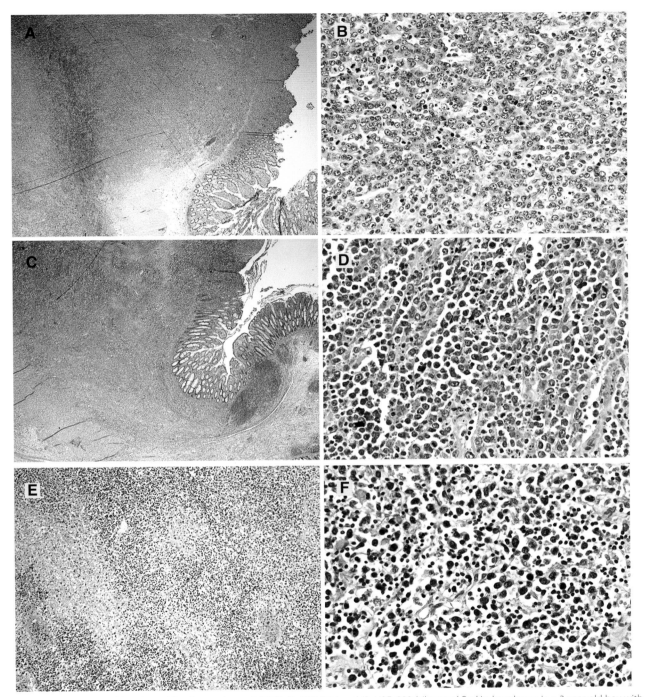

Figure 20.10 X-linked lymphoproliferative syndrome 1 (XLP). (A, H&E, 20x) and (B, H&E, 200x) Ileocecal Burkitt lymphoma in a 3-year-old boy with abdominal pain, harboring t(8;9) (q24.1; p13) with MYC rearrangement. When it "recurred" 3 years later, (C, 20x) and (D, 200x) there were only two analyzable metaphase cells, one normal and one with the more common t(8;14) (q24.1; q32). Both were EBV negative, but the recurrence was actually a genetically distinct second lymphoma. After attaining a complete remission following chemotherapy, he underwent autologous stem cell transplant. At age 9, he succumbed to fatal primary EBV infection complicated by hemophagocytic lymphohistiocytosis (HLH). (E, H&E, 100x) and (F, H&E, 400x) are autopsy images of a necrotic EBV-infected lymph node with many immunoblasts but no lymphoma. (G–J) Another patient with XLP1: This 4-year-old

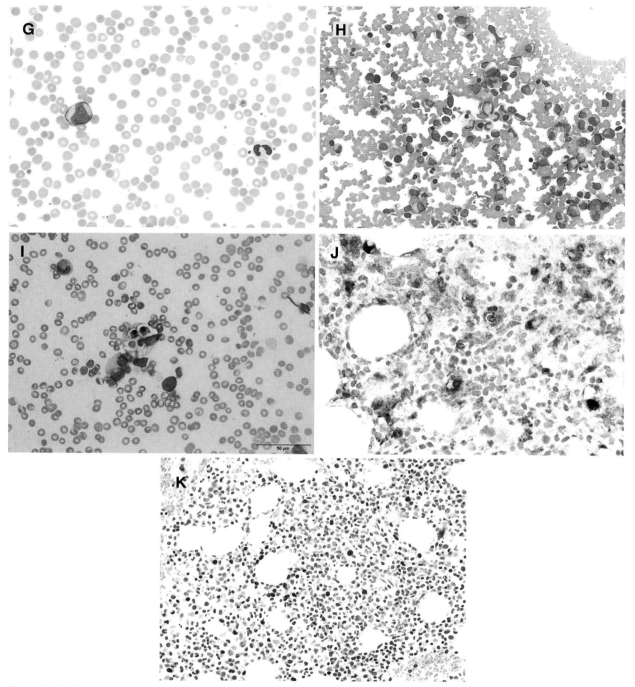

Figure 20.10 (cont.)

boy was initially diagnosed with and treated for Kawasaki disease. Because of persistent fever, viral studies were sent and he was found to have acute EBV infection. The peripheral blood smear showed leukocytosis with absolute lymphocytosis with many reactive lymphocytes (G, Wright-Giemsa, 400x), while the bone marrow (H, H&E, 200x) was remarkable for a prominent lymphoid component (T-cells > B-cells; cytotoxic/suppressor T-cells > helper T-cells), hemophagocytosis (H and I) and (J, CD68 immunostain, 400x), and occasional EBV-positive nuclei (K, EBER CISH, 200x).

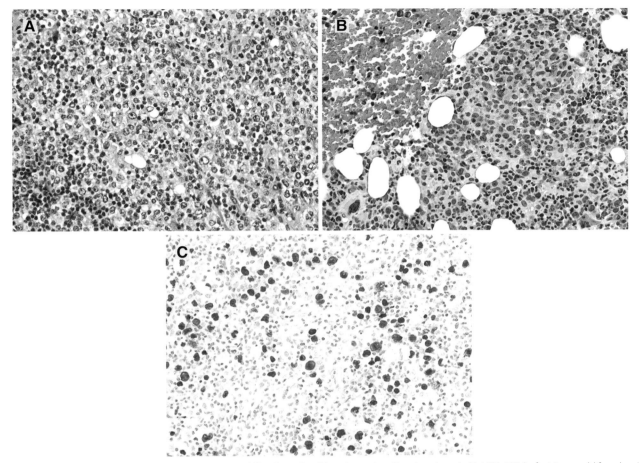

Figure 20.11 Ataxia telangiectasia (AT). EBV-positive diffuse large B-cell lymphoma in axillary lymph node (A, H&E, 200x) of a 13-year-old female with history of AT. Lymphoma was present in the bone marrow at diagnosis (B, clot section, H&E, 200x), and recurred several months later after treatment (C, 200x, EBER ISH).

malignancy observed in patients with WAS and is often of the B-cell NHL subtype. The overall incidence of malignant lymphoma in one study of 50 Wiskott-Aldrich patients was approximately 20% [25].

References

1. Kratz CP, Stanulla M, Cavé H. Genetic predisposition to acute lymphoblastic leukemia: Overview on behalf of the I-BFM ALL Host Genetic Variation Working Group. Eur J Med Genet. 2016; 59(3): 111–15.

2. Tran H, Nourse J, Hall S, Green M, Griffiths L, Gandhi MK. Immunodeficiency-associated lymphomas. Blood Rev. 2008; 22(5): 261–81.

3. Shah S, Schrader KA, Waanders E, Timms AE, Vijai J, Miething C, et al. A recurrent germline PAX5 mutation confers susceptibility to pre-B cell acute lymphoblastic leukemia. Nat Genet. 2013; 45(10): 1226–31.

4. Churchman ML, Qian M, Te Kronnie G, Zhang R, Yang W, Zhang H, et al. Germline genetic IKZF1 variation and predisposition to childhood acute lymphoblastic leukemia. Cancer Cell. 2018; 33(5): 937–48.

5. Hock H, Shimamura A. ETV6 in hematopoiesis and leukemia predisposition. Semin Hematol. 2017; 54(2): 98–104.

6. Rampersaud E, Ziegler DS, Iacobucci I, Payne-Turner D, Churchman ML, Schrader KA, et al. Germline deletion of ETV6 in familial acute lymphoblastic leukemia. Blood Adv. 2019; 3(7): 1039–46.

7. Noetzli L, Lo RW, Lee-Sherick AB, Callaghan M, Noris P, Savoia A, et al. Germline mutations in ETV6 are associated with thrombocytopenia, red cell macrocytosis and

predisposition to lymphoblastic leukemia. Nat Genet. 2015; **47**(5): 535–8.

8. Valdez JM, Nichols KE, Kesserwan C. Li-Fraumeni syndrome: A paradigm for the understanding of hereditary cancer predisposition. Br J Haematol. 2017; **176**(4): 539–52.

9. Comeaux EQ, Mullighan CG. TP53 mutations in hypodiploid acute lymphoblastic leukemia. Cold Spring Harb Perspect Med. 2017; 7(3): a026286.

10. Brown AL, de Smith AJ, Gant VU, Yang W, Scheurer ME, Walsh KM, et al. Inherited genetic susceptibility to acute lymphoblastic leukemia in Down syndrome. Blood. 2019; **134**(15): 1227–37.

11. Lim MS, Straus SE, Dale JK, Fleisher TA, Stetler-Stevenson M, Strober W, et al. Pathological findings in human autoimmune lymphoproliferative syndrome. Am J Pathol. 1998; **153**(5): 1541–50.

12. Xie Y, Pittaluga S, Price S, Raffeld M, Hahn J, Jaffe ES, et al. Bone marrow findings in autoimmune lymphoproliferative syndrome with germline FAS mutation. Haematologica. 2017; **102**(2): 364–72.

13. Lucas CL, Chandra A, Nejentsev S, Condliffe AM, Okkenhaug K. PI3Kδ and primary immunodeficiencies. Nat Rev Immunol. 2016; **16**(11): 702–14.

14. Dulau Florea AE, Braylan RC, Schafernak KT, Williams KW, Daub J, Goyal RK, et al. Abnormal B-cell maturation in the bone marrow of patients with germline mutations in PIK3 CD. J Allergy Clin Immunol. 2017; **139**(3): 1032–5.e6.

15. Kuehn HS, Ouyang W, Lo B, Deenick EK, Niemela JE, Avery DT, et al. Immune dysregulation in human subjects with heterozygous germline mutations in CTLA4. Science. 2014; **345**(6204): 1623–7.

16. Lo B, Fritz JM, Su HC, Uzel G, Jordan MB, Lenardo MJ. CHAI and LATAIE: New genetic diseases of CTLA-4 checkpoint insufficiency. Blood. 2016; **128**(8): 1037–42.

17. Niehues T, Perez-Becker R, Schuetz C. More than just SCID: The phenotypic range of combined immunodeficiencies associated with mutations in the recombinase activating genes (RAG) 1 and 2. Clin Immunol. 2010; **135**(2): 183–92.

18. Riaz IB, Faridi W, Patnaik MM, Abraham RS. A systematic review on predisposition to lymphoid (B and T cell) neoplasias in patients with primary immunodeficiencies and immune dysregulatory disorders (inborn errors of immunity). Front Immunol. 2019; **10**: 777.

19. Coffey AJ, Brooksbank RA, Brandau O, Oohashi T, Howell GR, Bye JM, et al. Host response to EBV infection in X-linked lymphoproliferative disease results from mutations in an SH2-domain encoding gene. Nat Genet. 1998; **20**(2): 129–35.

20. Gaspar HB, Sharifi R, Gilmour KC, Thrasher AJ. X-linked lymphoproliferative disease: Clinical, diagnostic and molecular perspective. Br J Haematol. 2002; **119**(3): 585–95.

21. Pachlopnik Schmid J, Canioni D, Moshous D, Touzot F, Mahlaoui N, Hauck F, et al. Clinical similarities and differences of patients with X-linked lymphoproliferative syndrome type 1 (XLP-1/SAP deficiency) versus type 2 (XLP-2/XIAP deficiency). Blood. 2011; **117**(5): 1522–9.

22. Amirifar P, Ranjouri MR, Yazdani R, Abolhassani H, Aghamohammadi A. Ataxia-telangiectasia: A review of clinical features and molecular pathology. Pediatr Allergy Immunol. 2019; **30**(3): 277–88.

23. Suarez F, Mahlaoui N, Canioni D, Andriamanga C, Dubois d'Enghien C, Brousse N, et al. Incidence, presentation, and prognosis of malignancies in ataxia-telangiectasia: A report from the French national registry of primary immune deficiencies. J Clin Oncol. 2015; **33**(2): 202–8.

24. Buchbinder D, Nugent DJ, Fillipovich AH. Wiskott-Aldrich syndrome: Diagnosis, current management, and emerging treatments. Appl Clin Genet. 2014; **7**: 55–66.

25. Cotelingam JD, Witebsky FG, Hsu SM, Blaese RM, Jaffe ES. Malignant lymphoma in patients with the Wiskott-Aldrich syndrome. Cancer Invest. 1985; **3**(6): 515–22.

Chapter 21

Mastocytosis and Myeloid Lymphoid Neoplasms with Eosinophilia

Karen M. Chisholm, Tracy I. George

Mastocytosis

Mastocytosis is defined as a clonal proliferation of neoplastic mast cells in one or more organ systems. It is broadly separated into two categories of cutaneous mastocytosis and systemic mastocytosis, of which the latter can include cutaneous involvement. In the 2016 World Health Organization (WHO) Classification of Tumours of Haematopoietic and Lymphoid Tissues, mastocytosis was separated into its own category due to its heterogeneous clinical manifestations ranging from spontaneously resolving skin lesions in pediatric cutaneous mastocytosis to highly aggressive malignancies such as mast cell leukemia with short survival and multiorgan involvement [1, 2].

While cutaneous mastocytosis is relatively common in pediatrics, bone marrow involvement is quite rare [3]. Detection of *KIT* D816V in peripheral blood of children with cutaneous mastocytosis using allele-specific quantitative polymerase chain reaction is predictive of systemic involvement with a sensitivity of 85.2% and specificity of 100%; this can be used to decide when to perform a bone marrow biopsy in children presenting with cutaneous mastocytosis [4]. Of course, not all children with systemic mastocytosis will have the *KIT* D816V mutation and thus other features, such as organomegaly, can help guide when to perform a bone marrow biopsy [5]. If the bone marrow is involved, the patient qualifies as having systemic mastocytosis as long as the single major and at least one minor criterion or three or more minor criteria of the following are met [6].

Major Criterion

Multifocal dense infiltrates of ≥15 mast cells in bone marrow and/or other extracutaneous organ

Minor Criteria

1. >25% of mast cells are spindle-shaped or have atypical morphology in bone marrow or other extracutaneous organ

Or

>25% of all mast cells in the bone marrow smears are immature or atypical
2. *KIT* codon 816 activating point mutations detected in blood, bone marrow, or other extracutaneous organ
3. Expression of CD25 with or without CD2 in mast cells in bone marrow, blood, or extracutaneous organ
4. Serum total tryptase persistently >20 ng/mL (exception is if there is an associated myeloid neoplasm)

Variants of systemic mastocytosis can be distinguished by the presence of B and C findings [6]:

"B" Findings (Disease Burden)	"C" Findings (Requiring Cytoreduction)
Bone marrow mast cell burden of >30% and serum total tryptase of >200 ng/mL	Bone marrow dysfunction caused by neoplastic mast cell infiltration with ≥1 cytopenia (absolute neutrophil count <1.0 × 10^9/L, hemoglobin <10 g/dL, and/or platelet count <100 × 10^9/L)
Signs of dysplasia or myeloproliferation in non-mast cell lineages with normal to slightly abnormal peripheral blood counts	Palpable hepatomegaly with impaired liver function, ascites or portal hypertension
Hepatomegaly, splenomegaly, or lymphadenopathy without impaired liver function or hypersplenism	Skeletal involvement with large osteolytic lesions/ pathologic fracture
	Palpable splenomegaly with hypersplenism
	Malabsorption with weight loss due to gastrointestinal mast cell infiltrates

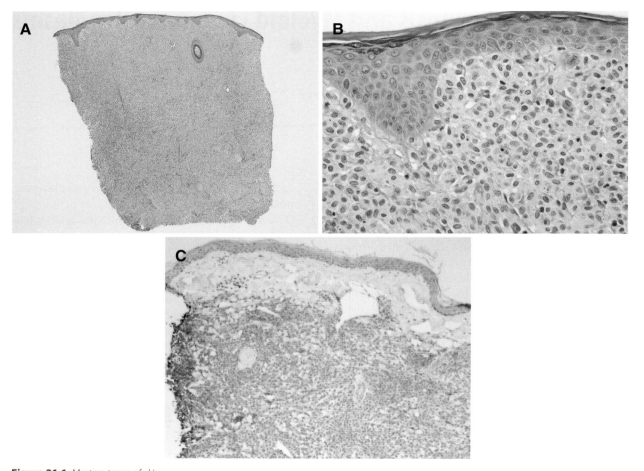

Figure 21.1 Mastocytoma of skin.

(A–C) This punch biopsy from a solitary nodule on a 2-month-old male illustrates the dense mast cell infiltrate occupying the entire dermis and extending to the limits of the biopsy (A, H&E, skin, 4x). Higher-power examination shows sheets of atypical mast cells with abundant eosinophilic cytoplasm and oval nuclei; fewer numbers of eosinophils are noted. Note the sparing of the epidermis (B, H&E, skin, 60x). CD25 highlights these mast cells (C, CD25, skin, 10x).

Cutaneous mastocytosis includes the following variants [3] (Figures 21.1–21.3):

1. Maculopapular cutaneous mastocytosis (includes urticarial pigmentosa)
2. Diffuse cutaneous mastocytosis
3. Mastocytoma of skin

Per the WHO classification, the variants of systemic mastocytosis include [6]:

1) Indolent systemic mastocytosis (≤1 B features, and no C findings)
2) Bone marrow mastocytosis (bone marrow only involved site)
3) Smoldering systemic mastocytosis (≥2 B findings but no C findings)

4) Systemic mastocytosis with an associated hematological neoplasm (typically acute myeloid leukemia [AML], myelodysplastic syndrome [MDS], myeloproliferative neoplasm [MPN], and MDS/MPN)
5) Aggressive systemic mastocytosis (≥1 C feature)
6) Mast cell leukemia (bone marrow with ≥20% mast cells)

In pediatrics, indolent systemic mastocytosis is one of the more common systemic mastocytosis variants (Figures 21.4 and 21.5). However, a few pediatric case series have reported systemic mastocytosis with associated AML with t(8;21), either with the diagnosis of leukemia [7–9] or after therapy commenced [10] (Figures 21.6 and 21.7).

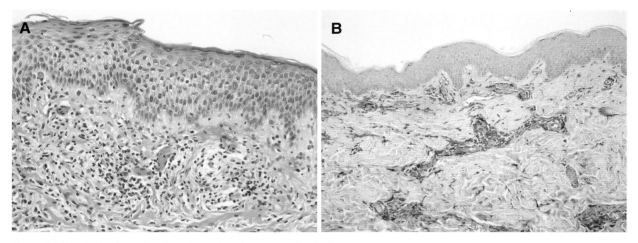

Figure 21.2 Urticaria pigmentosa/maculopapular cutaneous mastocytosis.

(A–B) This 4-year-old male presented with a macular rash that on biopsy shows an atypical infiltrate in the upper dermis consisting of spindle-shaped mast cells admixed with a few lymphocytes (A, H&E, skin, 30x). A corresponding tryptase immunostain highlights the scattered mast cells concentrated around vessels, but also scattered within the dermis (B, Tryptase, skin, 20x).

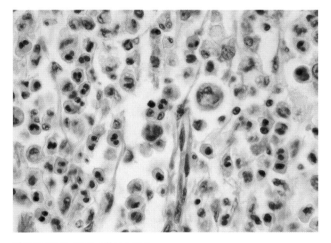

Figure 21.3 Mast cell sarcoma.

This 2-year-old child presented with a soft tissue mass eroding the skull base. Biopsy revealed sheets of pleomorphic cells (H&E, skull mass, 100x). A battery of immunohistochemical stains revealed a mast cell lineage including expression of tryptase (not shown). Mast cell sarcoma was diagnosed based on the extreme cytologic atypia in the tumor cells.

Chronic Eosinophilic Leukemia, Not Otherwise Specified

Chronic eosinophilic leukemia, not otherwise specified (CEL, NOS) is an MPN characterized by a clonal proliferation of eosinophils and defined per the 2016 WHO classification to meet five diagnostic criteria [11].

1. Eosinophil count $\geq 1.5 \times 10^9$/L
2. WHO criteria for other MPN, chronic myelomonocytic leukemia, and *BCR-ABL1*-negative atypical chronic myeloid leukemia (CML) not met
3. No rearrangement of *PDGFRA*, *PDGFRB*, or *FGFR1* genes, and no *PCM1-JAK2*, *ETV6-JAK2*, or *BCR-JAK2* fusion
4. Blasts <20% of cells in the peripheral blood and bone marrow;
   Inv(16)(p13.1.q22), t(16;16)(p13.1;q22), t(8;21)(q22; q22.1), and other diagnostic features of acute myeloid leukemia are not identified
5. Identification of a clonal cytogenetic or molecular genetic abnormality
   Or
   Blast cells represent $\geq 2\%$ of peripheral blood cells or $\geq 5\%$ of nucleated bone marrow cells

The eosinophils in this disorder can demonstrate abnormal granulation (regions of cytoplasm without granules), cytoplasmic vacuolization, nuclear hypo- or hyper-segmentation, and increased cell size. Due to the release of cytokines, enzymes, and other proteins from the eosinophils, end organ damage often occurs in CEL, NOS [11]. In pediatrics, CEL, NOS must be differentiated from idiopathic hypereosinophilic syndrome (iHES), the latter of which lacks clonality (Figure 21.8). Additionally, in cases without clonality and without end organ damage, the term *idiopathic hypereosinophilia* is employed. Secondary causes of eosinophilia need to be excluded.

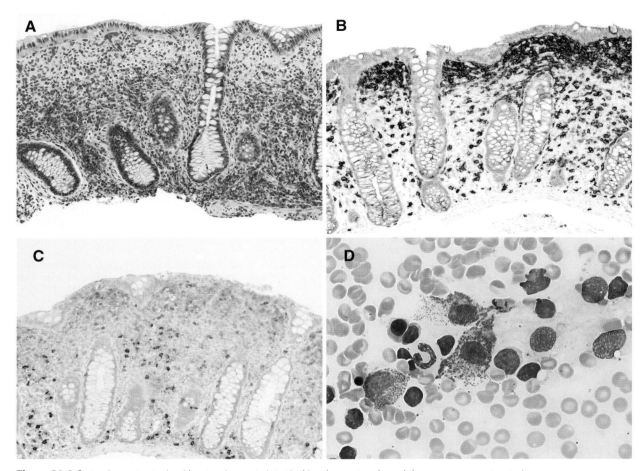

Figure 21.4 Systemic mastocytosis with extensive gastrointestinal involvement and occult bone marrow mastocytosis.

(A–D) This 5-year-old female presented with abdominal pain and diarrhea. Biopsy of the colon revealed a dense infiltrate of mast cells within the lamina propria with numerous eosinophils (A, H&E, colon, 20x).

Immunohistochemical stain for CD117 brightly marks the markedly increased mast cells present in a band-like infiltrate (B, CD117, colon, 20x). In contrast, a tryptase immunohistochemical stain is dim to negative in the mast cells in the area of the band-like infiltrate. The mast cells also marked for CD25 (not shown). For these reasons, CD117 is considered a better screening marker for mast cells in gastrointestinal biopsies (C, Tryptase, colon, 20x).

Interestingly, the bone marrow aspirate showed rare spindle-shaped mast cells, two of which are in the center of the image, that are hypogranular when compared to normal mast cells. Trilineage hematopoiesis was also present (D, Wright-Giemsa, bone marrow aspirate, 60x). The bone marrow biopsy, however, only showed rare normal round mast cells without aggregation (not shown).

Myeloid/Lymphoid Neoplasms with Eosinophilia and Rearrangement of *PDGFRA*, *PDGFRB*, or *FGFR1*, or with *PCM1-JAK2*

These myeloid and/or lymphoid neoplasms with the aforementioned gene rearrangements are clinically heterogeneous diseases. Most cases are associated with eosinophilia with cells that can have similar abnormalities to those seen in CEL, though there have been reports of cases without an eosinophil proliferation. At diagnosis, the neoplasm may present as a typical MPN, atypical CML, chronic myelomonocytic leukemia (CMML), CEL, AML, and/or a T- or B-lymphoblastic leukemia/lymphoma [12]. The cell of origin is a pluripotent lymphoid/myeloid stem cell [13]. In general, this category is defined by the presence of fusion products involving

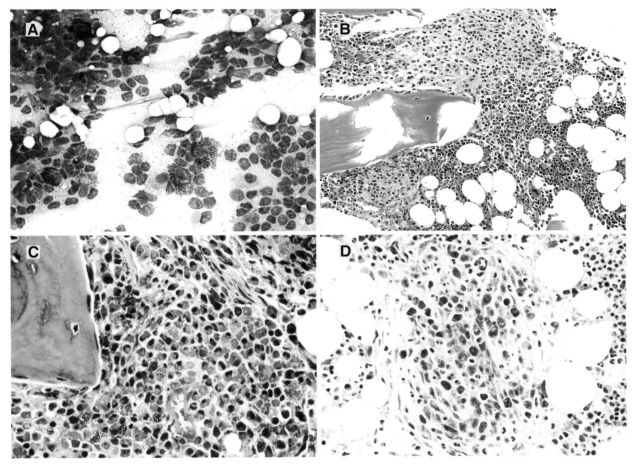

Figure 21.5 Indolent systemic mastocytosis.

(A–D) In bone marrow aspirates, mast cells are often identified within and directly adjacent to particles as shown in this aspirate from a 12-year-old male with a history of urticaria pigmentosa, increased mast cells in esophageal and stomach biopsies, and elevated tryptase >200 ng/mL. These mast cells have round to elongated nuclei and cytoplasm with many granules (A, Wright-Giemsa stain, bone marrow aspirate, 400x). In his bone marrow biopsy, paratrabecular aggregates of mast cells were identified, including some spindle-shaped forms, mixed with eosinophils and with associated fibrosis (B, H&E, bone marrow biopsy, 200x). The metachromatic granules in these mast cells were highlighted with Giemsa (C, Giesma, bone marrow biopsy, 400X) and toluidine blue stains (D, Toluidine blue, bone marrow biopsy, 400X).

PDGFRA, *PDGFRB*, *FGFR1*, or *PCM1-JAK2*. If such neoplasms with eosinophilia do not have rearrangements involving these genes, they are classified as CEL, NOS [11, 13].

Most cases with a *PDGFRA* rearrangement have a cryptic *FIP1L1-PDGFRA* fusion caused by a deletion of the *CHIC2* gene, leading to a constitutively activated tyrosine kinase; other cases may have a variant *PDGFRA* fusion or an activating mutation in *PDGFRA*. Peripheral eosinophilia is usually present, with a hypercellular marrow containing mature and immature eosinophils; dysplastic changes usually are not prominent and blasts are usually not increased [14–16]. Rare cases have presented without eosinophilia but with T-lymphoblastic leukemia or lymphoma [17] (Figure 21.9).

More than 30 genes have been identified to fuse with *PDGFRB* [18]. The only exception in this category is if the fusion partner leads to a *BCR-ABL1*-like B lymphoblastic leukemia, which would be classified as such. Only rare case reports of children with *PDGFRB* rearrangements in myeloid/lymphoid neoplasms have been published, with fusion partners including *CCDC88C*, *GOLGA4*, *BIN2*, and *TPM3* [19–21]. These cases have bone marrows with hypereosinophilia but without dysplastic features

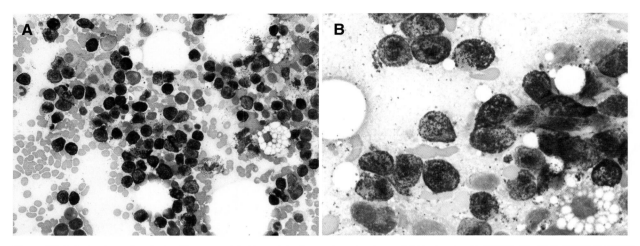

Figure 21.6 Systemic mastocytosis with an associated hematologic neoplasm (acute myeloid leukemia with t(8;21)(q22;q22.1); *RUNX1-RUNX1T1*).

(A–B) This 10-year-old male was diagnosed with AML with t(8;21). His end-of-induction bone marrow aspirate lacked evidence of residual AML, but did contain approximately 50% mast cells (A, Wright-Giemsa, bone marrow aspirate, 400x). On higher power, these mast cells were immature with elongated and indented nuclei, consistent with promastocytes (B, Wright-Giemsa, bone marrow aspirate, 1,000x). Flow cytometry showed that the mast cells expressed CD2, CD25, and bright CD117.

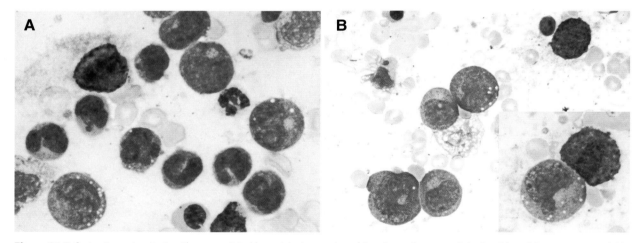

Figure 21.7 Systemic mastocytosis with an associated hematologic neoplasm (chronic myelomonocytic leukemia) evolving to acute myeloid leukemia with myelodysplasia-related changes.

(A–B) This bone marrow specimen is from a 12-year-old girl with a history of mixed germ cell tumor status post chemotherapy who developed asthma, tachycardia, and flushing. Her serum tryptase level was elevated. Due to pancytopenia, a bone marrow was performed that showed increased blasts and promonocytes meeting criteria for chronic myelomonocytic leukemia-2, as demonstrated in this image with increased atypical monocytes and promonocytes. In the upper left, an immature mast cell is present with a round shape and indented nucleus (promastocyte). At this time, mast cells were enumerated at 5% of total nucleated cells on aspirate and 10–15% by CD117 and tryptase immunohistochemistry with CD25 coexpression on the biopsy. *KIT* D816H was present and karyotype showed a complex karyotype with isochromosome 12p (A, Wright-Giemsa, bone marrow aspirate, 200x). Four months later, a subsequent bone marrow aspirate showed 24% blasts and promonocytes with 7% mast cells, now showing progression of this patient's associated hematological neoplasm to acute myeloid leukemia with myelodysplasia-related changes. The bone marrow aspirate shows increased blasts and blast equivalents with an immature mast cell in the upper right and in the inset (B, Wright-Giemsa, bone marrow aspirate, 125x; inset 200x).

(Figure 21.10). Neutrophilia and/or monocytosis may also be present. One case had a concurrent bone marrow MPN with nodal T-lymphoblastic lymphoma [20].

Myeloid/lymphoid neoplasms with *FGFR1* rearrangements, also known by 8p11 myeloproliferative syndrome, are heterogeneous diseases in pediatrics that can present

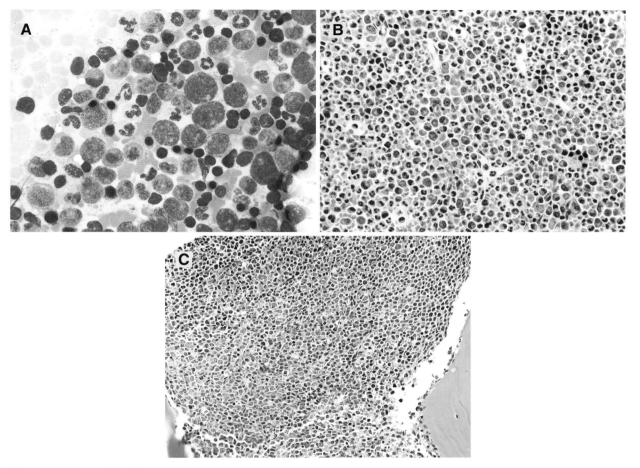

Figure 21.8 Hypereosinophilia.

(A) The aspirate smear from this 15-year-old female shows a marked marrow eosinophilia representing 30% of marrow elements, including mature eosinophils and eosinophilic precursors. Occasional dysplastic features including hypersegmentation were noted. All genetic testing was negative in this patient and the eosinophilia was favored to be reactive (Wright-Giemsa stain, bone marrow aspirate, 100x).

(B) The bone marrow biopsy from this 16-year-old female with a history of hypertensive crisis, chronic renal insufficiency, abnormal cardiac function, and persistent eosinophilia for more than 1 year revealed a hypercellular marrow with marked eosinophilia, including atypical forms with regions of sparse granules. Erythropoiesis and myelopoiesis were intact. After secondary causes of eosinophilia were excluded, she was diagnosed with idiopathic hypereosinophilic syndrome (H&E, bone marrow biopsy, 400x).

(C) Followed for five subsequent years, the female in Figure 21.8B developed more acute fatigue and anorexia. Her white blood cell count increased to 176.5×10^9/L and included 61% eosinophils with only 3% blasts. Bone marrow aspirates showed myeloid and eosinophilic hyperplasia with dysplasia, mild dyserythropoiesis, and increased myeloid blasts enumerated at 17%. On core biopsy, she had a hypercellular marrow with increased immature cells and eosinophils. Again, no genetic abnormalities were identified via karyotype, FISH, or molecular testing, so a diagnosis of CEL, NOS was rendered (H&E, bone marrow biopsy, 400x).

as MPN, MDS/MPN, AML, mixed phenotype acute leukemias, or T- or B-lymphoblastic lymphomas/leukemias. *FGFR1* has multiple fusion partners, including *BCR*, *ZMYM2* (also known as *ZNF198*), and *CNTRL* [22–26]. Pediatric cases have leukocytosis with eosinophilia with or without monocytosis or neutrophilia [23–26]. Such pediatric cases have demonstrated MPN, MDS/MPN,

CMML, atypical CML, and AML. T-lymphoblastic lymphomas more commonly occur with *ZMYM2-FGFR1* fusions [27].

Myeloid/lymphoid neoplasm with *PCM1-JAK2* is a provisional entity in the 2016 WHO classification, and can also include variant fusions such as *ETV6-JAK2* or *BCR-JAK2* [13]. These fusions result in a constitutively

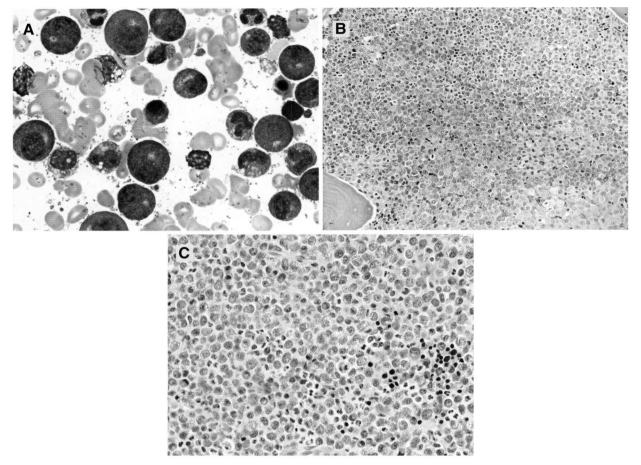

Figure 21.9 Myeloid and lymphoid neoplasm with *PDGFRA* presenting as T-lymphoblastic lymphoma.

(A–C) This 17-year-old male with a history of peripheral leukocytosis and eosinophilia (7.53×10^9/L) presented with recent weight loss and inguinal lymphadenopathy. Histologic evaluation of the lymph node biopsy revealed T-lymphoblastic lymphoma. Staging bone marrows showed a myeloid hyperplasia with many maturing eosinophils without an increase in lymphoblasts by morphology or flow cytometry (A, Wright-Giemsa, bone marrow aspirate, 1,000x). Bone marrow core biopsy was also hypercellular with a marked increase in eosinophils and left-shifted granulocytes (H&E, bone marrow biopsy, B – 200X, C – 400X). Fluorescence in situ hybridization on the bone marrow aspirate identified a deletion of 4q12 in 84% of cells, consistent with a *CHIC2* deletion leading to a *FIP1L1-PDGFRA* fusion product.

activated tyrosine kinase domain of JAK2. These neoplasms usually feature peripheral blood and bone marrow eosinophilia. While most cases have been in adults and include features of atypical CML, AML, and CEL, one pediatric case with acute erythroid leukemia has been described [28].

References

1. Arber DA, Orazi A, Hasserjian RP, Brunning RD, Le Beau MM, Porwit A, et al. Introduction and overview of the classification of myeloid neoplasms. In Swerdlow SH, Campo E, Harris NL, Jaffe ES, Pileri SA, Stein H, et al., eds. WHO classification of tumours of haematopoietic and lymphoid tissues. Lyon: IARC Press; 2017:16–27.

2. Vardiman JW, Brunning RD, Arber DA, Le Beau MM, Porwit A, Tefferi A, et al. Introduction and overview of the classification of the myeloid neoplasms. In Swerdlow SH, Campo E, Harris NL, Jaffe ES, Pileri SA, Stein H, et al., eds. WHO classification of tumours of haematopoietic and lymphoid tissues. Lyon: IARC Press; 2008:18–30.

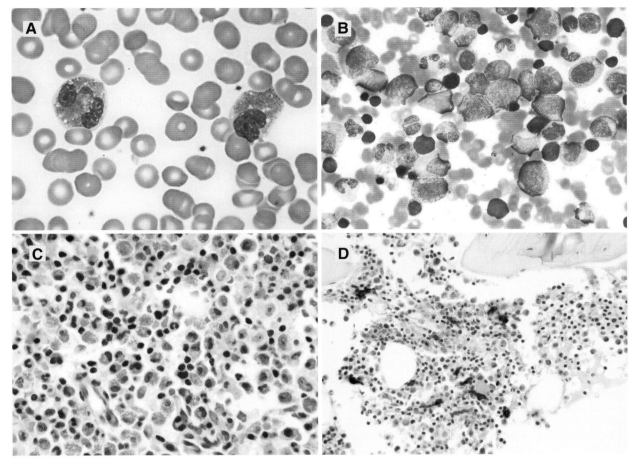

Figure 21.10 Myeloid neoplasm with *PDGFRB* presenting as chronic eosinophilic leukemia.

(A) This 3-year-old male presented with hepatosplenomegaly, a normal white blood cell count, mild normocytic anemia, and adequate platelet count, but an absolute eosinophilia of 1.43×10^9/L. The peripheral blood smear showed atypical mature eosinophils with an uneven distribution of eosinophilic granules, small cytoplasmic vacuoles, and abnormal nuclear lobation. FISH for *PDGFRB* showed a rearrangement in 6.5% of cells (Wright-Giemsa, peripheral blood, 200x).

(B) The bone marrow aspirate smear demonstrated trilineage hematopoiesis with increased eosinophils, including some large immature forms with monolobated nuclei. Rare forms with basophilic granules (harlequin cells) were noted. The M:E ratio was within normal limits (Wright-Giemsa, bone marrow aspirate, 100x).

(C) The bone marrow biopsy showed 90% cellularity with an increase in eosinophils amidst normal trilineage hematopoiesis (H&E, bone marrow biopsy, 100x).

(D) An immunohistochemical stain for tryptase highlighted scattered spindle-shaped mast cells without clusters. CD25 expression was also present (not shown). CD25-positive mast cells may be found in myeloid and lymphoid neoplasms with rearrangements of *PDGFRA*, *PDGFRB*, or *FGFR1* (tryptase, bone marrow biopsy, 50x).

3. Hartmann K, Escribano L, Grattan C, Brockow K, Carter MC, Alvarez-Twose I, et al. Cutaneous manifestations in patients with mastocytosis: Consensus report of the European Competence Network on Mastocytosis; the American Academy of Allergy, Asthma & Immunology; and the European Academy of Allergology and Clinical Immunology. J Allergy Clin Immunol. 2016; **137**(1): 35–45.

4. Carter MC, Bai Y, Ruiz-Esteves KN, Scott LM, Cantave D, Bolan H, et al. Detection of KIT D816V in peripheral blood of children with manifestations of cutaneous mastocytosis suggests systemic disease. Br J Haematol. 2018; **183**(5): 775–82.

5. Carter MC, Clayton ST, Komarow HD, Brittain EH, Scott LM, Cantave D, et al. Assessment of clinical findings, tryptase levels, and bone marrow histopathology in the

management of pediatric mastocytosis. J Allergy Clin Immunol. 2015; **136**(6): 1673–9 e3.

6. Horny H-P, Akin C, Arber DA, Peterson LC, Tefferi A, Metcalfe DD, et al. Mastocytosis. In Swerdlow SH, Campo E, Harris NL, Jaffe ES, Pileri SA, Stein H, et al., eds. WHO classification of tumours of haematopoietic and lymphoid tissues. Lyon: IARC Press; 2017:62–9.

7. Gadage VS, Kadam Amare PS, Galani KS, Mittal N. Systemic mastocytosis with associated acute myeloid leukemia with t (8; 21) (q22; q22). Indian J Pathol Microbiol. 2012; **55**(3): 409–12.

8. Johnson RC, Savage NM, Chiang T, Gotlib JR, Cherry AM, Arber DA, et al. Hidden mastocytosis in acute myeloid leukemia with t(8;21)(q22;q22). Am J Clin Pathol. 2013; **140**(4): 525–35.

9. Rabade N, Tembhare P, Patkar N, Amare P, Arora B, Subramanian PG, et al. Childhood systemic mastocytosis associated with t (8; 21) (q22; q22) acute myeloid leukemia. Indian J Pathol Microbiol. 2016; **59**(3): 407–9.

10. Mahadeo KM, Wolgast L, McMahon C, Cole PD. Systemic mastocytosis in a child with t(8;21) acute myeloid leukemia. Pediatr Blood Cancer. 2011; **57**(4): 684–7.

11. Bain BJ, Horny H-P, Hasserjian RP, Orazi A. Chronic eosinophilic leukaemia, NOS. In Swerdlow SH, Campo E, Harris NL, Jaffe ES, Pileri SA, Stein H, et al., eds. WHO classification of tumours of haematopoietic and lymphoid tissues. Lyon: IARC Press; 2017:54–6.

12. Patterer V, Schnittger S, Kern W, Haferlach T, Haferlach C. Hematologic malignancies with PCM1-JAK2 gene fusion share characteristics with myeloid and lymphoid neoplasms with eosinophilia and abnormalities of PDGFRA, PDGFRB, and FGFR1. Ann Hematol. 2013; **92**(6): 759–69.

13. Bain BJ, Horny H-P, Arber DA, Tefferi A, Hasserjian RP. Myeloid/lymphoid neoplasms with eosinophilia and rearrangement of *PDGFRA*, *PDGFRB* or *FGFR1*, or with *PCM1-JAK2*. In Swerdlow SH, Campo E, Harris NL, Jaffe ES, Pileri SA, Stein H, et al., eds. WHO classification of tumours of haematopoietic and lymphoid tissues. Lyon: IARC Press; 2017:72–9.

14. Farruggia P, Giugliano E, Russo D, Trizzino A, Lorenzatti R, Santoro A, et al. FIP1L1-PDGFRalpha-positive hypereosinophilic syndrome in childhood: A case report and review of literature. J Pediatr Hematol Oncol. 2014; **36**(1): e28–e30.

15. Rathe M, Kristensen TK, Moller MB, Carlsen NL. Myeloid neoplasm with prominent eosinophilia and PDGFRA rearrangement treated with imatinib mesylate. Pediatr Blood Cancer. 2010; **55**(4): 730–2.

16. Rives S, Alcorta I, Toll T, Tuset E, Estella J, Cross NC. Idiopathic hypereosinophilic syndrome in children: Report of a 7-year-old boy with FIP1L1-PDGFRA rearrangement. J Pediatr Hematol Oncol. 2005; **27**(12): 663–5.

17. Oberley MJ, Denton C, Ji J, Hiemenz M, Bhojwani D, Ostrow D, et al. A neoplasm with FIP1L1-PDGFRA fusion presenting as pediatric T-cell lymphoblastic leukemia/lymphoma without eosinophilia. Cancer Genet. 2017; **216–17**: 91–9.

18. Reiter A, Gotlib J. Myeloid neoplasms with eosinophilia. Blood. 2017; **129**(6): 704–14.

19. Abraham S, Salama M, Hancock J, Jacobsen J, Fluchel M. Congenital and childhood myeloproliferative disorders with eosinophilia responsive to imatinib. Pediatr Blood Cancer. 2012; **59**(5): 928–9.

20. Bielorai B, Leitner M, Goldstein G, Mehrian-Shai R, Trakhtenbrot L, Fisher T, et al. Sustained response to imatinib in a pediatric patient with concurrent myeloproliferative disease and lymphoblastic lymphoma associated with a CCDC88C-PDGFRB fusion gene. Acta Haematol. 2019; **141**(2): 119–27.

21. Hidalgo-Curtis C, Apperley JF, Stark A, Jeng M, Gotlib J, Chase A, et al. Fusion of PDGFRB to two distinct loci at 3p21 and a third at 12q13 in imatinib-responsive myeloproliferative neoplasms. Br J Haematol. 2010; **148**(2): 268–73.

22. Brown LM, Bartolo RC, Davidson NM, Schmidt B, Brooks I, Challis J, et al. Targeted therapy and disease monitoring in CNTRL-FGFR1-driven leukaemia. Pediatr Blood Cancer. 2019; **66**(10): e27897.

23. Chen X, Zhang Y, Li Y, Lei P, Zhai Y, Liu L. Biphenotypic hematologic malignancy: A case report of the 8p11 myeloproliferative syndrome in a child. J Pediatr Hematol Oncol. 2010; **32**(6): 501–3.

24. Dolan M, Cioc A, Cross NC, Neglia JP, Tolar J. Favorable outcome of allogeneic hematopoietic cell transplantation for 8p11 myeloproliferative syndrome associated with BCR-FGFR1 gene fusion. Pediatr Blood Cancer. 2012; **59**(1): 194–6.

25. Lv H, Hu S, Lu J, Zhai Q, Zhai Z, Du Z, et al. Precursor T-lymphoblastic lymphoma associated with t(8;9)(p11.2; q33): A case report and review of the literature. Acta Haematol. 2018; **139**(3): 176–82.

26. Wong WS, Cheng KC, Lau KM, Chan NP, Shing MM, Cheng SH, et al. Clonal evolution of 8p11 stem cell syndrome in a 14-year-old Chinese boy: A review of literature of t(8;13) associated myeloproliferative diseases. Leuk Res. 2007; **31**(2): 235–8.

27. Macdonald D, Reiter A, Cross NC. The 8p11 myeloproliferative syndrome: A distinct clinical entity caused by constitutive activation of FGFR1. Acta Haematol. 2002; **107**(2): 101–7.

28. Murati A, Gelsi-Boyer V, Adelaide J, Perot C, Talmant P, Giraudier S, et al. PCM1-JAK2 fusion in myeloproliferative disorders and acute erythroid leukemia with t(8;9) translocation. Leukemia. 2005; **19**(9): 1692–6.

Chapter

22

Histiocytic Lesions

Kudakwashe Chikwava

Introduction

Histiocytic disorders consist of many rare related and unrelated wide-ranging proliferations of cells supposedly derived from or sharing common immunophenotypes with macrophages (such as hemophagocytic lymphohistiocytosis) and dendritic cells (such as juvenile xanthogranulomas). These lesions can involve virtually any organ, resulting in an assortment of clinical presentations and prognostic outcomes that vary from localized incidental self-limiting lesions to multisystemic potentially fatal conditions that require chemotherapy or other aggressive treatments. Recent advances in our understanding of histiocytic lesions have shed new light on the pathophysiology of histiocytic disorders, revealing that many distinct entities have overlapping mutations of *BRAF* or other genes in the MAPK pathway [1]. In 2016, the Histiocyte Society proposed a revised classification system in which histiocytic disorders are sorted into five groups (summarized in Table 22.1) based on clinical, radiologic, histopathologic, immunophenotypic, and genetic/molecular characteristics [2]. This chapter roughly follows this new classification system to show and describe examples of lesions that represent the major groups of pediatric histiocytic lesions.

Langerhans Cell Histiocytosis

Langerhans cell histiocytosis (LCH) is a clonal proliferation of cells with an immunophenotype similar to Langerhans cells and shows Birbeck granules by electron microscopy. The cell of origin is now understood to be a myeloid progenitor cell in the bone marrow. The most commonly involved sites in localized LCH are bone followed by skin, lymph nodes, and lung. Multisystem disease has an additional preponderance for bone marrow, spleen, and liver. Diagnosis of LCH is based on identification of lesional cells that are large (20–25 μm) and oval, not dendritic like normal Langerhans cells or dermal interstitial dendritic cells. Nuclei are characteristically coffee-bean shaped,

Table 22.1 Summary of the Histiocyte Society's proposed revised classification of histiocytic lesions

1 **L (Langerhans) Group**
  – Langerhans cell histiocytosis (LCH)
  – Indeterminate cell histiocytosis (ICH)
  – Erdheim-Chester disease (ECD)
  – Mixed LCH-ECD

2 **C (Cutaneous and mucosal non-Langerhans cell histiocytoses) group**
  a. Cutaneous non-LCH
     i. Xanthogranuloma family
        – Juvenile xanthogranuloma
        – Adult xanthogranuloma
        – Solitary reticulohistiocytoma
        – Benign cephalic histiocytosis
        – Generalized eruptive histiocytosis
        – Progressive nodular histiocytosis
     ii. Non-xanthogranuloma family
        – Cutaneous Rosai-Dorfman disease
        – Necrobiotic xanthogranuloma
        – Other skin histiocytosis, not otherwise specified
  b. Cutaneous non-LCH with major systemic component
     i. Xanthogranuloma family
        – Xanthogranuloma disseminatum
     ii. Non-xanthogranuloma family
        – Multicentric reticulohistiocytosis

3 **R (Rosai-Dorfman disease [RDD]) group**
  a. Familial RDD
  b. Sporadic RDD
     – Classic (nodal) RDD
     – Extranodal RDD
     – Neoplasia-associated RDD
     – Immune disease-associated RDD
     – Unclassified RDD

4 **M (Malignant histiocytoses) group**
  a. Primary malignant histiocytosis
  b. Secondary malignant histiocytosis

5 **H (Hemophagocytic lymphohistiocytosis) group**
  a. Primary hemophagocytic lymphohistiocytosis (HLH)
  b. Secondary HLH
  c. HLH of unknown/uncertain origin [2]

Table 22.2 Hemophagocytic lymphohistiocytosis diagnostic criteria (2004 clinical trial)

1 **Genetic confirmation** of abnormality consistent with primary/familial HLH (*PRF1, NC13D, STXBP2, RAB27A, STX11, SH2D1A,* or *XIAP*) **or**

2 **Five or more of the following** criteria

Fever

Splenomegally

Cytopenias affecting 2 of 3 lineages
- Hemoglobin < 90 g/L (in infants <4 weeks: <100 g/L)
- Platelets < 100 × 10⁹/L
- Neutrophils < 1.0 × 10⁹/L

Hypertriglyceridemia or hypofibrinogenemia
- Fasting triglycerides >/= 3.0 mmol/L (i.e., >/= 265 mg/dL)
- Fibrinogen </= 1.5 g/L

Hemophagocytosis in bone marrow, spleen, or lymph node

Low or absent natural killer cell activity (according to local laboratory reference)

Increased ferritin >/= 500 mg/L

Increased soluble CD25 (i.e., soluble interleukin-2 receptor) >/= 2,400 U/mL [4]

Diagnosis of HLH requires either genetic confirmation or the presence of five of these eight criteria.

grooved, or appear folded with fine chromatin and inconspicuous nucleoli. Although mitoses are variable, there is usually no or minimal nuclear atypia. Cytoplasm is moderate and usually eosinophilic. The background of LCH lesions is variable and often shows few to numerous eosinophils. When numerous, the eosinophils frequently produce eosinophilic abscesses and Charcot-Leyden crystals. It is also not uncommon to find variable numbers of neutrophils in early lesions. Plasma cells tend to be sparse. With time, macrophages including multinucleated lesional cells and osteoclast-type giant cells accumulate. The appearance of LCH lesions also varies with the organ involved, as shown later in this chapter (Figures 22.1–22.5). Recent advances have shown that more than half of cases have mutations of *BRAF V600E*. Those that do not have *BRAF V600E* mutations appear to have some other mutations of the MAP2K1/ERK/ARAF pathway. Mortality is highest in patients who have involvement of so-called high-risk organs, which are the bone marrow, spleen, and liver.

Indeterminate Cell Histiocytosis

Indeterminate cell histiocytosis (ICH) is a very rare and poorly understood entity that bears histomorphologic similarities with but is distinct from LCH. It is thought to be a neoplastic proliferation composed of precursor cells of Langerhans cells. Patients typically present with multiple skin lesions (papules, nodules, or plaques) or, less commonly, enlarged lymph nodes or splenic disease. By definition, ICH lacks Birbeck granules. This absence of Birbeck granules is paralleled by negative staining with Langerin, allowing the stain to be used as a surrogate for electron microscopy. CD1a is positive and S100 is variable. The clinical outcome is highly variable, ranging from spontaneous regression to aggressive disease.

Erdheim-Chester Disease

Erdheim-Chester disease (ECD) is a histiocytic disorder characterized by disseminated lesions that resemble juvenile xanthogranuloma accompanied by distinctive lytic and sclerotic bone lesions. Although the average age at presentation is 55, pediatric cases have been reported. The supposed cell of origin is the dermal dendritic cell. Some studies have reported clonality and activating mutations of *BRAF V600E* have been demonstrated in >50% of cases, suggesting a close relationship to LCH. PI3KCA pathway gene mutations and *NRAS* mutations have been documented in 11% and 4% of cases, respectively. Erdheim-Chester disease lesions commonly affect bone and the cardiovascular system (95% and 50%, respectively). Less commonly involved are the retroperitoneal cavity and organs (kidneys, pancreas, and aorta) (30%), central nervous system and periorbital space (20 to 30%), and skin, especially eyelids (Figure 22.6).

Juvenile Xanthogranuloma

Juvenile xanthogranuloma (JXG) is the most common non-Langerhans cell histiocytosis. It consists of proliferations of cells with an immunophenotype consistent with dendritic cells. Most cases are cutaneous (solitary or multiple) or of deep soft tissue, with fewer involving systemic organs (central nervous system, orbital, hepatic, pulmonary, lymph node, and bone marrow disease). In the skin, JXG most commonly affects the head and neck. The skin lesions are commonly small papules and the soft tissue masses tend to be larger (Figure 22.7). Upper aerodigestive tract mucosa involvement often accompanies systemic organ involvement. Disseminated forms of JXG commonly occur by the age of 10 with nearly half presenting within the first year of life. Disseminated JXG is not believed to develop from solitary dermal lesions (Figure 22.8). There is known association with neurofibromatosis type 1 and it is not uncommon to find patients who have both LCH and JXG. No consistent cytogenetic

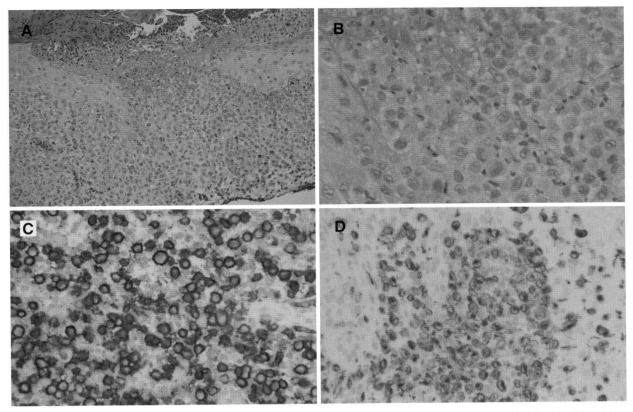

Figure 22.1 Cutaneous LCH. In skin clonal proliferations of LCH, cells show epidermotropism (a proclivity to involve the dermal-epidermal junction and papillary dermis). (a) This photomicrograph shows epidermotropism and secondary epidermal ulceration, another feature that may be seen in skin LCH. (b) The lesional LCH cells are large round to oval with characteristically coffee-bean-shaped or grooved nuclei. Varying numbers of eosinophils are often scattered in the background (400x). (c) CD1a immunohistochemical staining shows a characteristically strong membranous pattern (400x). (d) Langerin shows membranous and cytoplasmic staining with occasional paranuclear dots (400x). VE-1 immunohistochemical positivity (not shown here) suggests BRAF mutations.

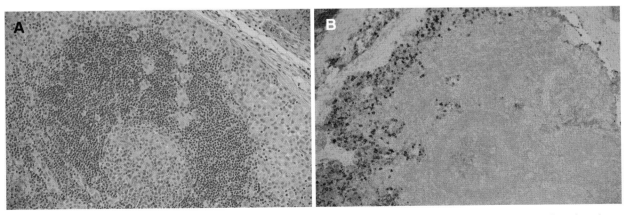

Figure 22.2 LCH involving lymph node. (a) Early lesions of nodal LCH involve the subcapsular sinuses. (b) CD1a shows LCH cells in the subcapsular sinus. Progressive disease will ultimately result in effacement of nodal architecture by paracortical extension.

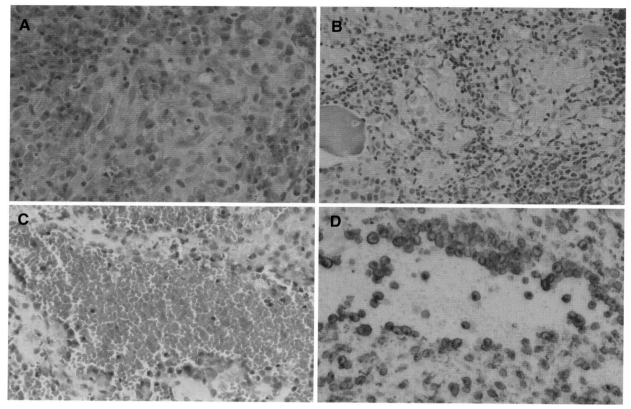

Figure 22.3 LCH involving bone. (a) LCH cells are obscured by a densely eosinophil-rich background. When eosinophils dominate, they form Charcot-Leyden crystals. (b) Involvement of the bone marrow space (as opposed to LCH limited to cortical bone), confers higher risk for recurrence, refractoriness to therapy, and death. These lesions, together with liver and spleen lesions, are classified as high risk. (c) Osseous LCH may show foci may show aneurysmal bone cyst-like areas. (d) This Langerin stain shows LCH cells lining an ABC-like cystic space. Frequently seen in osseous LCH (but not shown here) are CD1a and Langerin negative non-LCH multinucleated osteoclast-like giant cells.

or molecular genetic changes have been described and, unlike LCH and ECD, no mutations in *BRAF* have been identified in JXG. Most cases of disseminated JXG will resolve spontaneously; however, patients who have CNS disease may develop concomitant hemophagocytic lymphohistiocytosis with poorer outcome.

Reticulohistiocytoma

Reticulohistiocytoma (RH) is considered by some to be part of the JXG family of histiocytic disorders because of the significant overlap in histology and immunophenotype. Lesions may commonly involve skin as isolated cutaneous lesions, but may also involve mucous membranes and joint surfaces in cases of multicentric reticulohistiocytoma (Figure 22.9).

Rosai-Dorfman Disease

Rosai-Dorfman disease (RDD) is a rare and poorly understood histiocytic disorder that is also known as sinus histiocytosis with massive lymphadenopathy because of its typical clinical presentation and histologic appearance in lymph nodes. While many patients (40%) will have pure nodal presentation, others will have combined nodal and extranodal disease or purely extranodal disease. Most patients are children or young adults at presentation (mean age = 21 years) and a proclivity for males of African descent has been reported [3]. While the etiology of RDD is largely unknown, familial cases and cases with recurrent known mutations are described. Other cases have been associated with neoplasms and immune dysregulation. The familial cases have germline mutations

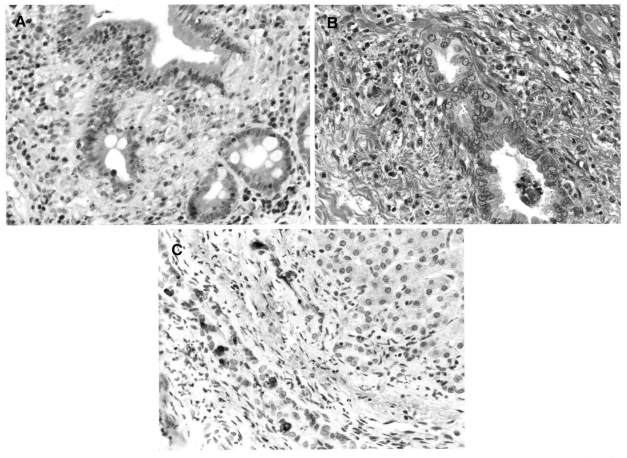

Figure 22.4 LCH involving the gastrointestinal tract. (a) Sheets of lesional cells mostly occupy the small bowel lamina propria. Occasional small nests or individual cells interpolate spaces between the surface or glandular epithelial cells and their basement membranes (600x). (b) Early liver lesions are notoriously subtle and often missed. LCH cells initially affect large caliber bile ducts causing sclerosing cholangitis and ultimately migrate peripherally within the biliary tree (600x). (c) CD1a stain is often required to highlight the inconspicuous LCH cells within the bile ducts interposed between the basement membrane and the biliary epithelial cells (600x). (d) More advanced liver cases show atypical histiocytic cells spilling into the lobules (600x).

of *SLC29A3* (the gene responsible for SLC29A3 spectrum of diseases) and *TNFRSF* (the FAS gene that causes autoimmune lymphoproliferative syndrome) (Figures 22.10–22.11).

Histiocytic Sarcoma

Histiocytic sarcoma (HS) is a rare malignant proliferation of cells with morphologic and immunophenotypic features of macrophages. Age at presentation ranges from infancy to old age. Primary cases arise de novo while other cases (secondary HS) follow lymphoma or leukemia, myelodysplasia, or germ cell tumor (especially malignant teratoma). To make the diagnosis of HS,

lesional cells must express at least one macrophage marker such as CD68, CD163, or lysozyme and be negative for markers of Langerhans cells (CD1a, and Langerin). An extended panel of immunohistochemical stains is required to rule out large-cell lymphomas and other malignancies such as melanoma and carcinoma (Figure 22.12).

Langerhans Cell Sarcoma

Langerhans cell sarcoma (LCS) is a high-grade malignant proliferation of dendritic histiocytes that have a Langerhans cell phenotype. Most cases arise de novo with very rare cases arising from prior LCH lesions or lymphoma. Most patients

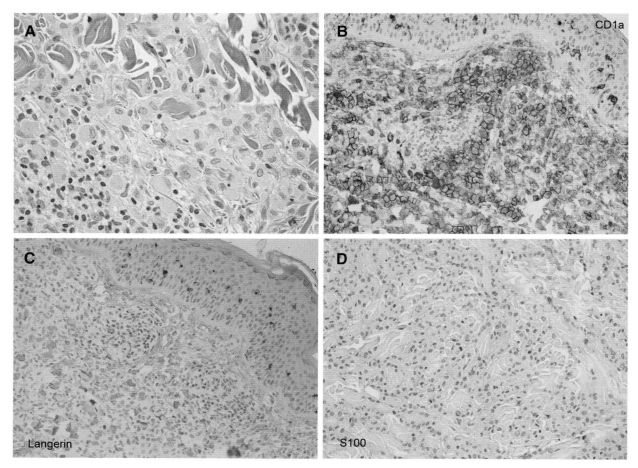

Figure 22.5 Skin lesions are usually dermal with extension into the subcutaneous tissues, unlike LCH, which is epidermotropic. (a) (600x) Lesional cells resemble LCH cells with irregular nuclear grooves and indentations. Cytoplasm is abundant and eosinophilic. No eosinophils are seen. In other cases, there may be spindling of cells. The mitotic rates are variable. Immunohistochemistry in this case shows lesional cells that are reactive with CD1a (b) (400x) but nonreactive with Langerin and S100 (c and d, 200x and 400x, respectively).

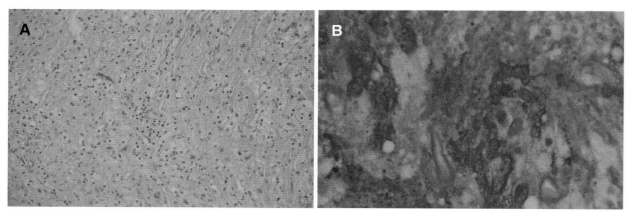

Figure 22.6 ECD involving the anterior mediastinum. (a) Lesions of ECD are characterized by infiltrations of histiocytes with abundant foamy/xanthomatous or sometimes eosinophilic cytoplasm and single small nuclei that lack atypia or prominent nucleoli. Touton-type giant cells, multinucleated cells with nuclei that form a horse-shoe shape and have cytoplasm that is foamy at the periphery and eosinophilic in the center, are often difficult to find. Abundant fibrosis (right side of picture) often accompanies the histiocytic infiltrates as do lymphocytes, plasma cells, and neutrophils (200x). (b) Similar to JXG family of lesions, ECD cells express macrophage markers including CD14, CD68, and CD163 as well as dendritic cell markers such as Factor 13a (shown here) (400x) and fascin. CD1a and Langerin are negative. Most cases are S100 negative with rare cases showing focal staining. Cases that have *BRAF* mutations may express immunoreactivity with VE1 stains.

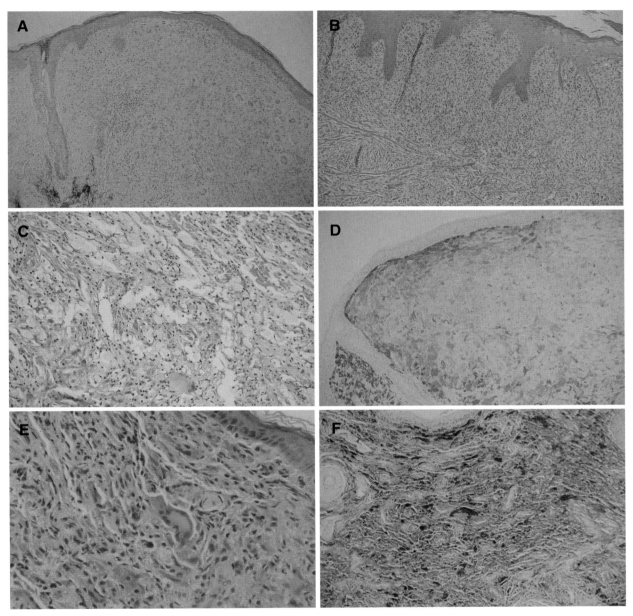

Figure 22.7 Cutaneous JXG. (a) Early lesions have small and oval histiocytes that have moderate amounts of faintly vacuolar cytoplasm and may have bland folded (but not complex) nuclei. Touton-type giant cells are seen in about 85% but not required for diagnosis (100x). (b) This early JXG lesion does not show Touton-type giant cells (200x). (c) In long-standing JXGs, some lesional cells accumulate fat and appear xanthomatous (400x). There may also be increased spindling of cells (not shown here) mimicking dermatofibroma. (d) Lesional cells show characteristic but variably strong reactivity for Factor 13a that is often more notable at the periphery of lesions (100x). Other stains that are positive include macrophage markers (CD14, CD68, and CD163). CD1a and Langerin are absent and S100 is either absent or low and variable in approximately 30% of cases. Several clinical and histologic variants of JXG are described, including hemosiderotic JXG (shown here), benign cephalic histiocytosis (multiple cutaneous lesions of head and neck), deep/soft tissue JXG, "giant" JXG (lesions > 2cm), and infantile systemic/disseminated JXG. (e and f) H&E and iron-stained sections of a hemosiderotic JXG (200x and 100x, respectively).

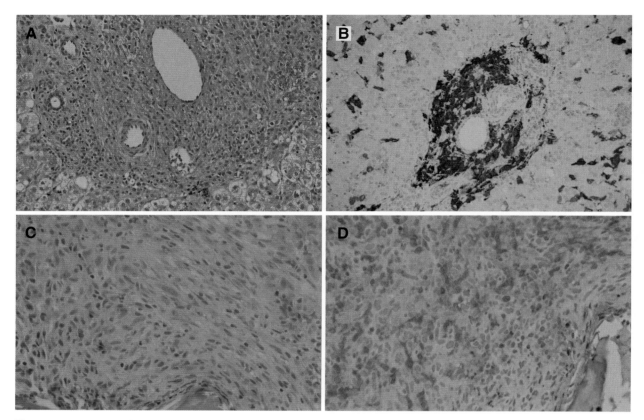

Figure 22.8 Disseminated JXG involving the liver and bone marrow. (a) Numerous medium-sized histiocytes without atypia mostly infiltrate the portal tracts without invading the bile ducts (100x). (b) Factor 13a stain highlights the histiocytic cells in the portal tracts as well as sinusoids (200x). Unlike LCH, liver involvement by disseminated JXG does not result in a sclerosing cholangitis. (c) Bone marrow space infiltrated by mostly spindle-shaped histiocytic cells. The lesional cells nuclei in this case are slightly pleomorphic with inconspicuous nucleoli. Touton-type giant cells are particularly rare in extracutaneous lesions and some cases may show significant fibrosis (200x). (d) Factor 13a stain highlights the histiocytic cells in the bone marrow space (200x).

are middle-aged, but pediatric cases have been reported. Most cases present as aggressive soft tissue or nodal tumors or as multiorgan involvement (spleen, liver, lung and bone marrow disease). Prognosis is often poor (Figure 22.13).

Hemophagocytic Lymphohistiocytosis

Hemophagocytic lymphohistiocytosis (HLH) includes a variety of immune disorders characterized by uncontrolled accumulation of activated macrophages and T-lymphocytes associated with upregulation of inflammatory cytokines. Whether familial or sporadic, HLH is often difficult to diagnose given its low incidence and inconsistent clinical features. Standard diagnostic criteria were established by the Histiocyte Society in 1994 with revisions in 2004. Primary HLH patients are usually infants or young children with a significant family history or known genetic etiology. However, adult presentations are being recognized more frequently. Long-term survival without hematopoietic stem cell transplant is unlikely in these patients. Infections (such as cytomegalovirus or Epstein-Barr virus [EBV]), malignancy, or vaccination may initiate the disease, but often the trigger is not apparent. Secondary HLH generally occurs sporadically mostly in older children or adults without a family history or a known genetic cause for HLH. Mortality from secondary HLH can be significant in the most florid forms and the risk of recurrence is poorly defined. Usually, an infection or some other medical condition is known to trigger the presentation.

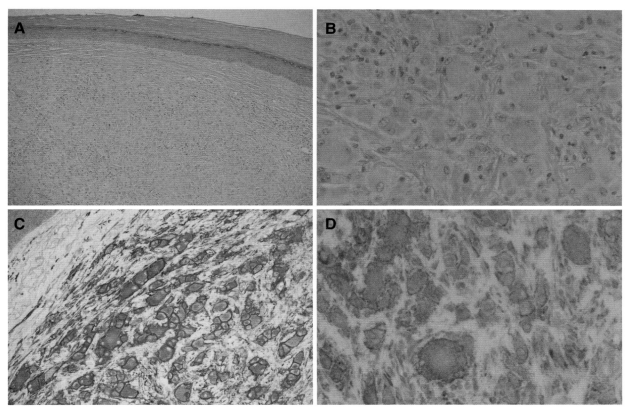

Figure 22.9 Solitary reticulohistiocytoma, cutaneous. (a) Skin RH lesions are predominantly dermal and may resemble JXG at low-power magnification (100x). (b) The lesional RH cell is very large (50–100 μm), with 1–3 eccentric, oval, or grooved nuclei and abundant, deeply eosinophilic glassy, periodic acid-Schiff (PAS)-positive, PAS with diastase resistant, cytoplasm (400x). Lesional cells are reactive with CD163 (c) and CD68 (d) (200x and 400x, respectively).

The most common offenders include EBV infection (EBV-associated hemophagocytic syndrome), cytomegalovirus, H5 N and H1N1 influenza, malignancy (malignancy-associated hemophagocytic syndrome), and rheumatologic disorders (macrophage activation syndrome). Less common triggers include lymphoproliferative disorders, intravenous alimentation, and multiple organ failure (Figure 22.14).

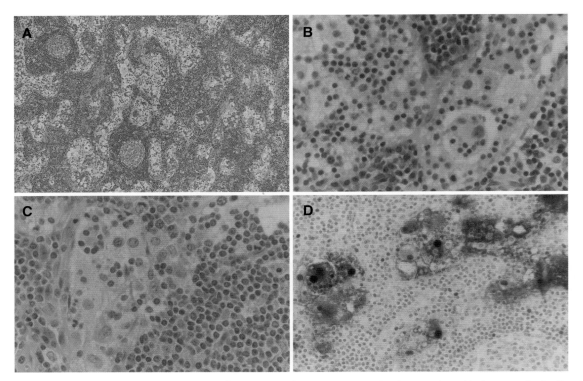

Figure 22.10 Nodal RDD. (a) Low-power magnification (100x) shows preservation of architecture but with sinuses markedly dilated by numerous large histiocytes with abundant pale to water-clear cytoplasm (b and c) (200x and 400x). The lesional cells are very large (>75 μm) with large eccentric hypochromatic nuclei containing single prominent central nucleoli. They also show emperipolesis (the presence/trafficking of intact leukocytes within cytoplasmic vacuoles) and the background has various inflammatory cells (plasma cells, mature lymphocytes, and neutrophils). (d) The lesional cells are strongly positive with S100, (400x) (as well as CD68 and CD163, but CD1a-negative). Nonreactive inflammatory cells within the vacuoles stand out.

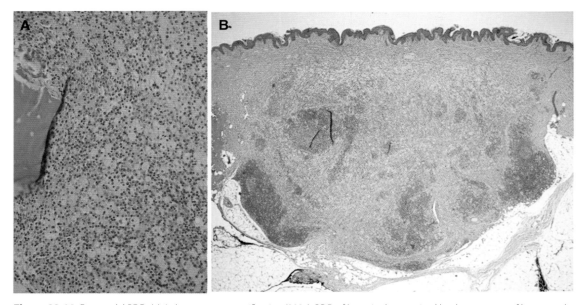

Figure 22.11 Extranodal RDD. (a) At low-power magnification (200x), RDD of bone is characterized by the presence of large numbers of foamy/lipid-containing macrophages with admixed lymphocytes and can be mistaken for xanthogranulomatous osteomyelitis. (b) (100x) In skin and soft tissues, RDD lesions simulate lymph nodes showing a "sinusoidal pattern" or a light and dark pattern of confluent aggregates of lesional histiocytic cells (light) and clusters of inflammatory cells (dark). Neutrophil-rich "suppuration" may confound the picture. Late or involuting lesions have fewer Rosai-Dorfman cells, more xanthoma cells, and spindled fibroblasts.

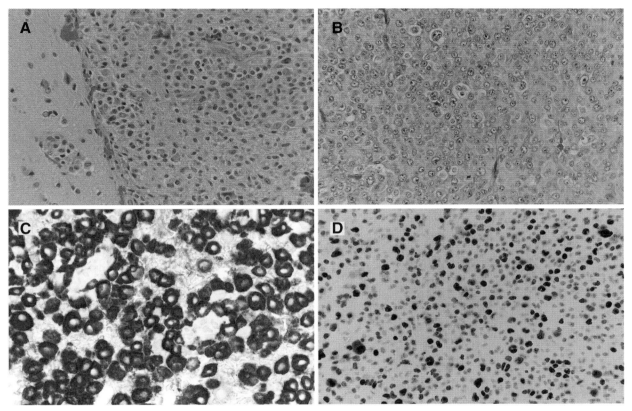

Figure 22.12 Histiocytic sarcoma. (a) This low-power photomicrograph (200x) shows infiltration of cortical brain tissue by large atypical histiocytic cells. Most histiocytic sarcomas are characterized by sheets of proliferating large non cohesive cells (>20 um). The lesional cells range from small and round to large and polygonal. Occasional spindle-shaped cells may be seen. Higher-power image (b) (400x) shows markedly pleomorphic vesicular nuclei with large prominent nucleoli. Hemophagocytosis is sometimes prevalent in tumor cells. The background of HS often shows variable numbers of inflammatory cells, including mature lymphocytes, plasma cells, eosinophils and non-neoplastic macrophages. (c) Lesional cells are reactive with macrophage marker CD163 (400x). (d) Lesional cells show a high proliferative index with Ki67 (200x).

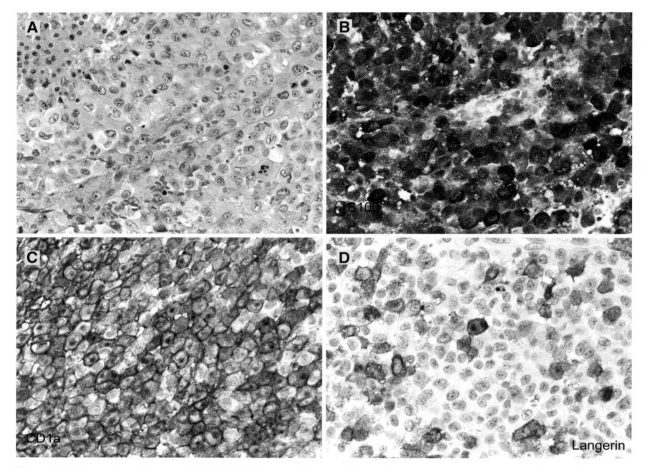

Figure 22.13 Langerhans cell sarcoma (LCS) (a) This highly aggressive tumor shows cells with nuclear features reminiscent of LCH cells. However, they have more pleomorphic nuclei, frequent and atypical mitoses, and fewer background inflammatory cells. This photomicrograph shows an abnormal mitosis (arrowhead) and a focus of necrosis (600x). (b and c) This case showed strong diffuse S100 and CD1a reactivity (600x). (d) Langerin staining is strong but focal (600x).

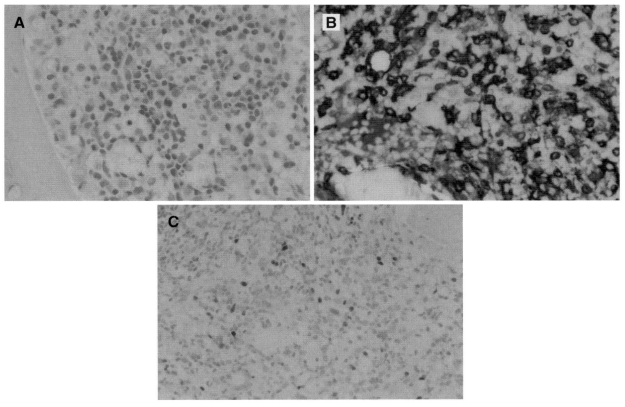

Figure 22.14 Secondary (EBV-induced) HLH. (a) Many macrophages infiltrate the marrow space and engulf apoptotic leukocytes and erythrocytes (hemophagocytosis) (600x). This phenomenon is neither sensitive nor specific for HLH and cannot be used insolation to make the diagnosis. (b) CD68 highlights many macrophages in the marrow space (400x). (c) EBV (EBER-1) in situ hybridization stain shows many positive cells in the marrow (200x).

References

1. Rollins BJ. Biology and genomics of LCH and related disorders. In Abla O and Janka G, eds. Histiocytic disorders. New York, Springer; 2018:53–71.

2. Emile JF, Abla O, Fraitag S, Horne A, Haroche J, Donadieu J, et al. Revised classification of histiocytoses and neoplasms of the macrophage-dendritic cell lineages. Blood. 2016; **127**(22): 2672–81.

3. Foucar E, Rosai J, Dorfman R. Sinus histiocytosis with massive lymphadenopathy (Rosai-Dorfman disease): Review of the entity. Semin Diagn Pathol. 1990; **7**(1): 19–73.

4. Henter JI, Horne A, Aricó M, Egeler RM, Filipovich AH, Imashuku S, et al. HLH-2004: Diagnostic and therapeutic guidelines for hemophagocytic lymphohistiocytosis. Pediatr Blood Cancer. 2007; **48**(2): 124–31.

Bone Marrow Manifestations of Systemic Diseases

Kristian T. Schafernak, Rachel A. Mariani, Nicole Arva, Jeffrey Jacobsen, Katherine R. Calvo

In this chapter, we illustrate a wide variety of conditions affecting the bone marrow not described in other chapters of this book. These include inherited or acquired anemias, bone marrow failure syndromes not described in the germline disorders, therapy-related changes, metastatic malignancy, and storage disorders.

Bone Marrow Failure Syndrome

Most of the bone marrow failure syndromes are included in Chapter 19, based on revised WHO classification. Here we include a few entities commonly seen in children.

Sideroblastic Anemia (Acquired and Constitutional)

Sideroblastic anemia refers plainly to an erythroid disorder with impaired heme biosynthesis and abundant "ring sideroblasts," which result when iron is abnormally deposited in the perinuclear mitochondria of erythroid precursors. Ring sideroblasts are seen in a variety of acquired conditions, including myeloid neoplasms and exposure to toxins/drugs and nutritional deficiency. Constitutional sideroblastic anemia can be X-linked due to missense mutations in *ALAS2* [1].

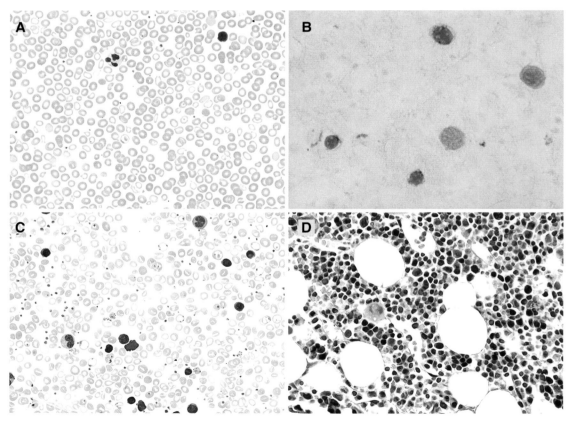

Figure 23.1 The blood smear (A: Wright-Giemsa, 400x) shows a dimorphic red blood cell population without history of transfusion. The bone marrow aspirate shows many ring sideroblasts (B: Prussian blue stain, 1,000x) and siderocytes containing Pappenheimer bodies (C: Wright-Giemsa, 100x). Erythroid hyperplasia is evident in the core biopsy (D: H&E, 200x).

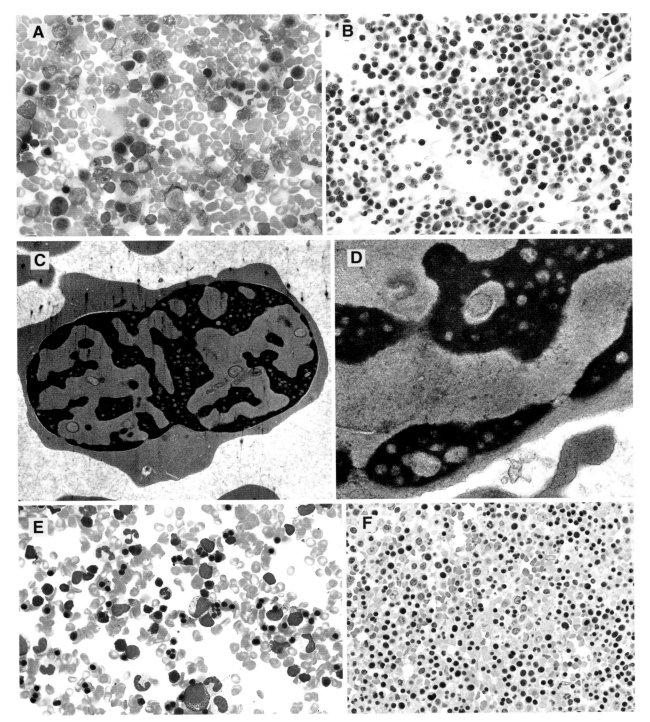

Figure 23.2 Congenital dyserythropoietic anemia (CDA). There are four types of CDA. Diagnosis includes bone marrow morphology and gene sequencing. Table 23.1 summarizes the features of the four types of CDA. Their marrows as in all types of CDA, show an erythroid hyperplasia. CDA type 1: (A: Wright-Giemsa stain; B: H&E, both at 400x), On electron microscopy (C and D), we can see partially fused erythroid precursors with unequal nuclei, but the most revealing feature is the electron-lucent "holes" imparting a spongy or "Swiss cheese" appearance to the dark-staining heterochromatin due to abnormal chromatin assembly. CDA type 2 is the most common CDA and tends to be diagnosed at a later age (5–30 years but on average 18–20 years). The marrow in these patients (E: Wright-Giemsa, 400x; F: H&E, 400x) shows normoblastic erythroid hyperplasia with binucleation, trinucleation, and multinucleation.

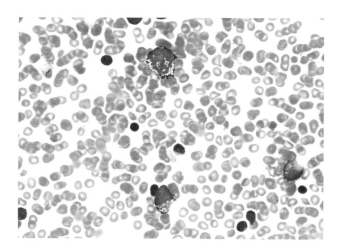

Figure 23.3 Pearson syndrome. Pearson marrow-pancreas syndrome is a rare congenital mitochondrial (mt) cytopathy due to mostly sporadic deletions of mtDNA, typically presenting during infancy with failure to thrive, often accompanied by pancreatic exocrine insufficiency and variable hepatic, renal, and endocrine failure. Hematologic manifestations include severe macrocytic sideroblastic anemia, neutropenia, and thrombocytopenia. Both myeloid and erythroid precursors display cytoplasmic vacuoles (Wright-Giemsa, 400x) [6]. Ring sideroblasts are also present (not shown). Prognosis is poor, with many succumbing before their fourth birthday, sometimes from lactic acidosis triggered by infection.

Therapy-Related Changes

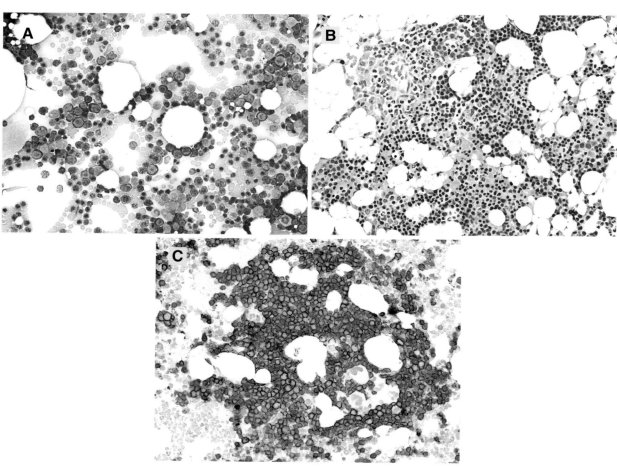

Figure 23.4 End of induction for lymphoblastic leukemia. In a post-therapy regenerative marrow, we typically see prominent erythroid hyperplasia (A: Aspirate smear, Wright-Giemsa, 400x). Sometimes, there is dyserythropoiesis in the form of megaloblastoid maturation and scattered erythroid progenitors displaying unequal nuclear budding. On the section, the erythroid precursors are in clusters (B: Clot section, H&E, 200x; C: CD71, IHC, 200x).

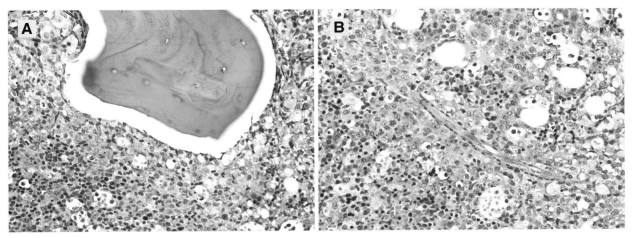

Figure 23.5 Colony-stimulating factor therapy effect. Normal trilineage hematopoiesis has normal topographic distribution; the immature myeloid precursors show paratrabecular and periarteriolar localization, normally forming a cuff that is one or two cells thick. This layer becomes a bit thicker when responding to an infection or in the setting of colony-stimulating factor therapy (A: Paratrabecular; B: Periarteriolar; H&E, 200x).

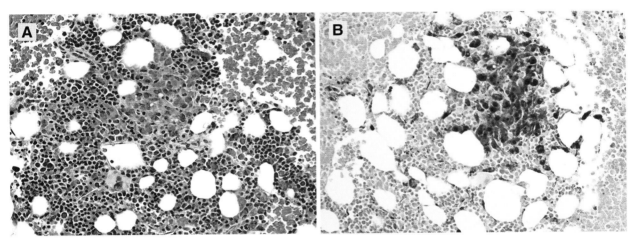

Figure 23.6 Iron excess. This patient developed iron overload from chronic transfusions (A: H&E of clot section, 200x; B: Prussian blue stain, 200x).

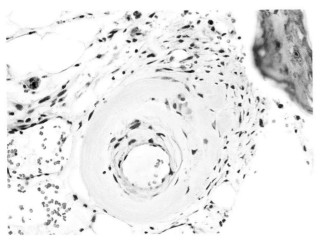

Figure 23.7 Radiation effect. Figure A (H&E, 200x): A blood vessel with intimal thickening and fibrosis of the vessel wall from a patient with pelvic Ewing sarcoma treated with systemic chemotherapy and radiation.

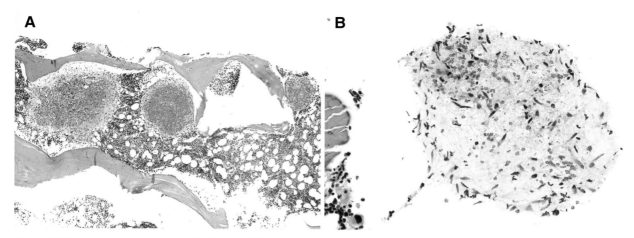

Figure 23.8 Bone marrow thrombosis. This 10-year-old boy underwent bone marrow examination for pancytopenia. The patient had been on tacrolimus for focal segmental glomerulosclerosis and tolerating it well since age 18 months, but it had been discontinued 2 weeks earlier due to concern for tacrolimus-induced refractory immune thrombocytopenia. The core biopsy shows multiple hemorrhagic nodules (A: H&E, 40x). There was also a non-hemorrhagic nodule consistent with organization of a thrombus (B: H&E, 200x). Tacrolimus and cyclosporin A have both been implicated in thrombotic microangiopathy [7].

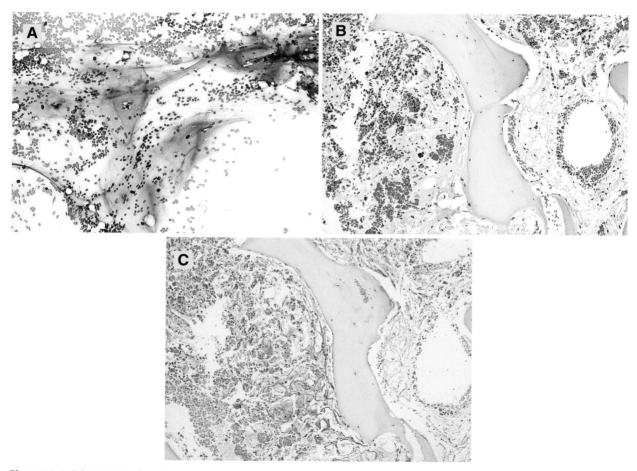

Figure 23.9 Gelatinous transformation/serous fat atrophy, most commonly seen after therapy such as chemoradiation. However, it can also be seen in anorexia nervosa, cachexia from chronic debilitating illnesses such as infections, malignancy, autoimmune disease, renal or heart failure, intestinal lymphangiectasia, and alcoholism [8]. A–C were from the bone marrow biopsy of a 16-year-old malnourished girl. The aspirate smear (A: Wright-Giemsa) shows amorphous bluish material. The core biopsy (B: H&E, 100x) has amorphous bluish, finely fibrillary/granular material with focal adipocyte atrophy, and patchy hematopoiesis. The amorphous material is composed of acid mucosubstances as demonstrated in C (Alcian blue, pH 2.5, 100x).

Stromal and Bone Changes

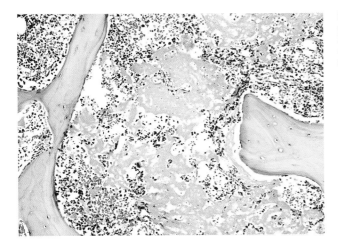

Figure 23.10 Aspiration artifact. A common artifact results from aspiration of marrow from the core biopsy; sometimes this happens because the biopsy is taken too close to where the aspirate had just occurred. Another cause is when negative pressure is applied. On the H&E section, one sees large areas of fibrin deposition (100x).

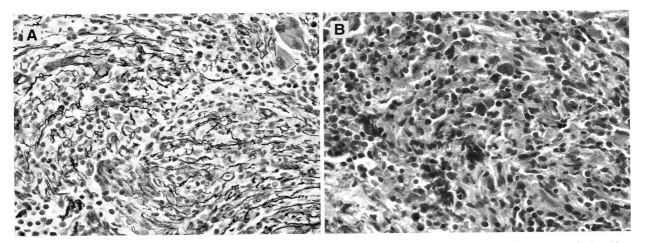

Figure 23.11 Autoimmune myelofibrosis. Autoimmune myelofibrosis is seen in patients with primary autoimmune diseases or serologic evidence of autoimmunity. This 12-year-old boy underwent bone marrow examination as an outpatient for neutropenia and anemia. The core biopsy was remarkable for a lymphohistiocytic infiltrate and "streaming" of cells. A and B show reticulin fibrosis on reticulin stain and collagen fibrosis with trichrome stain, respectively (400x). Cytogenetic finding was 47, XXY, consistent with Klinefelter syndrome. Individuals with Klinefelter's are at increased risk of autism and also at increased risk of "female-predominant" autoimmune diseases.

Bone Marrow Metastases

Neuroblastoma

Neuroblastoma (NBL) is the most common solid tumor in pediatric marrows. It is a neoplastic proliferation of neural crest cells that can arise anywhere along the sympathetic chain but commonly occurs in the adrenal gland. Current recommendations for standardization of bone marrow assessment and reporting in children with neuroblastoma from the international neuroblastoma criteria working group are published and generally accepted practice in pediatric pathology. Two bone marrow samples from at least two different sites should be

275

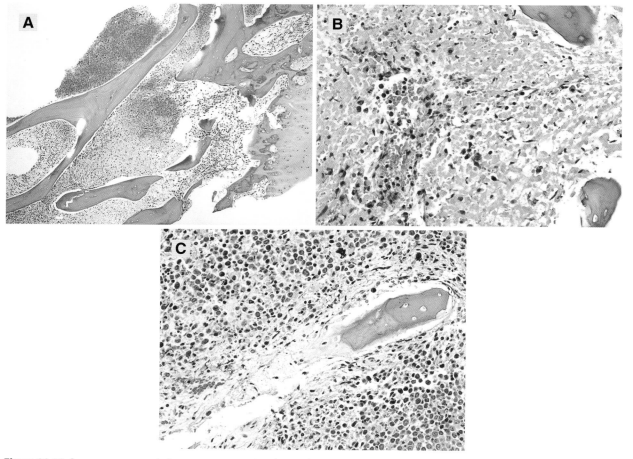

Figure 23.12 Bone marrow necrosis. Bone marrow necrosis with or without osteonecrosis is more common in site-directed biopsies than nondirected bone marrow specimens. The list of causes includes malignancy and infection among others [10]. A (H&E, 40x) is a directed pubic bone biopsy from a 6-year-old girl with sickle cell disease showing bone marrow necrosis. The biopsy was performed to exclude osteomyelitis. Images B and C come from a 7-month-old boy with circulating blasts. The initial bone marrow specimen (B, H&E, 200x) was completely necrotic. A second biopsy of the contralateral distal femur bone marrow biopsies (C, H&E, 200x) showed viable acute monoblastic leukemia.

analyzed. Metastatic tumor infiltration in bone marrow biopsies is estimated as the surface area occupied by neuroblastoma tumor as a percentage of the evaluable bone marrow Space on each biopsy (such as 0%, < 5%, > 5%, and so on) [14]. Immunohistochemistry is frequently used to improve detection in biopsies. Multiple sections (> 3) from all biopsies using a minimum of two antibodies is recommended [14]. Immunostains for NBL can be broadly categorized into three groups – group 1: neural markers, includes NSE (neuron-specific enolase), PGP9.5 (protein gene product 9.5), CD56 (neural cell adhesion molecule [NCAM]), chromogranin, and synaptophysin; group 2: neural crest markers include PHOX2B (paired-like homeobox 2B) and TH (tyrosine hydroxylase); group 3: NB84 that appears to be NBL-specific but whose exact function is yet unknown. For staging/restaging marrows, some practices rely on a combination of one neural marker like synaptophysin and one neural crest marker like PHOX2B, although there are no specific criteria.

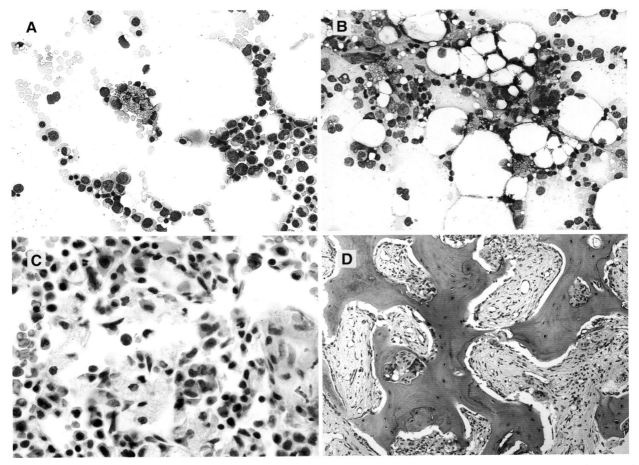

Figure 23.13 Cystinosis. Cystinosis is an autosomal recessive disorder resulting from mutations in the *CTNS* gene that cause cystine to form crystals in lysosomes, damaging the kidneys and/or corneas [11]. A and B (Wright-Giemsa) and C (H&E) depict colorless polygonal crystals in macrophages. Bone marrow core biopsy in either cystinosis or oxalosis will additionally show the stromal and bone changes of renal osteodystrophy (D: H&E), which shows irregular bone trabeculae, osteoblastic and osteoclastic proliferation, and stromal fibrosis.

Rhabdomyosarcoma

Rhabdomyosarcoma (RMS) is the most common soft tissue sarcoma seen in children and adolescents and the second most common solid tumor you will see in pediatric marrows [18, 19]. It is a tumor of skeletal myoblast-like cells. There are two major subtypes of RMS, embryonal and alveolar, which are characterized by different molecular mechanisms. RMS can metastasize to the bone marrow and mimic hematolymphoid neoplasms.

Ewing Sarcoma

Ewing sarcoma (ES) is an extremely aggressive tumor of bone and soft tissue that affects children and adolescents. It is composed of small round blue cells characterized by nonrandom chromosomal translocation producing fusion genes that produce aberrant transcription factors. The most common translocation is t(11;22)(qq24;q21), forming the gene fusion EWSR1::FLI1.

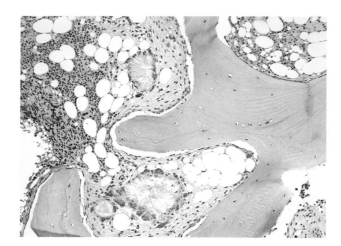

Figure 23.14 Oxalosis. Oxalosis refers to widespread tissue deposition of calcium oxalate in primary hyperoxaluria (PH). The crystals in oxalosis are very large and in bone marrow biopsies can be deposited in the stroma, where they are associated with a foreign body giant cell reaction, as well the bone matrix (H&E). Although not shown here, in aspirate smears, oxalosis crystals stack up to form long stringlike cords [12]. Case courtesy of Dr. Girish Venkataraman.

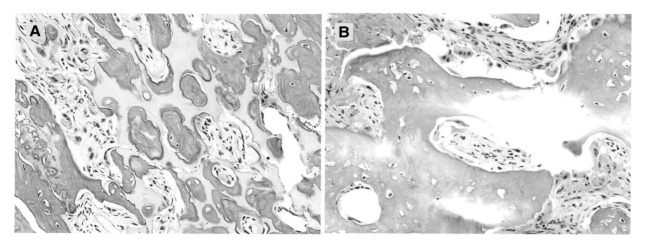

Figure 23.15 Osteopetrosis. (A and B: H&E) In osteopetrosis, excessive osteoblastic activity with decreased bone resorption (osteoclasts can be abundant but are functionally defective) leads to abnormally dense brittle bones prone to fracture [13]. Histologically, one sees markedly thickened bone that, with stromal fibrosis, obliterates the marrow space. As a result, leukoerythroblastosis can be observed in these patients. Inheritance can be autosomal recessive, autosomal dominant, or X-linked.

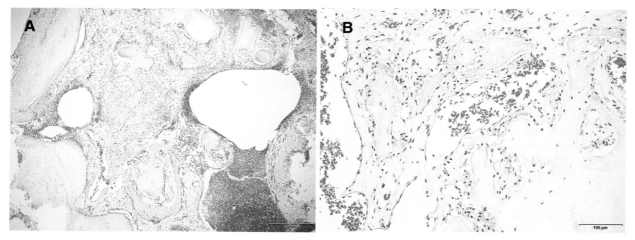

Figure 23.16 Gorham disease. Also known as vanishing bone disease, this is another rare bone disorder. It is characterized by bone resorption and replacement secondary to proliferation of thin-walled intraosseous vascular or lymphatic channels. It can be localized or spread to adjacent bone or soft tissue (A and B: H&E, 400x). Case courtesy of Dr. Silvia Bunting.

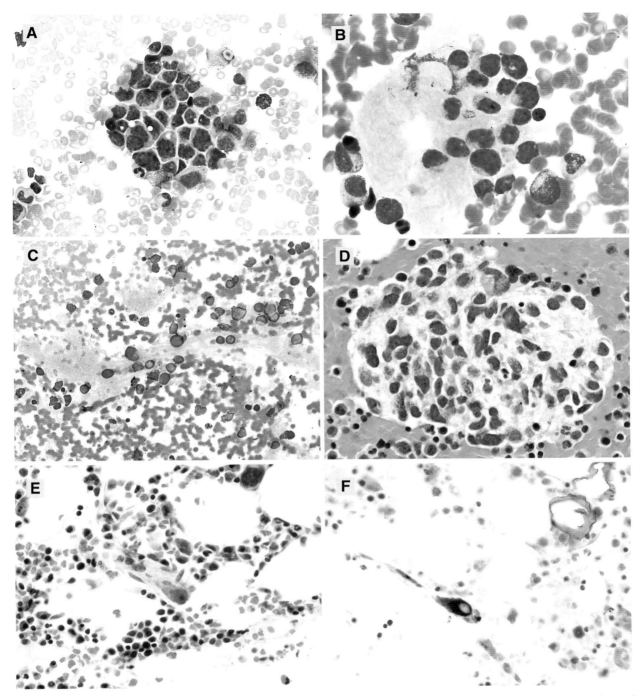

Figure 23.17 Neuroblastoma In bone marrow aspirate smears, tumor cells tend to be cohesive, in flat sheets, or in three-dimensional clusters (A: Wright-Giemsa stain, 400x). Sometimes they are set in neuropil, which has a fibrillar matrix (B: Wright-Giemsa, 400x), in contrast to disrupted granular megakaryocyte cytoplasm. Occasionally, the predominant pattern is that of individual tumor cells, which could potentially be misinterpreted as leukemic blasts, but recognizing the presence of neuropil will help practitioners avoid that pitfall (C: Wright-Giemsa, 200x). Note the stippled ("salt and pepper") chromatin pattern of the tumor cells in the clot section shown in D (H&E, 400x). Neuroblastoma cells can mature spontaneously or after therapy chemotherapy-induced maturation to ganglion cells (E: H&E, 400x; F: IHC, tyrosine hydroxylase, 400x), though this should not be assumed to confer a favorable prognosis. When maturing cells are present, they should be reported as differentiating neuroblastoma cells [14]. Rarely, NBL can be found in the placenta in a newborn [15]. G: (H&E, 200x) comes from the placenta of an infant born with congenital NBL; note tumor cells in the villous capillaries (fetal circulation). H (PGP9.5), I (synaptophysin), J (PHOX2B), K (TH), and L (NB84) were all taken at 400x on clot sections. PHOX2B shows nuclear staining and will be positive even in very undifferentiated cases of NBL. Please note that PHOX2B is also frequently expressed in pheochromocytoma and paraganglioma, whereas TH is more specific for NBL [16]. We also have non-myelinating Schwann cells that support neurites in the marrow, but the cell bodies of neurons (ganglion cells) are never a normal marrow finding [17].

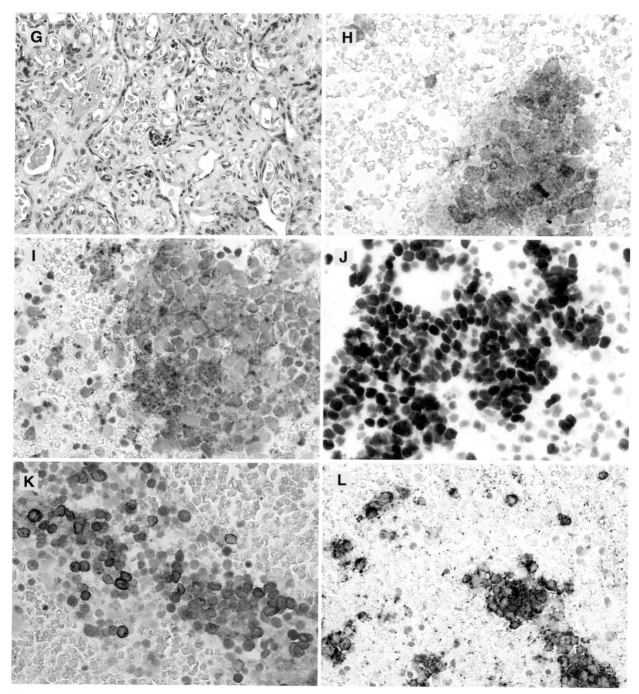

Figure 23.17 (cont.)

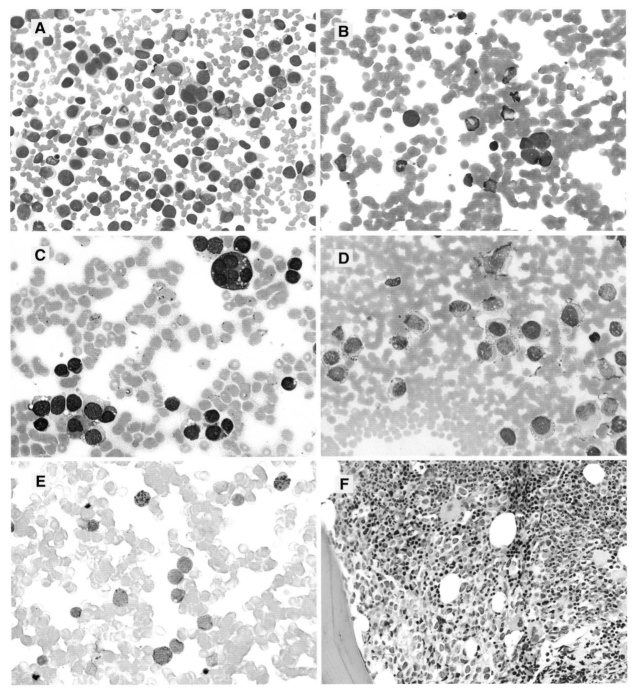

Figure 23.18 Rhabdomyosarcoma In bone marrow aspirate smears, RMS cells can be abundant and mostly discohesive (A: Wright-Giemsa stain), and could be mistaken for a hematopoietic neoplasm. It can be somewhat more cohesive (B: Wright-Giemsa, 400x), multinucleated (C: Wright-Giemsa, 400x), or vacuolated and reminiscent of Burkitt lymphoma/leukemia (D: Wright-Giemsa, 400x). The vacuoles contain glycogen rather than lipid (E: PAS positive, 400x) but negative on PAS/D stain (not shown). F and G (H&E, 200x) show pretreatment marrow from a girl with newly diagnosed RMS; note that, in G, the tumor cells are set in a fibrotic stroma that almost resemble the fibrillar neuropil of NBL. In a different case with a large multinucleated tumor giant cell, the tumor cells are positive for desmin (H, IHC, 400x) and myogenin (I, IHC, 400x). Rarely, alveolar RMS actually recapitulates alveoli in the lung, as in the bone marrow biopsy (J: H&E, 400x). With treatment, like in NBL, one can see maturation ("cytodifferentiation") [20].

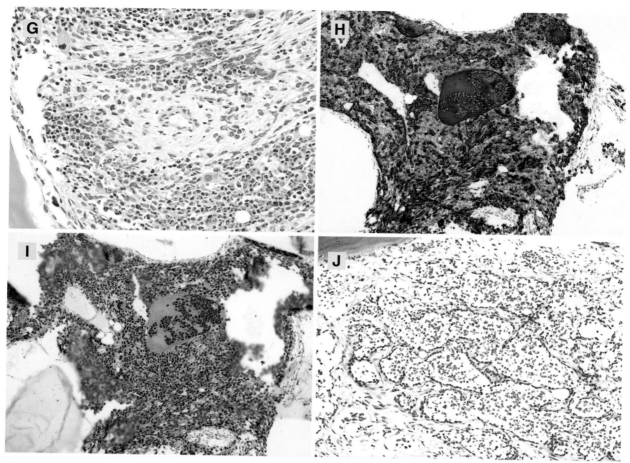

Figure 23.18 (cont.)

Desmoplastic Small Round Cell Tumor

Desmoplastic small round cell tumor (DRSCT) is a malignant mesenchymal neoplasm composed of small round cells in a background of stromal desmoplasia and is characterized by a recurrent translocation t(11;22)(p13; q12) resulting in the *EWSR1::WT1* gene fusion. It primarily affects children and young adults with a male predominance and presents with abdominal and peritoneal tumors. The cytologic features are similar to other small round cell tumors but its peculiar polyphenotypic immunoprofile with positivity for both epithelial and mesenchymal markers as well as nuclear staining for WT1 has led some to speculate whether the cell of origin/nearest normal counterpart might be a mesothelial or submesothelial cell [22, 23].

Retinoblastoma

Retinoblastoma is the most common ocular malignancy of childhood. It is an aggressive primitive neuroectodermal intraocular malignancy that affects

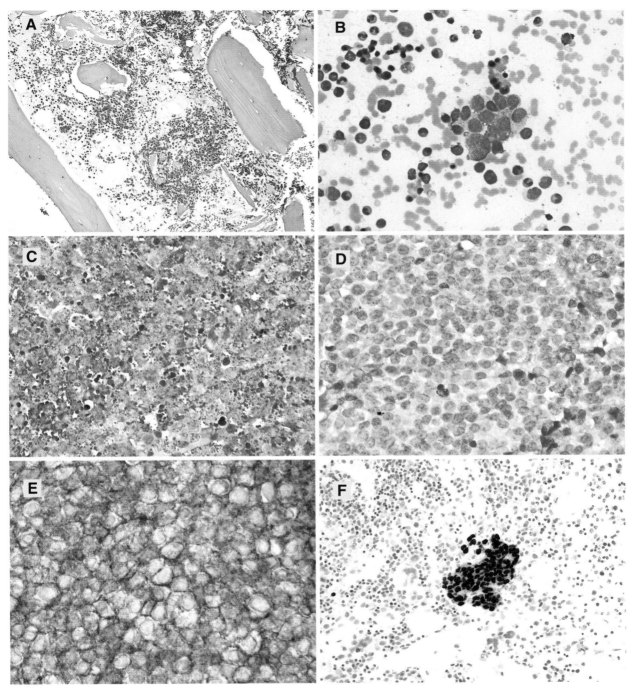

Figure 23.19 Ewing Sarcoma A: Bone marrow core biopsy (H&E) shows replacement by Ewing sarcoma. B: Touch imprint shows cohesive cluster of cells in the background of normal hematopoietic cells (Wright-Giemsa). C: cytoplasmic glycogen content (C: PAS, 400x; D: PAS with diastase digestion, 400x). Approximately 95% of cases show diffuse strong membranous staining for CD99 (E: IHC, 400x), but it is not specific as it could be positive in lymphoblastic leukemia/lymphoma. NKX2.2 (F: IHC, 200x) is a newer marker for ES. Because its specificity is only moderate, diagnostic specimens should be sent for molecular genetic confirmation [21].

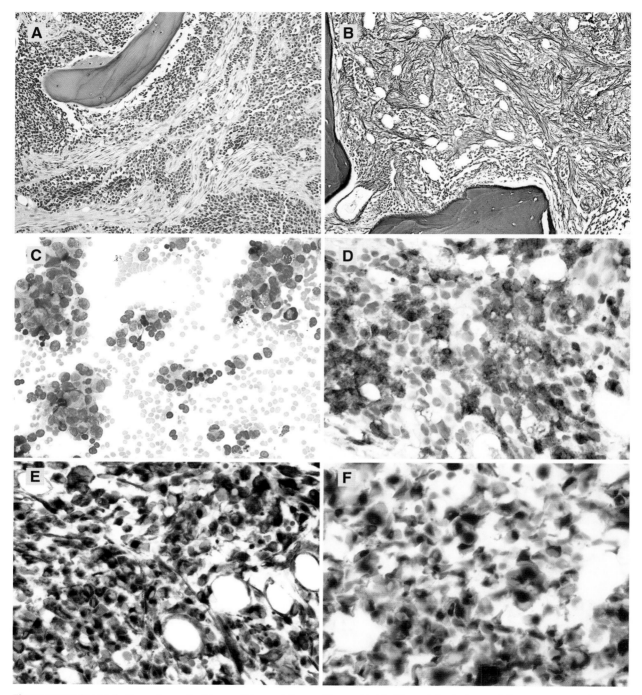

Figure 23.20 Desmoplastic small round cell tumor. This case is from a 15-year-old girl with an abdominal mass. A. Bone marrow core biopsy shows diffuse replacement by the tumor (H&E, 100x) set in a fibrotic stroma (B: reticulin stain, 100x). The bone marrow aspirate shows cohesive clusters of small round blue cells. Immunohistochemical stains show the tumor cells are positive for an epithelial marker (D: EMA, IHC, 400x), as well as mesenchymal markers, including vimentin (E, IHC, 400x) and desmin (F, IHC, 400x). Note the characteristic paranuclear dot-like staining in some of the cells.

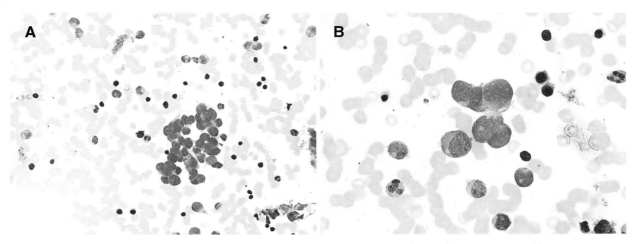

Figure 23.21 Retinoblastoma (A and B, Wright-Giemsa, 500x and 1,000x) Bone marrow involvement by metastatic retinoblastoma is uncommon, especially in developed countries [24]. Note rosette formation, scattered individual tumor cells, and the conformity of adjacent cell nuclei ("nuclear molding") in the bone marrow aspirate from this 2-year-old boy recently diagnosed with retinoblastoma.

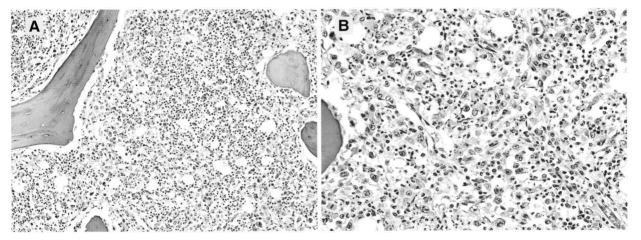

Figure 23.22 This is a 13-year-old boy with a 3- to 4-week history of intermittent colicky right upper quadrant abdominal pain and jaundice. Liver biopsy showed adenocarcinoma suggestive of cholangiocarcinoma or possibly of pancreatic origin. PET demonstrated widely metastatic disease, including bone marrow (A and B: H&E, 100x and 200x).

infants and young children and can be lethal. It is caused by mutations in the *RB1* gene, which was the first described tumor suppressor gene.

Carcinoma

Carcinomas are tumors of epithelial tissue from the skin or cells that line the inner or outer surface of organs. While carcinomas represent the lion's share of different cancer types in adults, carcinomas are rare in children.

Storage Diseases

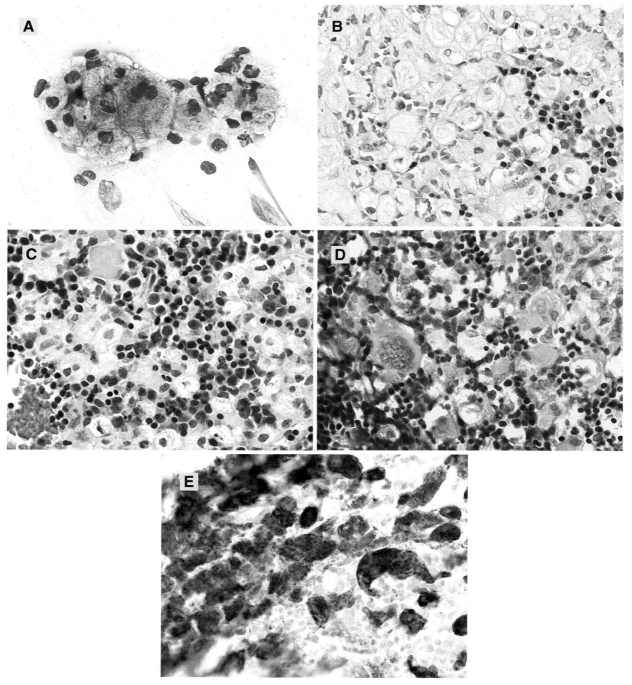

Figure 23.23 Gaucher disease. Type 1 (non-neuronopathic) Gaucher disease is an autosomal recessive storage disease caused by mutations in the glucocerebroside (*GBA*) gene. Gaucher cells accumulate in the liver, spleen, and bone marrow. In the bone marrow aspirate of this Ashkenazi Jewish teenage girl (A: Wright-Giemsa, 400x), these histiocytes show voluminous pale basophilic cytoplasm with striations or fibrillar appearance, resembling "wrinkled tissue paper" or "crumpled silk." Her bone marrow core biopsy (B: H&E, 400x) and clot section (C: H&E, 400x) were extensively involved. The Gaucher cells are positive on PAS (D: 400x) and tartrate-resistant acid phosphatase (TRAP) (E: IHC, 400x) stains, though the latter is seldom performed nowadays.

Table 23.1 Summary of the morphologic features of the 4 types of CDA [2–5]

	Type 1	Type 2	Type 3	Type 4
Inheritance	AR*	AR*	Familial AD* Sporadic AR*	AD/AR/X-linked*
Age at diagnosis	Birth to late adult	5–30 yo (average 18–20 yo)		
Gene affected	*CDAN1*	*SEC23B*	*KIF23*	*KLF1*
PB	Macrocytic	Normocytic		
	Reticulocytopenia	Reticulocytopenia		
Bone marrow	Erythroid hyperplasia	Erythroid hyperplasia	Erythroid hyperplasia	Erythroid hyperplasia
	Megaloblastic	Normoblastic		
	Intranuclear bridges	Bi/tri/multi-nucleation	Gigantoblasts up to 12 nuclei	Nonspecific dyserythropoiesis
EM	"Swiss cheese"			

* AR: autosomal recessive; AD: autosomal dominant.

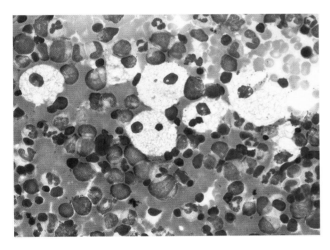

Figure 23.24 Niemann-Pick disease. Like in Gaucher disease, storage histiocytes accumulate in the liver, spleen, and bone marrow, sometimes with pulmonary involvement. Niemann-Pick disease is similarly an autosomal recessive disorder, with types A and B caused by mutations in the *SMPD1* gene while types C1 and C2 are due to mutations in the *NPC1* and *NPC2* genes, respectively. As depicted in the figure (Wright-Giemsa, 400x), these are foamy macrophages with fine round lipid-containing vacuoles and a "soap-bubble" appearance. Sometimes they are accompanied by sea-blue histiocytes (the latter predominate in Niemann-Pick disease type C, possibly reflecting slow conversion of sphingomyelin to ceroid). Niemann-Pick cells are positive for Sudan black B and oil red O.

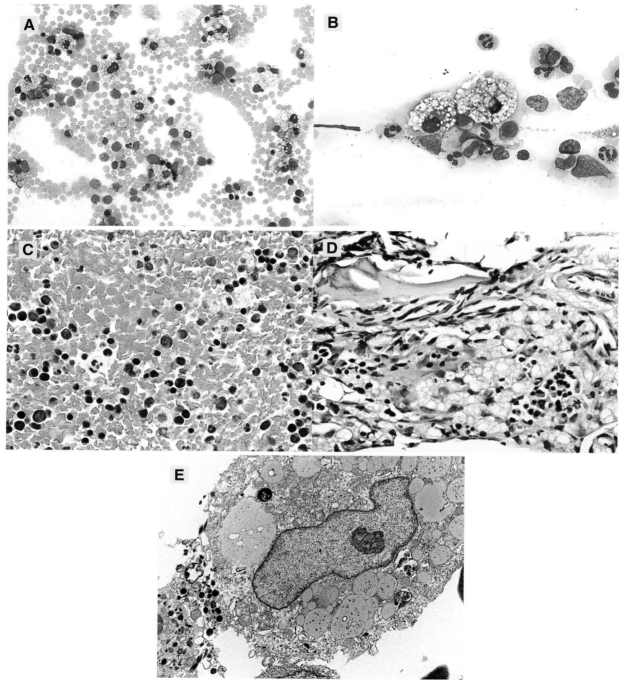

Figure 23.25 Wolman disease/lysosomal acid lipase deficiency. Wolman disease is an autosomal recessive inborn error of lipid metabolism caused by mutations in *LIPA* gene. It presents in infancy with massive infiltration of the liver, spleen, and other organs by foamy macrophages containing cholesteryl esters and triglycerides [25] (B: bone marrow aspirate, Wright-Giemsa, 400x; C: clot section H&E, 400x; D: core biopsy H&E: 400x). Oil red O and Cain's Nile blue would be positive. Ultrastructurally (E), one sees peculiar lipid inclusions.

Heavy Metal Toxicity/Deficiency

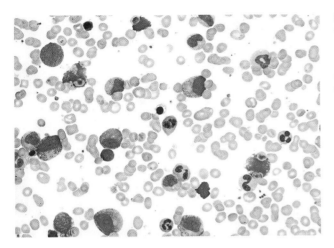

Figure 23.26 Arsenic toxicity can be seen in APL patients on As_2O_3 and all-*trans* retinoic acid, or ATRA [26] or accidental or intentional poisoning [27]. The case shown here involved a boy whose symptoms and signs were puzzling but always seemed to improve after his multiple admissions. The bone marrow biopsy shows isolated dyserythropoiesis. A random urine sample was sent for heavy metals testing and showed that the urine arsenic concentration was >20x the upper limit of normal.

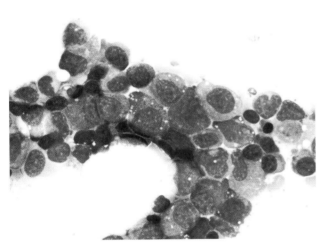

Figure 23.27 Copper deficiency/zinc excess. Copper is an essential trace element like iron, required for normal cell growth and metabolism. Copper deficiency can result from inadequate dietary intake or excess zinc intake. The patient could present with cytopenia or neuropathy. In the bone marrow, you will see vacuolization of myeloid and erythroid precursors (Wright–Giemsa stain, 1,000x, kindly provided by Dr. Silvia Bunting). There is dyspoiesis and variable numbers of ring sideroblasts, which can mimic MDS [28].

References

1. Porwit A, McCullough J, Erber WN. Blood and bone marrow pathology. 2nd ed. Edinburgh: Churchill Livingstone/Elsevier; 2011.

2. Proytcheva MA. Diagnostic pediatric hematopathology. Cambridge: Cambridge University Press; 2011.

3. Renella R, Wood WG. The congenital dyserythropoietic anemias. Hematol Oncol Clin North Am. 2009; **23**: 283–306.

4. Wickramasinghe SN, Wood WG. Advances in the understanding of the congenital dyserythropoietic anemias. Br J Haematol. 2005; **131**: 431–6.

5. de-la-Iglesia-Iñigo S, Moreno-Carralero MI, Lemes-Castellano A, et al. A case of congenital dyserythropoietic anemia type IV. Clin Case Rep. 2017; **5**: 248–52.

6. Bain BJ, Clark DM, Wilkins B. Bone marrow pathology. 4th ed. Chichester: Wiley-Blackwell; 2010.

7. Obut F, Kasinath V, Abdi R. Post-bone marrow transplant thrombotic microangiopathy. Bone Marrow Transplant. 2016; **51**: 891–7.

8. Boutin RD, White LM, Laor T, et al. MRI findings of serous atrophy of bone marrow and associated complications. Eur Radiol 2015; **25**: 2771–8.

9. Foucar K, Reichard K, Czuchlewski, D. Bone marrow pathology. 3rd ed. Chicago: ASCP Press; 2010.

10. Wool GD, Deucher A. Bone marrow necrosis: Ten-year retrospective review of bone marrow biopsy specimens. Am J Clin Pathol. 2015; **143**: 201–13.

11. Busuttil DP, Liu Yin JA. The bone marrow in hereditary cystinosis. Br J Haematol. 2000; **111**: 385.

12. Foucar K, Viswanatha DS, Wilson CS. Non-neoplastic disorders in bone marrow. Washington, DC: American Registry of Pathology in collaboration with the Armed Forces Institute of Pathology; 2008.

13. Orchard PJ, Fasth AL, Le Rademacher J, et al. Hematopoietic stem cell transplantation for infantile osteopetrosis. Blood. 2015; **126**: 270–6.

14. Burchill SA, Beiske K, Shimada H, et al. Recommendations for the standardization of bone marrow disease assessment and reporting in children with neuroblastoma on behalf of the International Neuroblastoma Response Criteria Bone Marrow Working Group. Cancer. 2017; **123**: 1095–1105.

15. Kume, A, Morikawa T, Ogawa M, et al. Congenital neuroblastoma with placental involvement. Int J Clin Exp Pathol. 2014; **7**: 8198–204.

16. Hung YP, Lee JP, Bellizzi AM, et al. PHOX2B reliably distinguishes neuroblastoma among small round blue cell tumours. Histopathology. 2017; **71**: 786–94.

17. Maryanovich M, Takeishi S, Frenette PS. Neural regulation of bone and bone marrow. Cold Spring Harb Perspect Med. 2018; **8**: a031344.

18. WHO Classification of Tumours Editorial Board. Soft tissue and bone tumours. 5th ed. Lyon: IARC Press; 2020.

19. Husain AN, Stocker JT, Dehner LP. Stocker & Dehner's pediatric pathology. 4th ed. Philadelphia, PA: Wolters Kluwer; 2016.

20. Smith LM, Anderson JR, Coffin CM. Cytodifferentiation and clinical outcome after chemotherapy and radiation therapy for rhabdomyosarcoma (RMS). Med Pediatr Oncol. 2002; **38**: 398–404.

21. Hung YP, Fletcher CD, Hornick JL. Evaluation of NKX2-2 expression in round cell sarcomas and other tumors with EWSR1 rearrangement: Imperfect specificity for Ewing sarcoma. Mod Pathol. 2016; **29**: 370–80.

22. Goldblum JR, Folpe AL, Weiss SW. Enzinger and Weiss's soft tissue tumors. 6th ed. Philadelphia, PA: Elsevier Saunders: 2014.

23. Sampson VB, David JM, Puig I, et al. Wilms' tumor protein induces an epithelial-mesenchymal hybrid differentiation state in clear cell renal cell carcinoma. PLoS One. 2014; **9**: e102041.

24. Zacharoulis S, Abramson DH, Dunkel IJ. More aggressive bone marrow screening in retinoblastoma patients is not indicated: The Memorial Sloan-Kettering Cancer Center experience. Pediatr Blood Cancer. 2006; **46**: 56–61.

25. Ireland RM. Morphology of Wolman cholesteryl ester storage disease. Blood. 2017; **126**: 803.

26. Miller KP, Venkataraman G, Gocke CD, et al. Bone marrow findings in patients with acute promyelocytic leukemia treated with arsenic trioxide. Am J Clin Pathol. 2019; **152**: 675–85.

27. Burtis CA, Ashwood ER, Bruns DE. Tietz textbook of clinical chemistry and molecular diagnostics. 5th ed. Philadelphia, PA: Elsevier Saunders; 2012.

28. Gregg XT, Reddy V, Prchal JT. Copper deficiency masquerading as myelodysplastic syndrome. Blood. 2002; **100**: 1493–5.

Index

Please note: page numbers in **bold** indicate figures or tables.